Mathematics
and Statistics
in Anaesthesia

Steven Cruickshank

Consultant Anaesthetist,
Department of Anaesthesia,
Newcastle General Hospital,
Newcastle upon Tyne, UK

With cartoons by Douglas Whitby

OXFORD

UNIVERSITY PRESS

Great Clarendon Street, Oxford OX2 6DP

Oxford University Press is a department of the University of Oxford.
It furthers the University's objective of excellence in research, scholarship,
and education by publishing worldwide in

Oxford New York

Athens Auckland Bangkok Bogotá Buenos Aires Calcutta
Cape Town Chennai Dar es Salaam Delhi Florence Hong Kong Istanbul
Karachi Kuala Lumpur Madrid Melbourne Mexico City Mumbai
Nairobi Paris São Paulo Singapore Taipei Tokyo Toronto Warsaw

with associated companies in Berlin Ibadan

Oxford is a registered trade mark of Oxford University Press
in the UK and in certain other countries

Published in the United States
by Oxford University Press, Inc., New York

First published 1998
Reprinted 2000

A catalogue record for this title is available
from the British Library

Library of Congress Cataloging in Publication Data
Cruickshank, Steve
Mathematics and statistics in anaesthesia/Steven Cruickshank.
Includes bibliographical references and index.
1. Anesthesia–Mathematics.   2. Anesthesia–Mathematical models.
3. Anesthesia–Statistical methods.   4. Pulmonary gas exchange–Mathematical models. I. Title.
RD82.C78   1998   617.9′6′0151–dc21   97-53170

ISBN 0 19 262312 5 (pbk)
ISBN 0 19 262313 3 (hbk)

Printed in Great Britain
on acid free paper by
Bookcraft (Bath) Ltd., Midsomer Norton, Avon

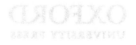

Key to icons

 This signifies a scaling or standardisation procedure

 This signifies an expression which may look complicated but is to be viewed as a 'package' which may appear in different guises. These are either the flux triplet or derivative packages.

 This signifies the approximation of a discrete variable by a continuous variable.

 This signifies the approximation of one discrete variable by another more convenient discrete variable.

 This signifies the approximation of a continuous variable by a discrete variable.

 Shaded titles indicate background or supplementary material.

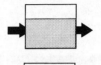 This signifies that steady-state conditions apply.

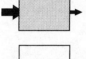 This signifies that input exceeds output and accumulation is occurring.

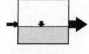 This signifies that output exceeds input and net elimination (negative accumulation) is occurring.

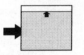 This signifies that output is zero and pure accumulation is occurring.

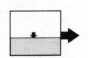 This signifies that input is zero and pure elimination is occurring.

Additional acknowledgements

The author would like to acknowledge, in addition to the forbearance of his family, in particular his son James who drew the 3-D diagrams and helped in many ways, and also Angus McNay, who read through the text and offered many suggestions for improvement.

Contents

Part 1 **Physiological and pharmacological modelling**

1.1.1 Introduction

The idea of modelling physiological processes by mathematics is an ambitious one.
Physiology is hugely complex and poorly understood in many aspects, but this
does not mean that we should just shrug our shoulders and give up. There are
things we can achieve and insights we can gain, but we must remain critical at all
times of what we do. The most important part of the process is the modelling, not
the mathematics. The intention in this book is to concentrate on the modelling
process, using simple examples and giving enough of the mathematical background for the solutions to be understood. The mathematical equations may look
quite impressive when written out, but if the model on which they are based is a
bad one, even clever manipulations of the equations will still produce nonsense;
garbage in—garbage out.

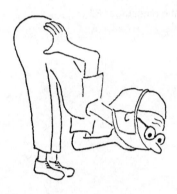

 A model is an attempt to mimic the *essential* features of some system. It therefore requires a simplification process whereby the important features are retained
and less important ones discarded. This process of sifting the essential from the
inessential is probably the most important part. It forces one to think carefully
about the factors involved in the behaviour of the system; in order to write an
equation, one needs to understand quite clearly what one means. The performance
of the model must be compared with the real system and any modifications introduced to make it approximate better to the real system.

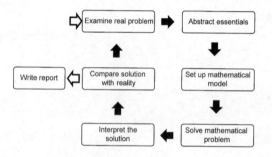

I have assumed a basic facility with simple algebraic operations and manipulation of equations. I have also assumed a knowledge of the elements of physics and
of physiology which any anaesthetist must know. Any deficiencies in these areas
should be remedied by reading the works listed in the bibliography.

 The theme of CO_2 physiology runs through the book. There are a number of reasons for this. First, it is a subject which is interesting and important in its own right
and illustrates many of the simplifying ideas involved in the construction of models.
Second, it provides an introduction to kinetic processes (i.e. changes with time)
which are fundamental to pharmacokinetics but which in that context seem to cause
such anguish to the examination candidate. Third, we are able easily and routinely to
measure changes in $PaCO_2$, either directly with blood gas analysis, or indirectly with
capnography. Since we manipulate levels of $PaCO_2$ in clinical practice every day, we
develop a 'feel' for how things change. We do not measure drug levels routinely in the
same way. Lastly, we can start with a very simple example which naturally illustrates
the modelling process without using complicated mathematics, and we can build
upon this simple model to consider more complex situations. Some of these models
and concepts then reappear in the section of the book devoted to statistics.

 The treatment is pictorial and graphical as far as possible. There is no attempt to
mathematical rigour or proof: I have merely tried to show that results are
'reasonable'.

1.1.2 The modelling process: physiological and statistical models

Anaesthetic trainees and their teachers are generally not very keen on the quantitative aspects of the basic sciences underlying clinical anaesthetic practice. The subjects of pharmacokinetics and statistics are particularly vilified, and enthusiasm for such subjects is viewed as a pitiable mental infirmity.

The difficulties in conveying the subjects of physiological and pharmacological models on the one hand, and of probability and statistics on the other, seem to be rather different. The process of mathematical modelling is a two-stage one; first the essential features of a system are abstracted into a model and this model is then used to construct equations. These equations must then be 'solved' to make the model usable. The physiological models can be understood relatively easily in a qualitative way, but the solution of the equations to which they give rise often requires mathematical skills and concepts that are unfamiliar or simply too advanced.

Conversely, the problem with understanding probability and statistics is that of understanding the models themselves; the mathematical manipulations involved are usually quite simple—summing, squaring, and so on. The models employ concepts that are inherently quite difficult and often demand the repeated application of the same ideas to the same problem. A perfectly logical and correct statistical statement can be made, for instance, that in repeated sampling 'the mean of the means is the mean'. This can lead to confusion. The problems are compounded by students trying to cram all of the unpleasant subjects in at the last minute before an exam. Retention of important ideas is usually quite minimal.

The process of learning these subjects is rather like respraying a car. For a perfect finish that does not fall off with the first bit of bad weather or a flying pebble, thin layers of lacquer must be applied carefully and allowed to cure before application of the next layer. Attempts to put the final thickness on in one go lead to an uneven and vulnerable finish. This book is designed so that it can be applied in small quantities at a time, over a prolonged period. Time should be allowed for the ideas to sink in before moving on to the next topic. To alter the analogy: graze, don't gorge.

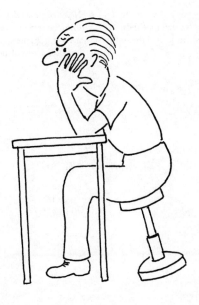

1.2.1 The input–output principle

The input–output principle (IOP) is an extremely simple yet astonishingly fertile idea in physiological modelling. The application of the principle is central to the quantitative approach to many physiological problems, and enables us to write equations which—if we can solve them—allow a more or less approximate description of the behaviour of the real physiological system. This book is more concerned with the modelling process than the details of the mathematical solution of the equations.

The IOP states that in any system in which a factor is being added to the system and removed from it, then

accumulation = input – output.

We shall use this simple idea numerous times to model real-life situations.

The IOP is very familiar from one's bank account. Although the principle is simple, we shall need to keep a close watch upon inputs and outputs of our systems. In steady states, which we deal with first, this is usually quite easy. In non-steady states we shall need to consider inputs and outputs over very small time intervals, although the modelling principle is identical. Often, we shall be quantifying the inputs and outputs of masses of substances, but at other times we model volumes or energy. We start with a couple of straightforward and familiar examples, and build on these to approach more complex situations.

The input–output principle

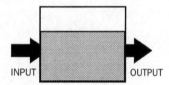

Steady State: Input = Output

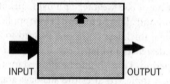

Positive Accumulation: Input > Output

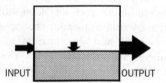

Negative Accumulation: Input < Output

Steady state. The input into the system is exactly balanced by the output and the system is in steady state. Accumulation is zero and the level in the system stays constant.

Positive accumulation (net gain). The input into the system exceeds the output and accumulation occurs. The level in the system rises.

Negative accumulation (net loss). The output from the system exceeds the input. There is a net loss from the system and the level falls: 'negative accumulation'.

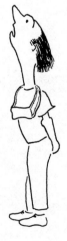

1.2.2   CSF flow and intracranial pressure

Cerebrospinal fluid (CSF) is secreted from the choroid plexus, circulates through the ventricular system and subarachnoid space, and is re-absorbed into the venous system by the arachnoid granulations. It is clear that, over any appreciable period, the uptake of CSF must be equal to the CSF production; input must equal output for the system to remain in steady state.

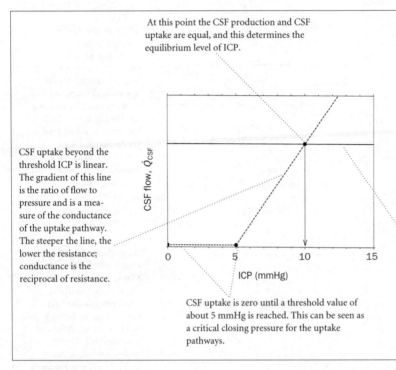

At this point the CSF production and CSF uptake are equal, and this determines the equilibrium level of ICP.

CSF uptake beyond the threshold ICP is linear. The gradient of this line is the ratio of flow to pressure and is a measure of the conductance of the uptake pathway. The steeper the line, the lower the resistance; conductance is the reciprocal of resistance.

CSF uptake is zero until a threshold value of about 5 mmHg is reached. This can be seen as a critical closing pressure for the uptake pathways.

CSF flows: input and output

Experiment has shown that CSF production is largely independent of intracranial pressure (ICP) as long as the cerebral perfusion pressure (CPP = mean arterial BP − ICP) remains above about 70 mmHg. On the other hand, the CSF re-absorption is dependent upon ICP; below a threshold value of about 5 mmHg, virtually no CSF uptake occurs, and as ICP increases above this threshold, the CSF uptake increases linearly.

CSF production is modelled as a constant quantity relative to ICP; whatever the value of ICP, we obtain the same CSF output. Various factors including anaesthetic agents may affect this level of production.

An empirical model

We need to make a number of points about what we have done. We have taken experimental data and abstracted what we believe to be the essential features: we have then incorporated them into a mathematical model version to describe how we think the real system might behave—at least approximately. The model is essentially an interpretation of what is obtained by experiment—it is empirical.

It is impossible that CSF production should remain actually constant (the same number of molecules each minute) and, anyhow, the constant production is dependent upon an adequate CPP. The model only applies under particular conditions and then only approximately.

Similarly, the zero uptake below the threshold value is not actually true—there is certain to be some uptake in this range. The uptake above this threshold will not be actually precisely linear either.

The model has taken the essentials of the system and used easily manipulated mathematical entities—constants and linear functions—to enable us to make approximate predictions about how such a system might behave in other circumstances. A model is always provisional—we can always hope to make it perform better.

Redrawn from: A. A. Artru Cerebrospinal Fluid Dynamics. In Clinical Neuroanesthesia. Edited by R. F. Cucciara, S. Black. J. D Michenfelder (2nd Edition) Churchill Livingstone. New York 1998. By kind permission of the publisher and Prof. Artru.

1.2.3　CSF dynamics

Varying the parameters

The general model that we have described can make predictions about the intracranial dynamics when we allow variation of the three parameters (2.4.1) involved—the CSF production rate, the threshold, and the gradient of the linear uptake.

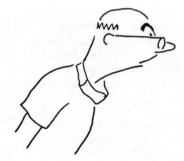

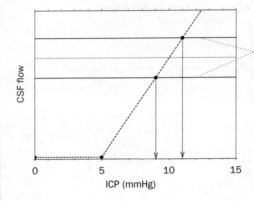

The production rate is constant in relation to ICP, but is affected by other factors. If the uptake function remains the same, any alteration in production level will affect the resulting equilibrium ICP. Volatile anaesthetics may increase the production and some intravenous anaesthetics may reduce it. Acetazolamide and frusemide reduce production.

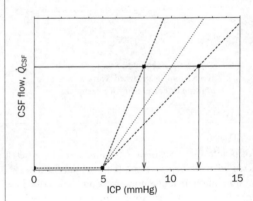

The gradient of the linear section of the uptake is steep if the resistance to flow is low. Volatile anaesthetic agents and subarachnoid haemorrhage for example may increase resistance and hence raise ICP. Low-dose opiates may reduce the resistance and hence increase the gradient of the uptake line and consequently reduce equilibrium ICP.

There is evidently plenty of scope for considering combinations of changing the three parameters and the effects that these would have on the resulting equilibrium ICP. This emphasizes that even a very simple abstracted model may have quite involved behaviour. Could we draw a single graph showing the dependence of ICP on the three factors involved? We cannot draw graphs of a variable (ICP) dependent upon more than two other variables (production, threshold, and gradient)—we can only portray them graphically by fixing one. We could, for example, draw a graph showing the effect of variation in production and gradient for a fixed threshold (2.11.1).

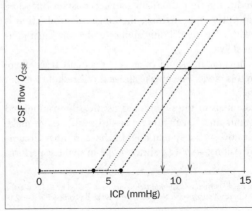

Variations in threshold level will also affect the equilibrium point. The threshold may be increased after subarachnoid haemorrhage and may contribute to hydrocephalus, which may occur in this condition.

1.3.1   Modelling steady states: $\dot{V}A$ and Pa_{CO_2}

We continue with a straightforward example that will form the basis of the more complex models that we shall develop later. The steady state relationship of alveolar ventilation $\dot{V}A$ and the Pa_{CO_2} is well known: increase the ventilation and the Pa_{CO_2} falls, reduce it and the Pa_{CO_2} rises. But what is the exact relationship and how can we model it? In order to start modelling we need to make some assumptions about the physiological problem. We want to describe the steady state Pa_{CO_2} which results from any chosen value of $\dot{V}A$ after the system has had time to 'settle down' from any change.

It is a good principle of mathematical modelling to move from the specific to the general in order to get a 'feel' for the problem. We will start with a specific problem; If the CO_2 production $\dot{V}_{CO_2}$ is 200 ml/min, what must be the $\dot{V}A$ which will result in a steady state Pa_{CO_2} of 5 kPa?

The model

We treat the lung as if it were a single uniform alveolar space or compartment with a steady flow through it of fresh gas—the alveolar ventilation $\dot{V}A$. These are severe simplifying modelling assumptions: we know that there are actually millions of individual alveoli and that ventilation is cyclical, not continuous.

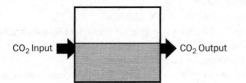

Steady state means that the level of CO_2 as measured by the Pa_{CO_2} remains constant; it does not vary with time. For steady state conditions to apply, the CO_2 input must equal the CO_2 output.

If the atmospheric pressure is assumed to be 100 kPa, then by Dalton's Law the alveolar fraction of CO_2 is $FA_{CO_2} = 0.05$. This means that 5% of the gas in the alveolar space is CO_2. Every time we remove 100 ml of this gas mixture from the space, we have eliminated 5 ml CO_2, and hence for each litre of $\dot{V}A$, 50 ml of CO_2 is removed. If the production is 200 ml/min and we are in steady state, then we must have a value of $\dot{V}A = 4$ l/min to ensure that input and output are equal.

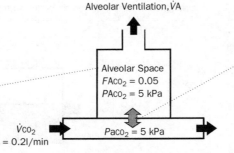

The alveolar membrane is very thin and CO_2 diffuses very rapidly, so that the gradient for P_{CO_2} across the membrane is assumed to be negligible. This enables us to equate PA_{CO_2} and Pa_{CO_2}, and to use the simple equivalence of pressure and content in a gas mixture as described by Dalton to determine alveolar CO_2 concentration.

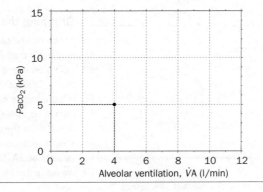

This calculation from the model gives us one point on the graph that relates $\dot{V}A$ and Pa_{CO_2}. When $\dot{V}A = 4$ l/min, $Pa_{CO_2} = 5$ kPa.

1.3.2   Modelling assumptions

We can carry out similar calculations for any chosen level of $PaCO_2$ assuming a constant production of $\dot{V}CO_2 = 200$ ml/min (0.2 l/min). For instance, if we work out the $\dot{V}A$ required to ensure a steady state $PaCO_2 = 2.5$ kPa, it is clear that $PACO_2$ must also be 2.5 kPa, and hence 2.5% of the alveolar ventilation will now be CO_2. Since 200 ml is 2.5% of 8 l, this must therefore be the required $\dot{V}A$. Similar calculation for $PaCO_2 = 10$ kPa demands $\dot{V}A = 2$ l/min.

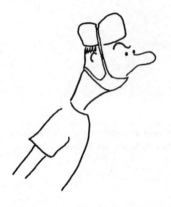

Abstracting the essentials: modelling assumptions

The process of creating a model involves the extraction of the essential features of the physiological system. Needless complexity is avoided in the first approach and the model is kept as simple as possible. Further refinement can be added later and quite complicated models built up.

The assumptions upon which the model has been constructed can be summarized as follows:

1. The lung behaves as a single uniform space or compartment.
2. Alveolar ventilation $\dot{V}A$ is a continuous, constant flow through this compartment.
3. CO_2 is produced at a constant rate of 200 ml/min.
4. Diffusion across the alveolar membrane is easy and rapid, so that $PaCO_2$ and $PACO_2$ can be considered equal.
5. Atmospheric pressure is constant, at $P_I = 100$ kPa.
6. Dalton's Law allows us to determine the alveolar fractional CO_2 concentration $FACO_2$ as a simple proportion.
7. Gas volumes are all measured at body temperature.

Evidently, not all of these assumptions are exactly true; the model is an approximation to reality. We wish to construct a model that behaves in a similar way to a real system in respect of the relationship of $\dot{V}A$ to $PaCO_2$. Pretending that the lung resembles an empty biscuit tin enables us to begin.

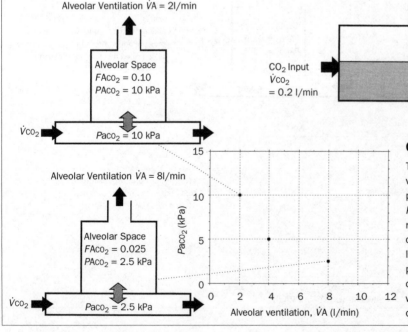

Graphing the solution

These simple calculations using our very basic model have given us three points on a graph of $\dot{V}A$ against $PaCO_2$. These points show that the relationship is non-linear—the points cannot be made to lie on a straight line. This is the graph of inversely proportional quantities (2.6). If we double the $\dot{V}A$, the $PaCO_2$ is halved; if we halve the $\dot{V}A$, the $PaCO_2$ is doubled.

1.3.3 Generalizing the model

We now need to generalize our model to obtain an expression which will describe the steady state PACO$_2$ that will result from any choice of $\dot{V}$CO$_2$ and $\dot{V}$A.

General model for PACO$_2$ determined by $\dot{V}$A and $\dot{V}$CO$_2$.

We apply the IOP. We assumed the CO_2 production to be constant and took a typical value of 200 ml/min (0.2 l/min) for our initial calculation. To allow consideration of other levels of CO_2 production, we denote this as $\dot{V}$CO$_2$ l/min. This is the input into the system.

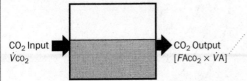

CO$_2$ Input
$\dot{V}$CO$_2$

CO$_2$ Output
[FACO$_2$ × $\dot{V}$A]

This is just the proportion of the total flow out of the alveolar space which is CO_2.

FACO$_2$ = PACO$_2$ / P_I. The alveolar CO_2 fraction FACO$_2$ is a ratio of pressures. It is a proportion—a dimensionless number.

Alveolar Ventilation $\dot{V}$A

The thin alveolar membrane and ready diffusibility of CO_2 allows us to write

$$F\text{ACO}_2 = \frac{P\text{ACO}_2}{P_I} \approx \frac{P\text{aCO}_2}{P_I}.$$

Alveolar Space
FACO$_2$
=
PACO$_2$ /100

$\dot{V}$CO$_2$

PACO$_2$

Equating input and output for steady state conditions, we have

$$\dot{V}\text{CO}_2 = \frac{P\text{ACO}_2}{P_I} \times \dot{V}\text{A}, \quad \text{which can be rearranged as}$$

$$P\text{ACO}_2 = \frac{\dot{V}\text{CO}_2 \times P_I}{\dot{V}\text{A}}.$$

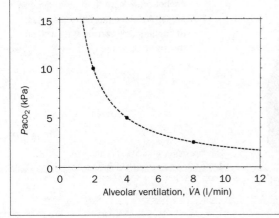

The graph shows the general relationship between $\dot{V}$A and PACO$_2$ for $\dot{V}$CO$_2$ = 0.2 l/min. The three original points that we calculated are shown. Generalization of the mathematical model enables us to draw the graph of all combinations of $\dot{V}$A and PACO$_2$ which satisfy the steady state condition for this level of CO_2 production.

The modelling equation; examining the solution

Note that we have used gas *volumes* to track *masses* of CO_2 added to and removed from the system. This is our first modelling equation. The expression that we have obtained is

$$P\text{aCO}_2 = P_I \times \frac{\dot{V}\text{CO}_2}{\dot{V}\text{A}}$$

This expression does not describe the actual variation of PACO$_2$ with $\dot{V}$A, it describes how the *model* behaves. This is an elementary point, but is easily forgotten. If the model is a good analogue of the real system, then the system will behave in an approximately similar fashion. If not, we need a better model.

It can often be helpful to regroup different elements of a mathematical expression to see better what is going on.

- $P\text{aCO}_2 = P_I \times \left[\dfrac{\dot{V}\text{CO}_2}{\dot{V}\text{A}} \right]$

The expression in brackets is a ratio of flows; it is a dimensionless number. It is the proportion of the atmospheric pressure P_I which is PACO$_2$ in the model.

- $P\text{aCO}_2 = \dfrac{1}{\dot{V}\text{A}} \left[P_I \times \dot{V}\text{CO}_2 \right]$

If P_I and $\dot{V}$CO$_2$ are fixed, then $P\text{aCO}_2 \propto 1/\dot{V}\text{A}$.
i.e. PACO$_2$ is inversely proportional to $\dot{V}$A and directly proportional to $\dot{V}$CO$_2$.

Variables and parameters

$\dot{V}A$ and $\dot{V}CO_2$ are both important in determining $PaCO_2$. In our initial consideration, we fixed the CO_2 production because we were primarily interested in establishing the relationship between $\dot{V}A$ and $PaCO_2$. We often fix a quantity for a set of calculations even though it is in principle able to vary. We 'ran' the model with certain values of $\dot{V}CO_2$ and obtained the family of curves. In this use, we treat $\dot{V}CO_2$ as a *parameter* of the model. When we look at the surface depiction below, we are looking at the simultaneous variation of $\dot{V}A$ and $\dot{V}CO_2$, and $PaCO_2$ is then viewed as a function of two variables (2.11). The model is the same; it all depends upon what we want to look at. We shall see the use of parameters in probability distributions later, where we obtain a family of distributions that differ only in the value of one or more determining parameters (3.2).

1.3.4   Surfaces and functions of two variables

We have constructed the graph of the relationship between $\dot{V}A$ and $PaCO_2$ for the particular $\dot{V}CO_2$ of 0.2 l/min. We can draw similar curves for other levels of production. All of the curves have the same basic shape and the effect of increasing production is to shift the curve upwards; for the same level of $\dot{V}A$, $PaCO_2$ is increased. This can be displayed as a family of curves on the graph, with each curve representing a different level of $\dot{V}CO_2$.

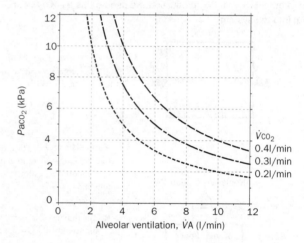

All possible combinations of $\dot{V}A$ and $\dot{V}CO_2$ and the resulting $PaCO_2$ must lie on the shaded surface. The value of the $PaCO_2$ is the vertical height above the base.

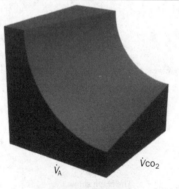

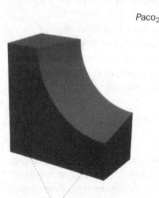

This slice or plane represents a fixed $\dot{V}CO_2$ and shows variation of $PaCO_2$ with $\dot{V}A$. It has the rectangular hyperbola profile of inversely proportional quantities. (2.8)

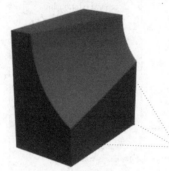

$PaCO_2$ as a function of two variables

Another way of depicting the relationship between $\dot{V}A$ and $\dot{V}CO_2$ in determining $PaCO_2$ is to construct a three-dimensional graph. This portrayal shows the resulting $PaCO_2$ from any combination of $\dot{V}A$ and $\dot{V}CO_2$. We can only use this for a function dependent upon two variables, since we cannot draw more than three dimensions. We could not show the effects of continuously varying P_i as well on the same diagram.

This face represents a fixed $\dot{V}A$ and shows the linear variation of $PaCO_2$ with $\dot{V}CO_2$. (2.5)

1.4.1   The same equations, different model

The gas laws are empirically derived descriptions of the behaviour of real gases. They are only approximately true for real gases and the laws break down seriously at extremes of temperature and pressure. They can be explained in terms of the kinetic theory of gases and thermodynamics, and modifications of the fundamental model have been made to improve the correspondence with reality; for example, Van der Waals' equation. The purpose of introducing them here is that they give rise to a model which is identical to that which we have just developed from first principles in describing the relationship of $\dot{V}A$ and $Pa{CO_2}$.

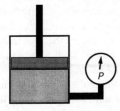

Boyle's Law. The volume of a gas at constant temperature is inversely proportional to the pressure: $V \propto 1/P$.

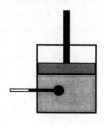

Charles' (or Gay-Lussac's) Law. The volume of a gas at constant pressure is directly proportional to the absolute temperature: $V \propto T^\circ \text{K}$.

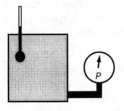

Alternatively, the pressure of a gas at constant volume is directly proportional to the absolute temperature: $P \propto T^\circ \text{K}$.

The ideal gas laws

These are combined into the general gas law or equation of state for a perfect gas:

$$PV = nRT,$$

where R is the universal gas constant and n is the number of moles of gas, i.e. a measure of mass. Further details can be found in texts of physical chemistry.

We can use the same surface depiction as before in the relationship of $\dot{V}A$, $\dot{V}{CO_2}$ and $Pa{CO_2}$. This time, all possible values of P, V and T must lie on the shaded surface. The equations can be seen to have the same form, with one directly proportional variable and one inversely proportional variable. These describe the behaviour of a fixed mass of n moles of gas.

If volume V is held constant, then pressure P varies directly with temperature. This is seen in the horizontal slice here (constant V).

$$P = T\left[\frac{nR}{V}\right].$$

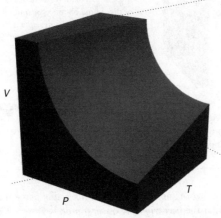

If pressure P is held constant, then volume V varies directly (i.e. linearly) with temperature $T^\circ \text{K}$:

$$V = T\left[\frac{nR}{P}\right].$$

If temperature is held constant, the volume and pressure vary inversely. This is Boyle's Law:

$$V = \frac{1}{P}[nRT].$$

1.5.1 Flux and fluxoids

Consider a pipe carrying a solution of salt at concentration 1 g/l, flowing at a rate of $\dot{Q} = 10$ l/min. We collect the effluent from the pipe for 10 min in a bucket. How much salt have we collected? The answer is trivially easy—100 g, which we obtain quite easily by multiplying the three quantities together:

concentration × flow × time = mass.

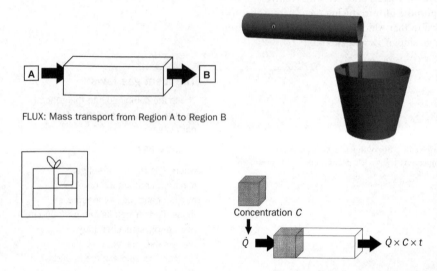

FLUX: Mass transport from Region A to Region B

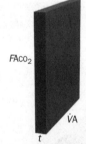

Concentration C

$\dot{Q}$ → $\dot{Q} \times C \times t$

We have transferred a mass of salt from one end of the pipe to the other, and the magnitude of this mass is given by the triplet product above, which is termed the *flux*. Flux is a transfer of a quantity from one region to another. We shall normally be concerned with mass transfer, but we shall also model one example of an energy flux.

In modelling the simple problem of steady state Pa_{CO_2} and $\dot{V}A$, we were also dealing with a question of mass-transfer. CO_2 is being transferred from the alveolar space to the atmosphere, and we worked out the quantity of CO_2 transferred (i.e. eliminated) by considering the flow ($\dot{V}A$) over a period of 1 min and the fractional CO_2 concentration, FA_{CO_2}. In this case we are measuring the mass of CO_2 in terms of a volume at assumed constant physical conditions—this is justified by reference to the general gas law, $PV = nRT$. If P and T are constant, V is directly proportional to n, the number of moles—i.e. the mass—of gas (1.4.1). We shall meet this flux package [Concentration × Flow × Time = Mass] in various contexts in the modelling examples.

Fluxoids

Since flux is calculated by multiplying three quantities together, we may represent masses transferred as the volumes of three-dimensional figures, the axes of which are *concentration*, *flow*, and *time*. The Pa_{CO_2}. and $\dot{V}A$ relationship can be used to illustrate this.

FA_{CO_2}

$\dot{V}A$

t

We consider a period of 1 min and assume constant $\dot{V}A$ and $\dot{V}_{CO_2}$. If we are in steady state, then FA_{CO_2} (and hence Pa_{CO_2}) must be unchanging with time by definition. This means that the 3-D figure must have a flat top and hence be a cuboidal structure. The volume of the cuboid obtained by multiplying the magnitude of its three dimensions must represent a mass. Since we are in steady state, this must be the same as the CO_2 production, $\dot{V}_{CO_2}$.

There are three axes. The vertical axis is fractional alveolar CO_2 concentration (FA_{CO_2}) which our modelling assumptions allow to be directly proportional to Pa_{CO_2}. The horizontal axis is time in minutes. The axis projecting into the paper is the flow axis, in this case $\dot{V}A$.

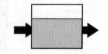

We shall call such structures that represent the flux or mass-transfer *fluxoids*: a silly name may help to fix the idea. We should imagine such a structure whenever we encounter the flux triplet [Concentration × Flow × Time = Mass]. All fluxoids with flat tops represent steady state conditions. If the top surface is curved, they represent a time-dependent process. Fluxoids will enable us to understand the more complicated problems of non-steady states more easily and see the physiology through the equations.

1.5.2 CO_2 flux: $Paco_2$ and $\dot{V}A$

CO_2 flux: $Paco_2$ and $\dot{V}A$

We can use the fluxoid idea to show quite easily how the inverse relationship of $Paco_2$ and $\dot{V}A$ arises. The IOP tells us that, for a steady state, we must have a minute CO_2 output equal to $\dot{V}co_2$. If we consider fluxoids with a time dimension of magnitude 1 min, then if the fluxoid has a flat top, the $Paco_2$ is not changing with time. For a constant output, the product of the other two dimensions, $Paco_2$ and $\dot{V}A$, must be a constant. The graph of $Faco_2$ (and hence of $Paco_2$, by the modelling assumptions) and $\dot{V}A$ is then simply the graph of all possible values of $\dot{V}A$ and $Faco_2$ which allow this fluxoid to have a volume equal to the minute CO_2 production $\dot{V}co_2$. This sounds more complicated than it is.

How does the presence of CO_2 in the inspired gas affect the model? The CO_2 input is now from two sources and we can balance input and output for steady states and obtain

$$\dot{V}co_2 + \dot{V}A \times Fico_2 = \dot{V}A \times Faco_2$$

which can be rearranged as

$$Faco_2 = \frac{\dot{V}co_2}{\dot{V}A} + Fico_2$$

This tell us that for a fixed $\dot{V}A$, The $Faco_2$ and hence the $Paco_2$ are simply raised by the value of $Fico_2$ ($Pico_2$) in the inspired gas. The fluxoid now sits on a platform of height $Pico_2$.

If we require the $Paco_2$ to remain constant at 5kPa despite rebreathing say 1%CO_2 mixture ($Fico_2 = 0.01$), then we must increase $\dot{V}A$ such that the upper fluxoid block has a height 4kPa. The required $\dot{V}A$ is now 5 l/min. ($\dot{V}co_2 = 0.2$ l/min.)

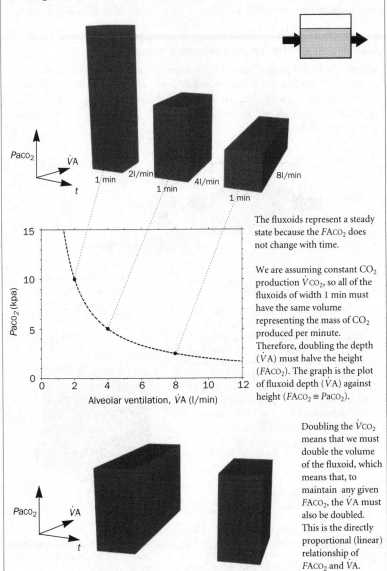

The fluxoids represent a steady state because the $Faco_2$ does not change with time.

We are assuming constant CO_2 production $\dot{V}co_2$, so all of the fluxoids of width 1 min must have the same volume representing the mass of CO_2 produced per minute. Therefore, doubling the depth ($\dot{V}A$) must halve the height ($Faco_2$). The graph is the plot of fluxoid depth ($\dot{V}A$) against height ($Faco_2 \equiv Paco_2$).

Doubling the $\dot{V}co_2$ means that we must double the volume of the fluxoid, which means that, to maintain any given $Faco_2$, the $\dot{V}A$ must also be doubled. This is the directly proportional (linear) relationship of $Faco_2$ and $\dot{V}A$.

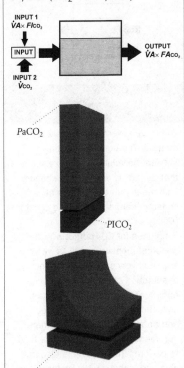

Breathing a CO_2-containing mixture elevates the homeostasis surface so that it sits on a platform of height $Pico_2$.

1.5.3   Cardiac output $\dot{Q}$ by CO_2 flux

The Fick principle is a well-known physiological modelling approach to measurement of blood flows. The Fick principle can be stated as follows:

During any interval of time, the quantity of a substance entering a compartment in the inflowing blood must equal the sum of accumulation within that compartment and the quantity leaving in the efferent blood.

This is evidently a statement about inputs and outputs and is a particular case of the more general IOP which specifically refers to blood flows. However, we wish to keep our concept of flow in mass transfer processes very general so that we can use the same ideas in diverse circumstances; flux is the more fundamental concept. The Fick principle can be demonstrated by the example of cardiac output measurement using CO_2, and we shall see that the principle of mass transfer is identical to the alveolar ventilation example and numerous others that we shall meet.

Cardiac output by the Fick principle using CO_2

We use the fluxoid picture again. This time the concentration is the CO_2 content of the blood. We consider a time interval of 1 min *during which time the system is assumed to be in steady state*, i.e. the cardiac output $\dot{Q}$ l/min is constant. $\dot{V}CO_2$ is constant. The usual axis system is employed but this time the flow axis represents cardiac output.

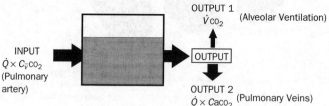

OUTPUT 1
$\dot{V}CO_2$ (Alveolar Ventilation)

INPUT
$\dot{Q} \times C_{\bar{v}}CO_2$
(Pulmonary artery)

OUTPUT

OUTPUT 2
$\dot{Q} \times CaCO_2$ (Pulmonary Veins)

The CO_2 input into the system in the afferent blood in 1 min is the volume of the whole block. The system here is the lung.

Problems with the CO_2 method

There are several problems with this method. The equation relating $\dot{V}CO_2$ to the volume of a box assumes that the box *is* actually box-shaped. This means an assumption of constant cardiac output and constant $[C_{\bar{v}}CO_2 - CaCO_2]$, i.e. steady state conditions for CO_2 output over the period of measurement. As we shall see, it is very easy to violate this assumption of steady state conditions for CO_2 output. Expired gas collection and analysis is tedious and open to inaccuracy, and measurements take a considerable time to perform. The method is also invasive and, although it is no longer used in practice, illustrates the Fick principle well.

The volume of the upper block is the mass difference of the CO_2 delivered to the lung and that taken away in the efferent blood, and must therefore be the quantity removed from the lung by alveolar ventilation. We measure this directly by collecting expired gas and calculating the minute production $\dot{V}CO_2$ and thus obtain the volume of the upper block. By measuring its height, the difference between $CaCO_2$ and $C_{\bar{v}}CO_2$, we can calculate the cardiac output $\dot{Q}$.

$$\dot{Q} \times (C_{\bar{v}}CO_2 - CaCO_2) \times 1 = \dot{V}CO_2,$$

which rearranges as

$$\dot{Q} = \frac{\dot{V}CO_2}{(C_{\bar{v}}CO_2 - CaCO_2)}.$$

To give an example, using typical values for $CaCO_2$ = 0.48 litres per litre of blood, and $C_{\bar{v}}CO_2$ = 0.52 litres per litre of blood, and $\dot{V}CO_2 = 0.2$. $\dot{Q} \times (0.52 - 0.48) = 0.2$, which gives $\dot{Q} = 5$ l/min.

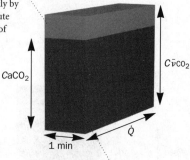

$CaCO_2$

$C_{\bar{v}}CO_2$

$\dot{Q}$

1 min

The CO_2 output from the system in the efferent blood in 1 min is the volume of the lower block.

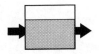

1.5.4 $\dot{Q}$ by O$_2$ uptake

The Fick method using CO_2 can be modified by using O_2 uptake instead of CO_2 output. Although this has many of the same disadvantages as the CO_2 method, the assumption of steady state conditions for O_2 uptake is more reliable than that for CO_2 output. The method still involves measurement over appreciable periods—a few minutes—during which cardiac output and uptake must be assumed to be constant. It does not lend itself to rapid repeated measurement in sick patients and has been superseded by the thermodilution method (1.6.2).

Cardiac output using Fick principle and O$_2$ uptake

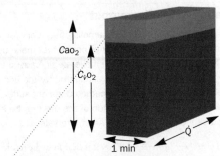

This is an identical diagram to the previous one, except that the top block now represents the mass of O_2 taken up over a period of 1 min. This can be measured directly. The O_2 uptake, $\dot{V}O_2$ can be much more reliably assumed to be constant than can CO_2 output in the former method. Excess O_2 uptake beyond requirement is limited by saturation of haemoglobin, and uptake below requirement rapidly manifests itself as hypoxia. We equate the uptake of O_2 with the volume of the top block fluxoid [flow × (concentration difference between arterial and venous) × time].

$$\dot{Q} \times (CaO_2 - C\bar{v}O_2) \times 1 = \dot{V}O_2,$$

which rearranges as

$$\dot{Q} = \frac{\dot{V}O_2}{(CaO_2 - C\bar{v}O_2)}.$$

(Alveolar Ventilation) INPUT 1 $\dot{V}O_2$

INPUT

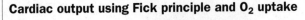

OUTPUT
$\dot{Q} \times CaCO_2$
(Pulmonary veins)

(Pulmonary artery) INPUT 2 $\dot{Q} \times C\bar{v}O_2$

Fick methods

Both of these Fick methods are quite easy to understand, because assumed steady-state conditions apply and we are calculating volumes of boxes—assumed regular solid objects. We have concentrated on the fluxoid picture because this should enable us to see more easily what is going on when quantities are changing with time. Next, we look at the dye-dilution method of cardiac output measurement, and at the modern, easily performed but perhaps not quite so easily understood, thermodilution method.

1.6.1 $\dot{Q}$ by dye-dilution

The Fick methods for cardiac output determination involving O_2 uptake and CO_2 output are clearly steady state methods. The universally applied method in clinical practice now is thermodilution using a cardiac output computer. This is a development of the older dye-dilution method in which a dye is injected rapidly into the pulmonary artery and its concentration in blood drawn intermittently from a peripheral artery over the ensuring minute or so is determined. Alternatively, blood was drawn at constant rate from the artery and passed through a densitometer chamber. A typical (simulated) record of the dye-dilution method is shown and it is evident that dye concentration is not in steady state.

Dye-dilution determination of cardiac output

A suitable dye, e.g. Indocyanine green, is used. The sampling frequency (or response time of the densitometer) limits the number of points that make up the record. The primary peak is followed by a secondary, smaller peak, caused by recirculation of the dye. The secondary peak must be eliminated for the accuracy of the method to be acceptable. The thermodilution method does not suffer in practice from either of these disadvantages. Elimination of the dye may be slow, which means that the method cannot be repeated at short intervals.

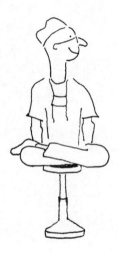

It is clear from the record that the dye concentration is changing with time, but the method allows only a limited resolution of sampling. We assume that the record would be a 'smooth' curve if only we could sample more frequently. We do not really know what goes on between the points that we actually measure.

By fair means or foul, we fit a smooth curve to these points and then calculate the area under the curve (AUC). In the days in which this method was used, this probably meant plotting the points, fitting a curve 'by eye', and counting squares on a piece of graph paper. Counting squares gives us a model of a stepped fluxoid changing with time.

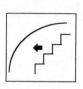

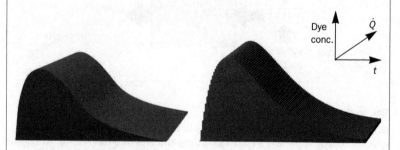

We imagine a smooth fluxoid like this one within the messy real data of a dye dilution run. We then consider this smooth structure to be constructed from a large number of flat topped fluxoid 'wafers'.

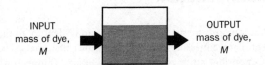

INPUT
mass of dye,
M

OUTPUT
mass of dye,
M

We know that a fluxoid has a volume equivalent to a mass. The substance that we are measuring is the dye and we know how much of this we have injected, M mg. After eliminating the secondary peak, the sum of the individual fluxoid volumes under the envelope of the smooth curve must be M. Since all of the dye has been 'removed', the dye input and output are equal.

Elimination of the secondary peak

Although this method is obsolete, it does illustrate important features. The recirculation of dye produces a second peak, which interferes with our assessment of the 'true' AUC and hence $\dot{Q}$. The decay phase of the record is well described by a single exponential process until the recirculation interrupts it. This portion of the curve can be treated to a linear transformation by plotting *log* concentration against time. Deviations from the linear regression line can be stripped (2.9.12) away and the 'pure' curve replotted, and hence the AUC calculated with the effects of recirculation removed.

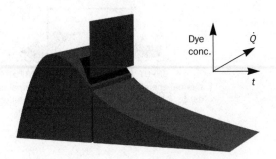

Dye
conc.

$\dot{Q}$

t

If we assume that the cardiac output is constant during the measurement (as we must do), then the sum of the fluxoid wafer volumes is the same as the sum of the areas of the individual faces (i.e. the approximate area under the curve) multiplied by the depth, $\dot{Q}$, the (supposedly constant) cardiac output.

$$M = AUC \times \dot{Q}$$
$$\dot{Q} = \frac{M}{AUC}$$

We shall encounter a number of other smooth fluxoids representing various quantities. We should imagine all of them to be constructed of many fluxoid wafers, thin enough to make the curve of the surface of the total fluxoid structure reasonably smooth. We can calculate areas of rectangles easily. This idea is the basis of that of the integral and areas under curves explained in (2.14.2). The mathematical technique of integration allows us to determine areas under curves of certain functions exactly using infinitely thin wafers. By numerical methods (2.16) we can work out areas under curves approximately, using a variety of techniques. The technique of the measurement method will determine how accurately we can measure an area under a curve—the thermodilution method of cardiac output measurement is capable of much greater resolution than the dye dilution method, so that we get a much smoother record.

1.6.2 $\dot{Q}$ by thermodilution

The principle of thermodilution measurement of cardiac output is identical to the dye-dilution method except that we measure flux of *energy* rather than mass. The method has a number of important advantages over dye-dilution. Temperature measurements are made by thermistor, and the area under the resulting curve is calculated by the cardiac output computer, to produce a value for cardiac output, and derived measures such as cardiac index and peripheral resistance, being displayed automatically.

Cardiac output $\dot{Q}$ by thermodilution

A known volume of cold saline at known temperature is injected at time $t = 0$. This saline is diluted in the cardiac output and causes the temperature of the blood passing the thermistor positioned downstream to fall. The equivalent quantity to the mass of dye is the *energy content difference* from the same volume of blood at body temperature.

INPUT
thermal energy
deficit

OUTPUT
thermal energy
restitution from
blood

This is a simulated idealized thermodilution record. The rapid response time of the thermistor gives a much smoother record than is achievable with dye dilution. This gives us much more confidence in fitting a 'smooth' curve—or allowing the computer to do so for us. Because the energy content of a small volume of cold saline is negligible compared with the total heat energy content of the tissues, this is equilibrated with the tissues and not discernible in recirculation, as is dye concentration. This means that the measurement can be repeated at short intervals. We *must* assume, however, that there is no equilibration with tissues other than blood during the measurement period itself.

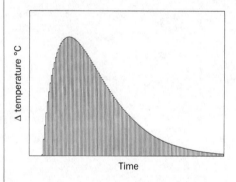

Time

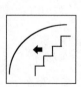

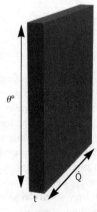

The fluxoid now no longer has a volume that is a *mass*, because the temperature difference is not a mass concentration. Temperature is, however, a measure of *energy* concentration and is related to the energy content of unit mass of substance by the specific heat, *s*.

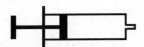

Energy content =
Mass × Specific Heat × Temperature difference from blood
$m \times s \times (\theta_{blood} - \theta_{saline})$

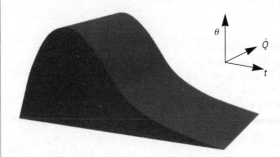

The volume of cold saline injected, m, is warmed to body temperature θ_{blood} by energy flow from the blood. The energy content difference of a syringe of cold saline at temperature θ_{saline} compared with blood is (volume × specific heat × change in temp), i.e. $m \times s_{saline} \times (\theta_{blood} - \theta_{saline})$, and this is the energy that must be acquired by the saline. s_{saline} is the specific heat, in Joules/kg/$T°$C. We treat this total energy change as the volume of our fluxoid.

We simply equate the energy content difference of the saline in the syringe with the total volume of the fluxoids.

$$m \times s_{saline} \times (\theta_{saline} - \theta_{blood}) = AUC \times s_{blood} \times \dot{Q}$$

If we assume the value for s to be the same for blood and saline and rearrange, then we have

$$\dot{Q} = \frac{m\left(\theta_{saline} - \theta_{blood}\right)}{AUC}.$$

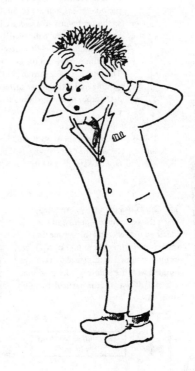

1.7.1   The Kety–Schmidt method for cerebral blood flow (CBF)

The measurement of cerebral blood flow (CBF) is accomplished using the same flux principles as cardiac output. The classical method is that of Kety and Schmidt, using N_2O uptake into the brain. More modern methods using radioactive isotopes such as [133]Xenon are merely modifications of the earlier method. The fluxoid idea should make this easy to understand.

Kety–Schmidt method

A low concentration (10–15%) of N_2O is inspired, and N_2O concentration c_{N_2O} vol.% measured at intervals in arterial blood, e.g. from radial artery cannula, and in the venous blood from the jugular bulb. The jugular bulb N_2O content is assumed to reflect the concentration of N_2O in the brain and to be unaffected by other tissues—a rather optimistic assumption. A typical simulated record is shown. We again assume that the measurements that we have are points on smooth curves—one for arterial Ca_{N_2O} and one for jugular venous Cjv_{N_2O}.

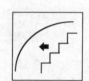

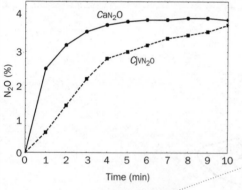

The rise in Ca_{N_2O} is governed by the pharmacokinetics of N_2O inhalation; details are available elsewhere. We assume a constant CBF throughout the period of measurement (c. 10–15 min), so this represents an average CBF over the period. We have the usual concentration–time–flow axis system, so volumes represent masses of N_2O. The total N_2O *flux* into the brain is the volume under the upper surface of the 3-D graph, where the flow axis is the CBF.

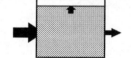

The flux *out of* the brain in the period is the volume under the lower surface. The volume of the strangely shaped piece between the upper and lower surface must be the quantity of N_2O left behind in the brain.

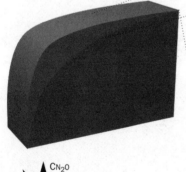

The Ca_{N_2O} and the Cjv_{N_2O} eventually reach the same value—at least in the idealized model—and this means that there is no further net uptake of N_2O. The brain is assumed at this stage to have equilibrated with the inflowing blood, so that it is 'full' of N_2O for the particular equilibrium Ca_{N_2O}.

The volume of this piece is again the sum of the volumes of fluxoids and is the area between the curves (ABC) multiplied by the CBF. This represents the mass of N_2O taken up by the brain: the mass of N_2O = $ABC \times \dot{Q}_{CBF}$.

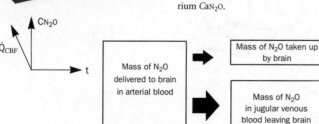

The new problem with this measurement method, compared with the otherwise similar cardiac output Fick measurements, is that we cannot directly measure the mass of N_2O taken up by the brain as we were able to measure O_2, CO_2, mass of dye, or energy content in the various methods for $\dot{Q}$. We need some more assumptions.

1.7.2 The Kety–Schmidt method and tissue capacitance

We know the equilibrium value for $C_{\text{a}N_2O}$ (and $C_{\text{jv}N_2O}$, as they are then the same). The brain tissue partial pressure of N_2O, $P_{\text{br}N_2O}$ is then assumed to be at equilibrium with $P_{\text{a}N_2O}$, the partial pressure in the arterial blood. The mass of N_2O stored in the brain for any given $P_{\text{a}N_2O}$ is determined by the solubility of N_2O in brain tissue.

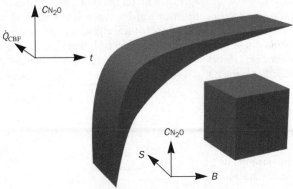

The volume of these two shapes must be equal since they both represent the mass of N_2O in the brain at equilibrium. We can generalize to another substance with a different value for S or a brain of different size B, or a different equilibrium value of C_{N_2O}. These alter the volume of the solubility cube.

$$\dot{Q}_{CBF} \times (ABC) = [C_{blood}N_2O/100\ \text{ml}] \times S \times B,$$

$$\dot{Q}_{CBF} = \frac{[C_{blood}N_2O/100\ \text{ml}] \times S \times B}{(ABC)}.$$

Since neither $\dot{Q}_{CBF}$ nor the brain mass is known, we must express $\dot{Q}_{CBF}$ in specific terms ml/min/100g brain tissue. For $S = 1$, we have

$$\frac{\dot{Q}_{CBF}}{B} = \frac{[C_{blood}N_2O/100\ ml]}{(ABC)}$$

Solubility and partition coefficients

We have a measure of the mass M of N_2O as the volume of the odd-shaped piece, but we have nothing to equate it to, because we do not know what the total mass of N_2O taken up by the brain is. What can we do about this?

The total mass of N_2O in the brain after equilibrium is $B \times S \times C_{\text{a}N_2O}$, where B is the volume of the brain: if the concentration in blood is measured per 100 ml, then B is in ml per 100 ml of tissue. This triplet can be displayed as a box, the volume of which is a mass. This box is not itself a fluxoid (no flow, no time) but can be equated with one, since both represent masses.

Solubility is characterized as the *partition coefficient* of N_2O. We can describe a ratio of volumes of N_2O in blood and brain at the same partial pressure, i.e. at equilibrium. The blood/brain partition coefficient S for N_2O is conveniently approximately unity. This means that we can measure the equilibrium content $C_{\text{a}N_2O}$ (ml per 100 ml of blood) and assume the same value for the brain tissue:

$$S_{\text{blood/brain}} = \frac{V_{\text{blood}}N_2O/100\ \text{ml}}{V_{\text{brain}}N_2O/100\ \text{ml}} = 1$$

at equilibrium.

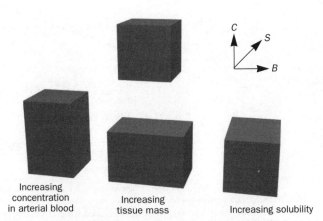

The volume of the box is the mass of substance stored in the tissue. This is dependent upon three factors, tissue mass, solubility, and concentration.

Tissue capacitance

The concept of tissue capacitance is quite useful. It is the product of the mass or volume of the tissue—the brain can hold more N_2O than the pituitary—and the solubility of the substance—the partition coefficient S. It is a measure of the *capacity* of a tissue to contain a substance; if the solubility is high, the blood/tissue partition coefficient is low (the tissue/blood coefficient is high) and the tissue can accommodate a large amount of the substance relative to blood. The actual quantity held in the tissue depends upon the concentration in the arterial blood and whether equilibrium has been reached.

1.8.1   **Apnoeic oxygenation**

The technique of apnoeic oxygenation is most frequently employed during the apnoea test in assessment of brain stem function in the intensive care unit. It has uses in anaesthesia where there is competition for the airway, e.g. in bronchoscopy or laryngoscopy, or in emergency when ventilation is impossible. In the technique, the intubated apnoeic patient—perhaps from muscle relaxants, perhaps because of brain stem destruction—is kept oxygenated by means of a catheter inserted through the tube into the trachea, through which oxygen is passed at about 4 l/min. No positive pressure is applied. Under ideal circumstances, adequate haemoglobin saturation can be maintained for a considerable period, measured in tens of minutes. How does it work and what are these ideal circumstances? As usual, the key to modelling is the IOP.

Pa_{CO_2} in apnoea

The endotracheal tube is open to the atmosphere and oxygen is simply insufflated down the tube. The lung volume under these conditions is held at the Functional Residual Capacity (FRC). We shall assume a value for FRC of 2 l. If there is no active ventilation, this volume is constant. We shall track input and output gas volumes in this space.

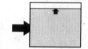

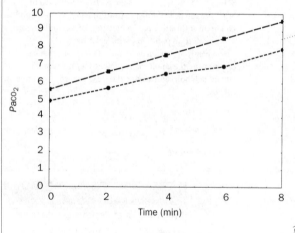

Since there is no alveolar ventilation and $\dot{V}_{CO_2}$ continues unabated, we expect the Pa_{CO_2} to rise. This graph shows the rise in Pa_{CO_2} measured in two patients undergoing apnoeic oxygenation (real data). The rate of rise of Pa_{CO_2} is remarkably constant—there is a convincing linear relationship between duration of apnoea and Pa_{CO_2}. In our modelling of apnoeic oxygenation, we shall assume a perfect linear relationship of Pa_{CO_2} with time, rising at 0.5 kPa/min. If we know the starting Pa_{CO_2}, we can calculate the Pa_{CO_2} at any time t in the ensuing period.

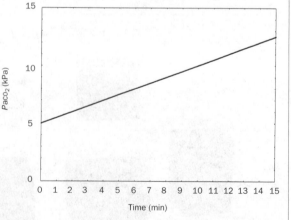

The gas in the FRC is in equilibrium with the CO_2 in the blood. As before, we assume a negligible gradient across the alveolar membrane, so that $PA_{CO_2} = Pa_{CO_2}$ at all times. The rate of rise of PA_{CO_2} is therefore also 0.5 kPa/min.

The rate of rise of Pa_{CO_2} is typically 0.3–0.7 kPa/min, although it will usually be lower in brain death (hypothermia, absent brain contribution to metabolism) when the apnoea test is required. The linearity is an observed, empirical relationship which is approximate and may not continue at extreme values of hypercapnia, but we adopt a perfect linear relationship as a model. The starting value of Pa_{CO_2} at time $t = 0$ will depend upon the pre-existing $\dot{V}_{CO_2}$ and $\dot{V}_A$, as we already know (1.3).

The airway is open to atmospheric pressure, so that the alveolar space is a constant volume, the FRC. Atmospheric pressure $P_I = 100$ kPa.

1.8.2 **FRC and distribution volume**

FRC and volume of distribution for CO_2

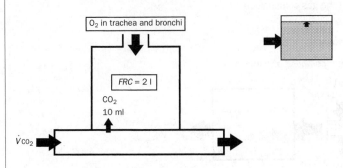

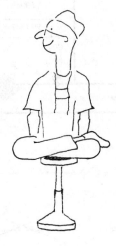

The $PaCO_2$ is rising according to our model at the rate of 0.5 kPa/min. The total pressure in the alveolar space, which is open to atmosphere, is 100 kPa. The $FACO_2$ is therefore rising at 0.005/min, i.e. 0.5% in 1 min. Since the total volume of the FRC is 2000 ml, then during each minute 10 ml CO_2 (0.5% of 2000 ml) is added to the FRC (Dalton's Law). If we have a CO_2 production of $\dot{V}CO_2 = 200$ ml/min, then 5% of it enters the alveolar space and 95% remains in the body water.

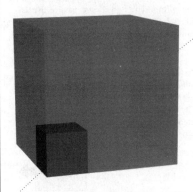

The $PaCO_2$ at any instant is assumed to be the same throughout the model—we are modelling the body as a single container or compartment. The alveolar space—the FRC—is a part of this compartment in which the $PaCO_2$ reflects that in the rest of the model, but in which—because of Dalton's Law—we can make direct calculation of the quantity of CO_2 entering.

Although CO_2 enters the alveolar space, because there is no alveolar ventilation, no CO_2 escapes from the system as a whole. The FRC is simply part of the larger 'compartment'. Since the $\dot{V}CO_2$ is constant with no removal and the rise in $PaCO_2$ linear, we need only have one compartment in our model. A constant quantity continuously added to a constant-volume container causes a linear rise in concentration if none escapes.

The rate of rise of $PaCO_2$ is linear and the magnitude of this rise in the model reflects the balance between the rate of CO_2 production $\dot{V}CO_2$ and the volume of the container to which it is being added. This volume is the volume of distribution for CO_2. The larger this volume is, the greater is its ability to 'mop up' the $\dot{V}CO_2$ and hence slow the rate of rise of $PaCO_2$.

We may be mildly surprised that $PaCO_2$, which is not a concentration, increases linearly with duration of apnoea, but we accept it with gratitude since it makes a model easy to construct. The volume of distribution is a notional container, an abstraction. It is simply viewed as a receptacle for the CO_2 that is contained within the body and cannot escape. It is, in effect, a proportionality constant which relates $\dot{V}CO_2$ and the resulting rise in $PaCO_2$. This demands that the proportionality constant should be measured in kPa/l.CO_2.

1.8.3   **Input and output in the FRC**

Tracking gas volumes in the FRC

The volume of the FRC is constant at 2000 ml and yet the gas composition within it is changing with time. Using the IOP we have

input gas volume = output gas volume,

i.e. the FRC gas *volume* is in steady state, while the gas *composition* within it is not.

Input. CO_2 enters the FRC at a rate of 10 ml/min. This is determined by the CO_2 production and the volume of distribution for CO_2 which, in turn, determines the rate of rise of $PaCO_2$ and hence of $PACO_2$.

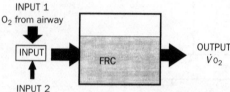

INPUT 1
O_2 from airway

INPUT   OUTPUT
FRC $\dot{V}O_2$

INPUT 2
CO_2 from
blood

Output. If we assume that the O_2 uptake $\dot{V}O_2$ is 200 ml/min, then this is the output from the FRC. There is thus a 190 ml discrepancy which must be made up by gas flowing in from the open airway. If we are filling the trachea and bronchi with oxygen through a catheter, then 100% oxygen will be drawn in by bulk flow—*not* diffusion—into the FRC. There is a gentle breeze in the airway as O_2 is 'sucked in' at the rate of 190 ml/min. This is in effect a 'passive alveolar ventilation'—it is ventilation without muscular effort and without CO_2 elimination.

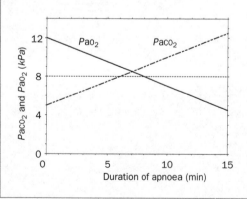

O_2 in trachea and bronchi

190 ml

FRC = 2 l

CO_2 O_2
10 ml   200 ml

If 190 ml of 100% O_2 is drawn into the FRC to replace the O_2 taken up each minute, then the imbalance between O_2 taken up and O_2 supplied is 10 ml/min—the 'space' required to accommodate the rising $PACO_2$. The rate of fall of PAO_2 in these circumstances is thus predicted by the model to be the same as the rate of rise of $PACO_2$—0.5 kPa/minute.

How long a duration of apnoea can be tolerated before the threshold of unacceptable hypoxia is breached depends upon the starting value of PAO_2, i.e. the degree of pre-oxygenation before the onset of apnoea. At a starting PaO_2 value of 12 kPa, the 8 kPa barrier would be breached after 8 min. The $PaCO_2$ would have risen to 9 kPa by this time for a starting value of 5 kPa.

We are quite naturally and easily here calculating $PaCO_2$ and PaO_2 values at any time t, from knowledge of the rate of change of each and the values at which we started (the onset of apnoea). Note also that we have tacitly assumed that PaO_2 and PAO_2 are identical. This is because we have a perfect lung model, with no possibility of $\dot{V}/\dot{Q}$ mismatch to give shunt. We have also ignored effects of nitrogen entering the alveoli from body stores if the PAN_2 is reduced.

1.8.4 **Effects of pre-oxygenation and O$_2$ concentration**

Changing the conditions; time to hypoxia

What happens if we modify the concentration of oxygen in the tracheo-bronchial tree—perhaps by insufflating insufficient oxygen so that air is drawn in? Suppose that the O$_2$ concentration is now 50%. There will still be 190 ml of gas flowing into the FRC by the bulk flow (passive ventilation) mechanism, but only 50% of this, i.e. 95 ml, will be O$_2$. The discrepancy in O$_2$ input and output in the FRC is now 105 ml/min—10 ml due to CO$_2$ and 95 ml to dilution of 100% O$_2$. The $F_{A}O_2$ thus falls by 105/2000/min—the equivalent of 5.25 kPa/min—more than tenfold the rate of fall when 100% O$_2$ is present in the airways.

Assuming a pre-oxygenation regime that has ensured a starting P_aO_2 of 50 kPa, the falls in P_aO_2 for O$_2$ concentrations of 100%, 50%, and 21% are seen. The leisurely fall (0.5 kPa/min) seen with 100% means that, according to the model, CO$_2$ toxicity would be a limiting factor to the duration of apnoea long before serious hypoxia occurred. Even with 21%, provided that pre-oxygenation has been efficient, about 5 min of apnoea is tolerable—the rate of fall is about 8 kPa/min. Hypoxia would be apparent before CO$_2$ toxicity in this case.

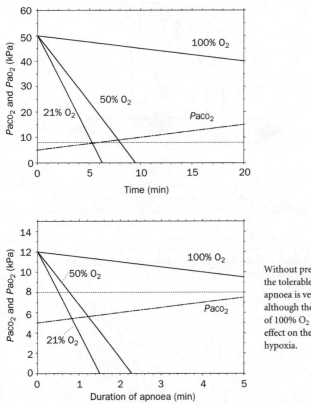

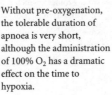

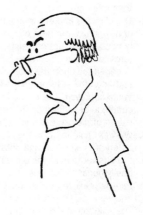

Without pre-oxygenation, the tolerable duration of apnoea is very short, although the administration of 100% O$_2$ has a dramatic effect on the time to hypoxia.

Think about the effects of the size of the FRC in governing the rate of fall of P_aO_2. The size of the FRC in relation to the $\dot{V}O_2$ is an important factor in determining the rate of fall; small babies with high $\dot{V}O_2$ relative to body mass and small FRC are particularly vulnerable to rapid onset of hypoxia.

Differential equations

This problem is an example of a simple *differential equation* arising from a model. It is so simple that we have had no difficulty in solving it using elementary arithmetic.

1. We obtained an expression for the *rate of change* of Pa_{O_2} with duration of apnoea. This arose from the modelling assumptions applied to an observed relationship of rise of Pa_{CO_2} during apnoea. This rate of fall of Pa_{O_2} was constant, but its magnitude—i.e. the slope—depended upon the concentration of O_2 in the tracheo-bronchial tree. A differential equation is one that describes the rate of change of the quantity in which we are interested. Many mathematical models give rise to differential equations, most of them rather more difficult to solve than this one.

2. The clinically important question of how long a duration of apnoea is possible without crossing the threshold of unacceptable hypoxia depended upon the rate of fall and upon the starting Pa_{O_2}—the *initial condition*. The initial condition depended upon the extent of pre-oxygenation.

3. We were able to *solve* the differential equation and obtain the answer to our problem quite easily because the rate of fall of Pa_{O_2} is predicted to be constant and we knew the starting value. The solution of a differential equation is another equation that describes the value of the quantity at any time—in our case the actual Pa_{O_2} as a function of time. The solution is a linear equation because a constant rate of change describes a linear (2.5) relationship—the rate of change is the gradient of the line (2.12.).

4. Most differential equations which arise in practice are much more difficult to solve than this one and many are actually impossible. The important point to note is that the model based upon physiology gives rise to a differential equation that needs a mathematical method for solution. In this book we concentrate on the *modelling process* and only outline the principles of the *mathematical methods* involved in the solution of the physiological problems.

1.8.5   **Apnoeic oxygenation and differential equations**

Review of the model

The simple model has given us a quantitative idea of the effects of varying the conditions in apnoea. The determining factors are as follows:

(1) the size of the FRC;
(2) the CO_2 production, $\dot{V}_{CO_2}$ and volume of distribution;
(3) the O_2 consumption, $\dot{V}_{O_2}$ and hence the respiratory quotient, *RQ*;
(4) the extent of pre-oxygenation;
(5) the concentration of O_2 provided in the airway.

Gas is drawn into the FRC by a bulk flow which effectively acts as a passive alveolar ventilation. This occurs because CO_2 is 'mopped up' by the body fluids and controls the rate of rise of Pa_{CO_2}, ensuring only a small volume delivery into the FRC.

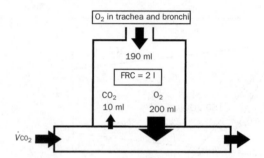

The FRC, although a gas-containing space containing a mixture of gases and therefore subject to Dalton's Law, is effectively treated as a subspace of the CO_2 volume of distribution since it has at all times the same P_{CO_2} as the rest of the body. This is built into the modelling assumptions—CO_2 produced is treated as instantly and uniformly distributed throughout the volume of distribution. Of course this is unrealistic, but it enables us to solve the practical problem, which is to obtain a useful estimate of tolerable apnoea times under different circumstances.

1.9.1 Pre-oxygenation: washing out the nitrogen

As we have already seen, the technique of pre-oxygenation can be of literally vital importance. The process involves replacing the nitrogen in the lung with oxygen so that the oxygen store is augmented, and we have already seen the effectiveness of this. But how rapidly do we expect to be able to achieve the replacement of nitrogen with oxygen? We can model this as an extension of the models that we have already encountered. Although details of technique (e.g. the ability to maintain an air-tight seal with a face mask) will have an important influence, it is useful to have a semi-quantitative idea of how rapidly changes in concentration occur under ideal conditions. This turns out to be a simple matter requiring only application of a 'rule of thumb' (and some mild mental arithmetic) if the underlying processes are understood; and, very importantly, the ideas are transferable to many other analogous circumstances. Although there are some equations to work through, these come straight from the model, and other models that we construct are made in a similar and fairly stereotypical way. If you work carefully through this one, the rest should be quite straightforward.

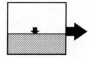

Modelling nitrogen removal from the lung in pre-oxygenation.

We start with a discrete model and assume an even simpler alveolar model than before (1.3.2) with an FRC volume = 2 l and a $\dot{V}A$ of 4 l/min. We simplify by assuming no input of N_2 into the alveolar space—we are going to ignore N_2 stored in tissues for the moment. An initial $FA_{N_2} = 0.80$ is assumed for convenience. Unlike the model in (1.3.2) however, we will examine *discontinuous* ventilation.

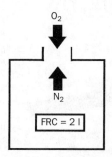

- If all of the minute $\dot{V}A$ was taken in a single breath, what would the resulting FA_{N_2} be? The mass of N_2 contained in 2 l of FRC is now contained in 2 + 4 = 6 l of FRC + $\dot{V}A$, so that the resulting fraction is 33% of 0.8 = 0.264. $FA_{N_2} = 0.264$ after 1 min.
- If the $\dot{V}A$ were split into two, 2 l breaths, the first breath would mix with an equal volume of FRC and the resulting FA_{N_2} would be 50% of 0.8 = 0.4. The second breath would then halve this value in turn, so that, after 1 min, the FA_{N_2} would have fallen to 0.2. Each value is 50% of the previous one.
- If we split the $\dot{V}A$ into four 1 l breaths, the sequence of FA_{N_2} would be 0.8, 0.53, 0.36, and 0.24, to arrive at 0.16 after 1 min. Each value is 66% of the previous one.
- If we split the $\dot{V}A$ into eight 0.5 l breaths, the sequence of FA_{N_2} would be 0.8, 0.64, 0.51, 0.41, 0.33, 0.26, 0.21, and 0.17, to arrive at 0.13 after 1 min. Each value is 80% of the previous one.

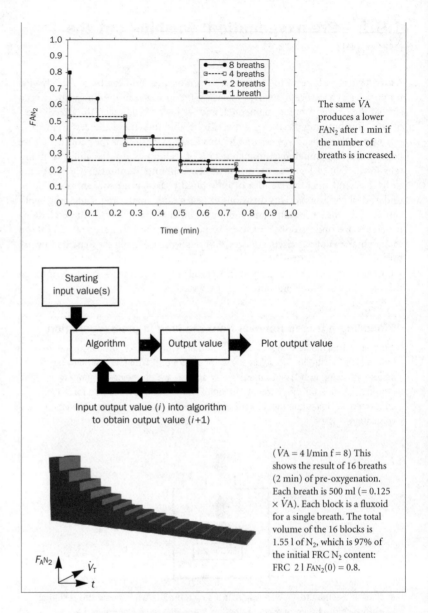

The same $\dot{V}A$ produces a lower FAN_2 after 1 min if the number of breaths is increased.

($\dot{V}A = 4$ l/min f = 8) This shows the result of 16 breaths (2 min) of pre-oxygenation. Each breath is 500 ml (= 0.125 $\times \dot{V}A$). Each block is a fluxoid for a single breath. The total volume of the 16 blocks is 1.55 l of N_2, which is 97% of the initial FRC N_2 content: FRC 2 l $FAN_2(0) = 0.8$.

What we have done is to calculate the dilution breath-by-breath by taking the output value for FAN_2 at the end of the previous breath as our input for the calculation for the next breath. This method is a bit tedious to carry out, although quite easy on a calculator, or we can programme a computer to do it for us. It is at least mimicking the discrete nature of tidal ventilation. This type of calculation is an example of an iterative process called a recurrence relation, in which the output from one stage provides the input to the next calculation. We shall need recurrence relations later (2.16.1). What is the limit of this process as we split the constant $\dot{V}A$ into more and more smaller breaths?

1.9.2 **Discrete and continuous models**

We used a recurrence relation to calculate successive values of FAN_2; each value was a fixed proportion of the previous one and we saw the effect of apportioning the fixed $\dot{V}A$ into a larger number of breaths—the FAN_2 value after 1 min diminished as the number of breaths increased. We now see what happens when we continue this process of chopping up the fixed $\dot{V}A$ into an infinite number of breaths, i.e. a continuous flow. As usual, we need the IOP.

IOP and N$_2$ washout

We will consider a continuous flow of $\dot{V}A$, as we did in (1.3). We will look at what happens in an arbitrary small time interval δt and we should find the fluxoid idea helpful. Since the FAN_2 is changing with time, we will denote its value at time t as $C(t)$ i.e. C for concentration. This will then tie in with other models involving changing concentrations. Alveolar fraction is a proportional concentration.

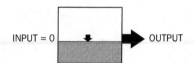

INPUT = 0   OUTPUT

Input. We are administering only 100% O_2, so that the input of N_2 is zero. The contribution from N_2 washout from tissues is ignored. Input = 0.

Output. The loss of N_2 from the lung is entirely due to $\dot{V}A$ and the removal in the small interval δt is given by the flux triplet [Flow × Concentration × Time]. The problem is that the concentration $C(t)$, i.e. FAN_2, is changing with time, so that it is not the same at the end of the interval as it was at the beginning.

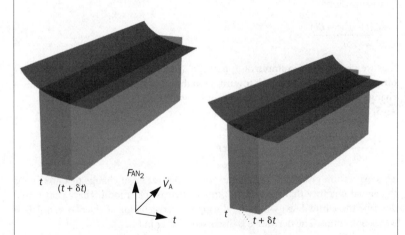

Output. Although the N_2 concentration is changing with time, if the interval is very small, the change in concentration during the interval will not be very large compared with the absolute value of $C(t)$ at any instant—we will make only a small error by ignoring the change during the interval.

output in $\delta t \approx \dot{V}A \times C(t) \times \delta t$.

If we make δt very small indeed, this approximation becomes better (2.12.1). The stepped approximation will get closer and closer to the true curved surface.

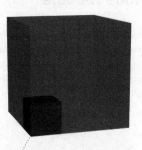

accumulation = input − output:

accumulation in $\delta t \approx 0 - \dot{V}_A \times C(t) \times \delta t$
$$\approx -\dot{V}_A \times C(t) \times \delta t$$

But this negative accumulation is the total loss of N_2 which takes place from the whole FRC in δt. The *change in fractional concentration within the FRC* over the interval δt which results from this elimination is thus given by

$$[C(t) - C(t + \delta t)]\, V_{FRC}$$

the change in the concentration multiplied by the volume in which that concentration change takes place.

Equating these, we obtain

$$[C(t) - C(t + \delta t)]\, V_{FRC} = -\dot{V}_A \times C(t) \times \delta t.$$

This can be rearranged as

$$\frac{C(t) - C(t + \delta t)}{\delta t} = -\frac{\dot{V}_A}{V_{FRC}} C(t).$$

Concentration is a measure relating mass to a specific volume eg g/l. In this case, fractional concentration F_{AN_2} tells us what proportion of each litre of FRC is N_2 eg $F_{AN_2} = 0.8$ means 800 ml of each litre is N_2 (using N_2 volume as a measure of mass). If we need to know the total quantity removed to equate with the IOP relationship, we need to multiply the specific concentration change in a litre by the volume of the compartment in which this change takes place – here the $V_{FRC} = 2$ l.

The expression

$$\frac{C(t) - C(t + \delta t)}{\delta t}$$

that we obtain is an example of a 'package' (like the flux 'package') we shall see often. As we allow δt to shrink towards zero this becomes the instantaneous rate of change of concentration with time denoted by $C'(t)$.

As $\delta t \to 0$,

$$\frac{C(t) - C(t + \delta t)}{\delta t} = C'(t) = -\frac{\dot{V}_A}{V_{FRC}} C(t).$$

This expression gives us $C'(t)$, the *first derivative* or rate of change of $C(t)$. $C(t)$ is the actual quantity that we want to know—that is the smooth curve that would describe the fall of F_{AN_2} with time during pre-oxygenation if alveolar ventilation were continuous. The derivative is discussed further in (2.12).

In equating the mass accumulation from the IOP with the concentration change, we must multiply by the total volume of the compartment in which the concentration change (per unit volume) takes place.

1.9.3   The model equation and the solution

N₂ washout: a differential equation

Our model has given us an equation for $C'(t)$, the rate of change of the FA_{N_2} at any time t. Does this equation make sense and can we solve it?

This is the function notation for the rate of change of $C(t)$. This is the gradient of a tangent to the solution curve at any value of t.

This term is the ratio of the alveolar ventilation $\dot{V}_A$ (gas flow) to the FRC volume V_{FRC} (volume of the system). It is always positive since $\dot{V}_A$ and V_{FRC} are both positive quantities. The term is large if the $\dot{V}_A$ is high relative to the size of the FRC. The rate of change will thus be rapid for high $\dot{V}_A$ and small FRC. This makes sense; a waterfall washes out a rockpool more quickly than a stream does a reservoir.

$$C'(t) = -\left[\frac{\dot{V}_A}{V_{FRC}}\right] C(t)$$

The expression has a negative sign, and hence the rate of change is negative and the concentration is falling. These accord with our expectations.

The expression has a large value when $C(t)$ is large; this means that the rate of change is greater at the beginning of the wash-out than towards the end of the process. The rate of change is thus proportional to the prevailing N_2-concentration $C(t) = (FA_{N_2})$. What we really want to know is not the rate of change, $C'(t)$ but the actual value of the function at any time t, $C(t)$.

The solution function is a washout exponential function (2.9.7). This is the time-dependent function for our smooth approximation to the N_2 washout problem.

The solution equation is

$$C(t) = A e^{-\left\{\frac{\dot{V}_A}{V_{FRC}}\right\}t}.$$

or alternatively

$$C(t) = A \exp\left[-\left\{\frac{\dot{V}_A}{V_{FRC}}\right\}t\right]$$

A is an arbitrary constant of integration which allows us to determine the starting conditions for the process. Since $\exp(0) = 1$, when $t = 0$, the function takes value A. In this case $A = C(0) = FA_{N_2}(0) = 0.8$, the starting value for FA_{N_2}.

The term in curly brackets is the rate constant and its magnitude determines the rate of the change of the function. The rate constant has negative sign, so the function is declining in value. The rate constant is the scaling factor that modifies t. This is the ratio of flow ($\dot{V}_A$) to the volume of the container it is washing out (V_{FRC}).

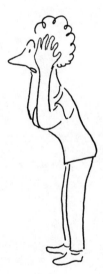

The solution function is a function the rate of change of which at any time t is given by the above differential equation. Details of how the solution arises are given in (2.15.2).

The solution function is shown together with the discrete eight-breath washout pattern. The solution to the differential equation shows the limit to which the process we applied in splitting up the fixed $\dot{V}A$ tends if continued. It is clear that even with eight breaths we shall make only a small error by modelling the discrete process by a continuous approximation. The value for $C(1)$, i.e. the FAN_2 at the end of 1 min, is 0.108, compared with the discrete prediction of 0.136. The benefits of using an easily manipulated function are great, as we shall see.

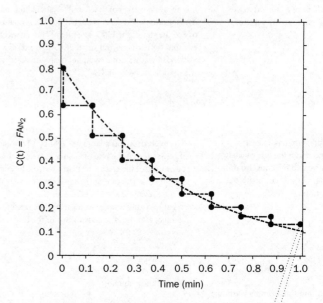

The solution function is a simple washout exponential. Details of exponential functions are given in (2.9). $C(0)$, the value at time $t = 0$, i.e. at the start of the pre-oxygenation, is A (note that any number raised to the power zero = 1). In our example, this is $FAN_2 = 0.8$. A is an arbitrary constant, which appears because we have integrated the differential equation to obtain our solution function (2.12., 2.13). Choice of A determines the initial condition.

1.9.4 N₂ washout and O₂ wash-in

O₂ wash-in

According to our model, the process of denitrification of the FRC by pre-oxygenation means replacing N₂ 'ml for ml' by O₂. This means that we do not have to produce a separate differential equation for FA_{O_2} as a function of time; we can simply use the N₂ washout to construct the O₂ wash-in curve—what is not N₂ is O₂. The justification for this procedure is ultimately Dalton's Law and the general gas law.

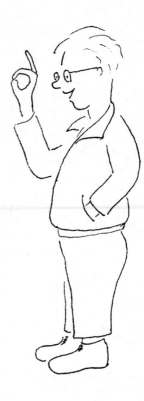

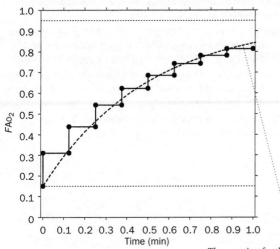

We consider only three gases [$FA_{N_2} + FA_{O_2} + FA_{CO_2} = 1$]; $FA_{CO_2} = 0.05$. We assume a starting $FA_{O_2} = 0.15$ and use an 'upside down' version of the N₂ wash-out curve. This predicts an $FA_{O_2} = 0.84$ after 1 min. The discrete (eight-breath) function is shown for comparison.

The equation for this wash-in function is

$$FA_{O_2}(t) = 0.15 + 0.8\left(1 - e^{-\left\{\frac{\dot{V}_A}{V_{FRC}}\right\}t}\right)$$

$\dot{V}_A = 4$ l/min.
$V_{FRC} = 2$ l.

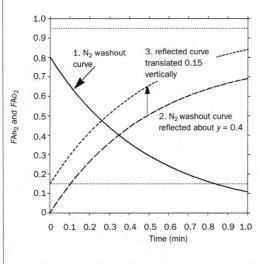

The exponential term within the bracket is exactly the same as the N₂ washout—the rate of the process is the same, as it must be. This is subtracted from 1; at $t = 0$ the exponential term equals 1, so the bracketed term is zero. This gives a starting $FA_{O_2} = 0.15$, as we need.

We have produced an equation that looks much more complicated than the FA_{N_2} one only because we are moving between $FA_{O_2} = 0.15$ and $FA_{O_2} = 0.95$—the old and the new equilibrium levels; the 'business part' is identical to the FA_{N_2}. This is merely a translation and reflection (2.3) of the same curve as FA_{N_2} (1.9.3).

In the graph: 1. N₂ washout curve; 2. N₂ washout curve reflected about y = 0.4; 3. reflected curve translated 0.15 vertically.

The O₂ wash-in function

This looks much more complicated than the equation for the N₂ wash-out, but we can take it apart:

$$F_{A O_2}(t) = 0.15 + 0.8\left(1 - e^{-\left\{\frac{\dot{V}_A}{V_{FRC}}\right\}t}\right)$$

As t increases, the exponential term declines towards zero, so that this second term approaches a limiting value of $FA_{O_2} = 0.8$. The whole expression tends to a limiting value of $0.15 + 0.8$; $FA_{O_2} = 0.95$. This is the alveolar fraction to which the system 'aspires', the equilibrium value for the model system. The remaining $FA = 0.05$ is for the FA_{CO_2}.

N$_2$ washout: examining the assumptions

In constructing our differential equation, we made assumptions the justification of which is perhaps dubious. We assumed, firstly, that the alveolar space behaved as a simple container washed through by a constant flow and, secondly, that there was no input of N$_2$ into the alveolar space, i.e. that the only N$_2$ to be removed is that present in the FRC at time $t = 0$. Neither of these assumptions is completely justifiable. The tissues of the body contain an appreciable quantity of N$_2$ which is removed via the lung if a N$_2$-free mixture is respired; this process is, however, much slower than the removal from the alveolar space. The washout from the alveolar space is also more complex than we have assumed: even in healthy patients there is evidence of a concurrent, slower process of washout from less well-ventilated parts of lung. In obstructive airway disease, this is exaggerated and the N$_2$ washout curves can be analysed to establish the degree of ventilatory disturbance. The appropriateness of a particular model is determined by the practical use to which it needs to be put. We are interested in determining approximately how rapidly we may expect to replace the N$_2$ in the lung to increase O$_2$ stores.

As a semi-quantitative model for application to acute changes, this is an acceptable start. N$_2$ washout from tissues is considered in (1.13.6).

1.10.1   **Standardizing the rate**

The rate of the exponential process in the N_2 washout was determined entirely by the ratio of flow ($\dot{V}A$) to volume ($VFRC$). No other factors are important in the simple model. We can standardize any simple wash-in or washout exponential process in which there is a flow $\dot{Q}$ into a container of volume V, by a device, the time constant τ. *The time constant is the time required for the flow to fill the container.* What constitutes the flow and what the container is will vary from circumstance to circumstance, but the principle remains intact. The time constant enables us to use a 'rule of thumb' to estimate the magnitude of the change that has occurred.

The time constant

In moving from one equilibrium level to another by a simple exponential process (this means that only a single exponential term is involved), the rate of the process is determined only by the exponent $\dot{Q}/V$ in the term $\exp\left[-\frac{\dot{Q}}{V}t\right]$ (2.9.). Whenever this becomes an integer value, we have values for the proportional change that we can memorize. The rate constant $\dot{Q}/V$ has units of '1/time', e.g. 2/min, which was the constant for our $\dot{V}A/VFRC$; this means that the system volume would be filled by the $\dot{V}A$ every 30 s. The reciprocal (upside-down version) of the rate constant $V/\dot{Q}$ has units of 'time' and is the *time constant* τ; this value of τ answers the question 'how long does it take for the flow to fill the container?' The proportion of the change that has occurred or is still to occur is shown in the table below. The origin of the table is explained in (2.9.9).

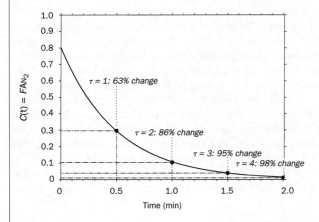

Applied to the N_2 washout curve, we have $\dot{Q} = \dot{V}A = 4$ l/min and $V = VFRC = 2$ l, so the time constant is 0.5 min; it would take this long to fill the system with the flow.

- After 0.5 min ($\tau = 1$), 63% of the change between starting value 0.8 and equilibrium value 0 has occurred. FAN_2 must therefore be approximately 0.504.

- After 1 min ($\tau = 2$), the FAN_2 value is 14% of 0.8 = 0.108.

- After 1.5 min ($\tau = 3$), the FAN_2 value is 5% of 0.8 = 0.04.

- After 2 min ($\tau = 4$), the FAN_2 value is 2% of 0.8 = 0.016.

Similar calculations on the O_2 wash-in require us to take into account the different start and finish point, but the proportional change in each time interval is always the same.

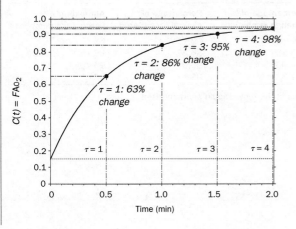

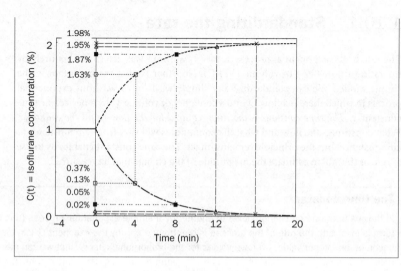

The time constant is a standardization procedure, so that we can do rapid, rough and ready estimates of the proportional change that we expect to have occurred. For instance, in the anaesthetic circle system with absorber, when changing volatile agent concentrations in response to clinical circumstance, it can help to have an approximate idea of how rapidly we might expect concentration within the circuit to change. This will depend upon the fresh gas flow ($\dot{Q} = $ FGF) and the volume of the system V (which will include the absorber, the tubing, and the patient FRC). Ignoring leaks, and uptake or discharge by circuit components and by the patient (big simplifying assumptions), we can make approximate predictions on the concentration of, say, isoflurane in the circuit as a function of time. Suppose that we are at equilibrium at time $t = 0$, and change the isoflurane concentration vaporizer setting from 1% to 2%, with FGF = 2 l/min and a system volume $V = 8$ l; $\tau = 4$ min. Concentrations are predicted to change as shown in the graph. The decay curve that we obtain for turning the vaporizer from 1% to off instead is also shown. Remember that this takes no account of absorption (or delivery) of isoflurane by the patient or circuit components; these will slow the rate of the process, so the graph shows the most rapid change that the ideal system would achieve—real life will be slower still. If we need to speed things up, we can turn up the FGF.

Number of time constants	Percentage of change remaining	Percentage of change completed	Approximate percentage completed
1	36.79	63.21	63
2	13.53	86.47	86
3	4.98	95.02	95
4	1.83	98.17	98

The approximate values in the table should be memorised

1.11.1   **More time-dependent processes**

We constructed a model for the steady state $PaCO_2$ that results from any CO_2 production $\dot{V}CO_2$ and alveolar ventilation $\dot{V}A$ (1.3). This model described the level at which the $PaCO_2$ 'settles down' after any change, but did not attempt to predict how the system behaves in moving from one steady state to another. This is our next task, and we should discover that we have done most of the hard work already with the N_2 washout/O_2 wash-in example.

The IOP formed the basis of the steady state model. We were able to assume that in equilibrium conditions the input of CO_2 into the system necessarily balanced the output from the lungs. In the apnoeic oxygenation model (1.8), we were able to model a non-equilibrium system starting from an empirical observation of a linear rise in $PaCO_2$ in apnoea. This entailed the idea of an idealized compartment which contained the CO_2, and the size of which determined the rate of rise of $PaCO_2$ for any given $\dot{V}CO_2$. The 'compartment' is an abstraction, although a simple and intuitive one. A single compartment and the model prediction that no CO_2 can escape—there is a flow of gas down the airway into the lung which prevents any egress of CO_2—meant that the rate of change of $PaCO_2$ was linear and the model easy to solve.

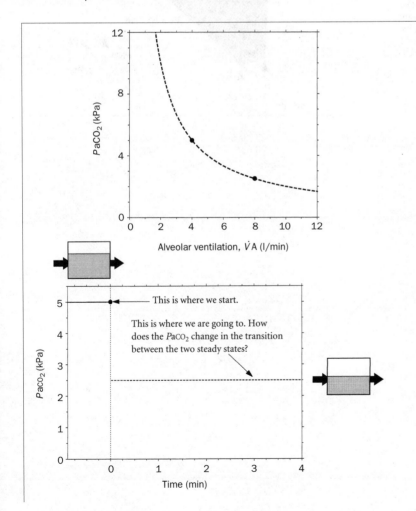

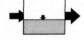

Modifying the steady state $\dot{V}A$ – $PaCO_2$ model

Suppose that we have a steady state $\dot{V}CO_2 = 0.2$ l/min. $\dot{V}A = 4$ l/min and hence $PaCO_2 = 5$ kPa. We then increase the $\dot{V}A$ abruptly to 8 l/min. We know from the steady state model that the $PaCO_2$ will settle at 2.5 kPa. For the $PaCO_2$ to fall to the lower level, there must be a reduction in the mass of CO_2 in the compartment and hence, for the transition period, the CO_2 output will exceed the input. Once the $PaCO_2$ has fallen to 2.5kPa, the input and output are matched again and steady state conditions return.

This is a fluxoid from an arbitrary small time interval δt. The Pa_{CO_2} is falling during the interval because we have increased the $\dot{V}A$ but have not yet reached the new equilibrium level at which input and output are balanced. The output of CO_2 in this interval will, as usual, be the volume of the fluxoid. We can think of the fluxoid as being in three parts.

This rectangular part is the largest we can make with a flat top without encroaching on the curved upper surface. Its volume is easy to calculate if we know the Pa_{CO_2} at the end of the interval $(t + \delta t)$.

The bottom part is the constant rectangular solid the volume of which is the same as the $\dot{V}_{CO_2}$ in δt, i.e. $[\dot{V}_{CO_2} \times \delta t]$. It has height Pa_{CO_2} = 2.5 kPa—the level which, for a $\dot{V}A$ of 8 l/min, ensures removal of the continuing CO_2 production. This is the equilibrium part of the fluxoid. The rest of the fluxoid is the net removal of CO_2 during the interval in excess of production.

The top part is a small volume that sits on the rectangular fluxoids below. It has a curved upper surface, reflecting the fact that the Pa_{CO_2} is changing over the interval—it is lower at the end of the interval than at the beginning because Pa_{CO_2} is falling. The error that we would make in calculating the CO_2 output if we ignored this top part evidently depends upon the width of the interval that we consider and how much change there is in Pa_{CO_2} during that interval, since these together determine the volume of the top part.

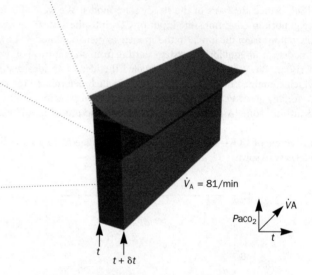

$\dot{V}_A = 8 l/min$

Pa_{CO_2} $\dot{V}A$ t

t

$t + \delta t$

1.11.2   The model equation

Constructing the differential equation

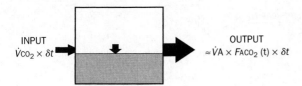

The IOP is applied as usual:
- CO_2 input in $\delta t = \dot{V}co_2 \times \delta t$
- CO_2 output in $\delta t \approx \dot{V}A \times FAco_2(t) \times \delta t$ (approximately)
- Accumulation = input − output in $\delta t = [\dot{V}co_2 - \dot{V}A \times FAco_2(t)]\,\delta t$

This is the same equation as for the steady state model, with the exception that $FAco_2(t)$ is now a time-dependent variable—it is changing over time.

We can equate this to the *concentration change* in CO_2 in δt taking place within the volume of distribution compartment D:[†]

$$[Cco_2(t + \delta t) - Cco_2(t)] \times D \approx [\dot{V}co_2 - \dot{V}A \times FAco_2(t)]\delta t.$$

Rearranging, we obtain

$$\frac{[Cco_2(t + \delta t) - Cco_2(t)]}{\delta t} \approx \frac{1}{D}[\dot{V}co_2 - \dot{V}A \times FAco_2(t)].$$

This looks a mess: what we want to know is $Paco_2(t)$, and we have an expression in terms of $Cco_2(t)$ and $FAco_2(t)$. How can we sort this out?

$FAco_2(t)$ is easy; by our modelling assumptions (1.3.2), $FAco_2(t) \approx Paco_2(t)/P_I$, which gives us

$$\frac{[Cco_2(t + \delta t) - Cco_2(t)]}{\delta t} \approx \frac{1}{D}\left[\dot{V}co_2 - \dot{V}A \times \frac{Paco_2(t)}{P_I}\right] = \frac{1}{P_I D}[P_I \times \dot{V}co_2 - \dot{V}A \times Paco_2(t)].$$

What about $Cco_2(t)$? If we return to the apnoeic oxygenation example for a moment, we remember that the $Paco_2(t)$ is rising linearly with time, which fact we used as justification for using a single compartment in our model. In apnoea there is no alveolar ventilation to eliminate CO_2, so that $\dot{V}A = 0$. The equation then becomes

$$\frac{[Cco_2(t + \delta t) - Cco_2(t)]}{\delta t} = \frac{\dot{V}co_2}{D}.$$

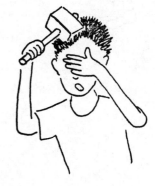

The LHS,

$$\frac{[Cco_2(t + \delta t) - Cco_2(t)]}{\delta t}$$

is the approximate rate of change of CO_2 concentration over the interval, and since in apnoea $Cco_2(t + \delta t)$ is greater than $Cco_2(t)$, this is a positive quantity—the concentration is rising. Since both $\dot{V}co_2$ and D are constants, this predicts a constant rise of $Cco_2(t)$ in apnoea, i.e. it predicts a linear relationship.

[†]D actually has units Volume CO_2/unit concentration change and is only notionally a 'volume'. It is a proportionality constant that relates concentration change which results from adding a mass of CO_2 (measured as a volume). Concentration change is small for any given added CO_2 mass, if D is large.

Empirical observation indeed showed a linear rise in $Paco_2(t)$ with apnoea (1.8.1), so we can replace $Cco_2(t)$ by $Paco_2(t)$ as long as we introduce a proportionality constant k to convert from concentration to partial pressure. Therefore, the extreme of step change in ventilation—apnoea—has reduced the equation to

$$\frac{[Paco_2(t + \delta t) - Paco_2(t)]}{\delta t} \approx \left[\frac{k}{P_I \times D}\right] P_I \times \dot{V}co_2,$$

and since we can measure the $\dot{V}co_2$ we can calculate a value for k/P_ID), which we shall denote by $1/D^*$:

$$\frac{[Paco_2(t + \delta t) - Paco_2(t)]}{\delta t} \approx \left[\frac{k}{P_I \times D}\right] P_I \times \dot{V}co_2 = \left[\frac{1}{D^*}\right] P_I \times \dot{V}co_2.$$

D^* is a composite proportionality constant (a fudge factor, if you prefer) which is performing the role of compartment volume, but contains information about the distribution volume, atmospheric pressure, and the relationship of the CO_2 concentration to the partial pressure within the system. It achieves a considerable abstraction of real physical and physiological variables into a single figure. It has the units of volume. This is a typical modelling simplification of reality—we can always examine the consequences of the simplification later. D^* can be estimated for a typical $\dot{V}co_2 = 0.2$ l/min and a rate of rise in apnoea of 0.5 kPa/min as 40 l.

We can now incorporate this D^* into our (non-apnoeic) modelling equation. This is an expression for the rate of change of $Paco_2$ over the small time interval δt:

$$\frac{[Paco_2(t + \delta t) - Paco_2(t)]}{\delta t} \approx \left[\frac{1}{D^*}\right] [P_I\dot{V}co_2 - \dot{V}A \times Paco_2(t)].$$

If we take the limit as $\delta t \to 0$, we obtain the modelling differential equation:

$$[Paco_2(t)]' = \frac{1}{D^*}[P_I\dot{V}co_2 - \dot{V}A \times Paco_2(t)]$$

This is the instantaneous rate of change of $Paco_2$ at any time, t.

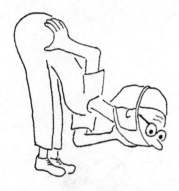

1.11.3   The solution function

Examining the solution

We modelled the step change in $\dot{V}A$ and obtained a differential equation describing the rate of change of $Paco_2$:

$$(Paco_2(t))' = \frac{P_I \times \dot{V}co_2}{D^*} - \frac{\dot{V}A}{D^*} \times Paco_2(t).$$

This expression is in two parts—one a constant term, which gives us the rate of rise in apnoea, and the other containing $Paco_2(t)$ itself, showing that the rate of change is proportional to the prevailing level of $Paco_2$. This is the condition for an exponential process (2.9) and so we expect an exponential term to appear in the solution. Remember that 'solution' means that this equation has a gradient at any point that is described by our modelling differential equation.

The solution is (2.15)

$$Paco_2(t) = \frac{\dot{V}co_2 \times P_I}{\dot{V}A} - A\ \exp\left\{-\frac{\dot{V}A}{D^*}t\right\}$$

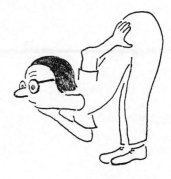

The solution has two parts: this part has no time-dependent term in it and is in fact the same as the equation that we obtained in (1.3.3). It is only dependent upon $\dot{V}A$, $\dot{V}co_2$ and P_I, as was our first model. It is the *equilibrium solution*—the state in which the system 'settles down' after the perturbation of a change in $\dot{V}A$. Note that there is no equilibrium solution for $\dot{V}A = 0$ since we cannot divide by zero. This makes sense; $Paco_2$ always rises in apnoea.

This part of the solution is time-dependent: it is the *transient term*, which describes how $Paco_2$ changes with time between the starting value and the new equilibrium value. A is an arbitrary constant to fix the starting point. Remember that $\exp(0) = 1$, so at the onset of the process when $t = 0$, the transient term has value A. When t is large, the term diminishes towards zero. Note also that $\dot{V}A$ appears in *both* the equilibrium and the transient parts of the solution. $\dot{V}co_2$ only appears in the equilibrium part—it has no influence on the rate of change, but only on the level in the 'long run'.

Note that, whatever the initial $Paco_2$, the *proportional change* in passing from the $Paco_2(0)$ to the new equilibrium is always the same and is governed by the rate constant (1.10.1). The rate constant is dependent upon $\dot{V}A$, the flow factor in the process. Since we are changing $\dot{V}A$, we expect to see different rates of change occurring depending upon the level of ventilation.

The rate constant is $\{\dot{V}A/D^*\}$, which is the ratio of the flow $\dot{V}A$ to the volume of the container that it is washing through, represented by D^*. This time, it is not the FRC which is the 'container' as it was in the N_2 example, where we ignored N_2 in the tissues, but the whole of D^* (whatever D^* might be). The FRC is now simply acting as a 'window' into the whole CO_2 storage system in the uniform compartment D^*.

If we now return to our example; we have a steady state $\dot{V}CO_2 = 0.2$ l/min. $\dot{V}A = 4$ l/min and hence $PaCO_2 = 5$ kPa. $D^* = 40$ l. We then increase $\dot{V}A$ abruptly to 8 l/min. We know from the steady state model that $PaCO_2$ will settle at 2.5 kPa:

$$PaCO_2(t) = \frac{\dot{V}CO_2 P_1}{\dot{V}A} + A \ \exp\left\{-\frac{\dot{V}A}{D^*}t\right\} = \frac{0.2 \times 100}{8} + 2.5 \ \exp\left\{-\frac{8}{40}t\right\}.$$

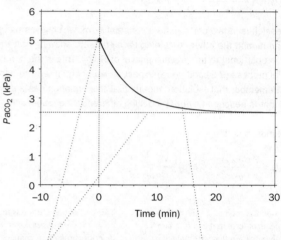

Starting $PaCO_2$ is 5 kPa, and after the process has settled down, the $PaCO_2$ is 2.5 kPa. The equilibrium term for $\dot{V}A = 8$ l/min does indeed predict a level of 2.5 kPa. At $t = 0$, $5 = 2.5 + A \exp\{0\}$, so $A = 2.5$ kPa for this particular example.

$PaCO_2(t)$ follows a simple exponential washout from the starting value to the new equilibrium value. The rate constant is predicted to be $\dot{V}A/D^* = 8/40$. This gives a time constant τ of 5 minutes.

The lesson we learn here is that solution function consists of two parts:
- the equilibrium solution that we established with modelling assumptions and only simple arithmetic in (1.3).
- the transient term which has a rate constant (and hence time constant, τ) determined by the flow/volume $\dot{V}A$ and D^*. The magnitude of the term at $t = 0$, arbitrary constant A, is simply the (signed) difference in the start and finish equilibrium levels obtained from the steady-state model.

The elaborate derivation and solution of the differential equation of this and similar models can be by-passed with a little physiological insight and familiarity with time constants.

1.11.4 Increasing and decreasing V̇A

Paco₂: going upwards and going downwards

The solution function tells us that the rate of the transition from one equilibrium to another is dependent upon V̇A:

$$Paco_2(t) = \frac{\dot{V}co_2 P_I}{\dot{V}A} + A\, \exp\left\{-\frac{\dot{V}A}{D^*}t\right\}.$$

In our example, we expect therefore that when we restore the original $\dot{V}A = 4$ l/min after we have settled down at the new equilibrium value $Paco_2 = 2.5$ kPa, the return transition to $Paco_2 = 5$ kPa, will be slower—the rate constant is halved from $8/D^*$ to $4/D^*$. The fluxoid idea explains to us why this *must* be so.

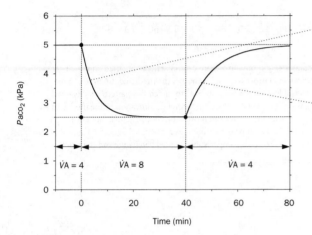

The transition from $\dot{V}A = 4$ l/min to $\dot{V}A = 8$ l/min produces a rapid fall in $Paco_2$ from 5 to 2.5 kPa.

The transition from $\dot{V}A = 8$ l/min to $\dot{V}A = 4$ l/min produces a more leisurely rise in $Paco_2$, from 2.5 back to 5 kPa. The time constant τ is $4/40 = 10$ minutes

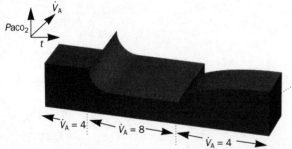

The front face of this fluxoid representation forms the graph above.

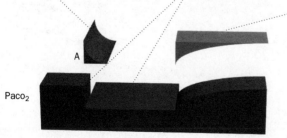

This piece is a fluxoid and its volume represents the net loss of CO_2 mass to the system in reaching the new equilibrium.

These are the equilibrium fluxoids for $\dot{V}A = 4$ l/min and $\dot{V}A = 8$ l/min. They each have a flat top and hence represent steady state conditions. (1.5.2.)

This piece is not there; it is a 'ghost' fluxoid. The steady state fluxoid has height 5 kPa for $\dot{V}A = 4$ min. This is the level required for removal of the continuing $\dot{V}co_2$. What is *not* there in the output for equilibrium conditions must be retained within the system. For the system to return to its former state, the same mass of CO_2 lost in moving to the lower equilibrium $Paco_2$ level must be restored. The volume of this 'ghost' fluxoid must therefore be the same as the 'real' one A. Since the depths ($\dot{V}A$) are in a ratio of 2 : 1 and the volumes are the same, the areas of the fluxoid faces must be in ratio 1 : 2. This means that they cannot have the same rate constant. In fact, the ratio of rate constants must be 2 : 1 as our solution predicts; since these are exponential functions, the areas of the faces are also in the same ratio (2.14.4). This is what the equations predict.

Data from a single subject showing the transition from high $\dot{V}A$ to low and back again. It is clear that the rates of the processes are different. Solid circles: At $t = 0$ total ventilation changed from 3.3 l/min to 14 l/min. Open circles show the changes following the reversion to total ventilation of 3.3 l/min.

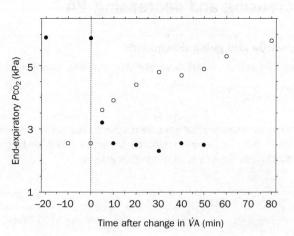

The real data $FE'CO_2(t)$ measured here cannot actually be fitted convincingly to a single exponential process model, although the predicted difference in the rates is discernible. Our model is not able to match this pattern exactly—we might be able to improve the fit with a further modification of the model, or we might find that with more data and more subjects and actually measuring $PaCO_2$ we might show a closer approximation to our model behaviour. Or not: the modelling process requires comparison of model behaviour and the real model.

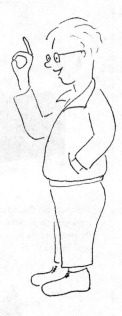

Redrawn from: Applied Respiratory Physiology. 4th edition. J. F. Nunn. Butterworth. London. By kind permission of the publisher and Prof. Nunn.

1.12.1   Modelling pulmonary air embolism

Pulmonary air embolism (PAE) is a danger in various operative procedures, notably during surgery on cervical spine or structures in the posterior fossa carried out in the sitting position. There are various methods of detecting when this has occurred. One of the long-established methods is end-tidal CO_2 ($FE'CO_2$) monitoring; the occurrence of venous air embolism is associated with a fall in the level of CO_2 in the end-tidal breath, and this is displayed on capnography. We shall model the effects of PAE on the CO_2 economy of the body, by building on the steady state and step change in $\dot{V}A$ models. We shall make some sweeping simplifying assumptions but still end up with a model that is considerably more complex than the previous ones we have met.

This problem forms an extended modelling project to show how quite complicated situations can be broken down into separate simpler problems.

Air embolism: the model

Air enters the venous side of the circulation and is carried through the heart and into the pulmonary vessels, where it obstructs the normal passage of blood through the alveolar capillaries and interferes with pulmonary gas exchange. We will not attempt any modelling of cardiac 'air lock' and the ensuing collapse of cardiac output; we are concerned only with the much commoner phenomenon of 'sieveing' of air bubbles by the pulmonary capillaries when modest amounts of air enter the venous circulation.

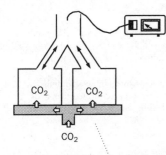

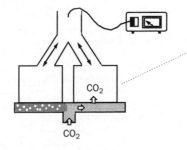

After the occurrence of the PAE, bubbles are present in the vessels feeding a portion of the alveolar space. Evidently, if all of the vessels are blocked, there is no pulmonary blood flow, gas exchange ceases, and death ensues rapidly. Usually, a modest proportion of the alveoli cease to take part in gas exchange. We shall measure the magnitude of the embolus by the *proportion of the total alveolar ventilation* VA_{tot} which is deleted by the PAE.

The previous models of steady state and step change in $\dot{V}A$ for modelling have required only a single homogeneous alveolar space—represented by an ideal alveolus. This is not sufficient for the PAE problem—we shall need two compartments in the total alveolar space. This diagram shows the model before the occurrence of the PAE when both alveolar compartments are behaving identically and ideally. CO_2 produced by metabolism is transported in the blood to the alveolar membrane where CO_2 exchange takes place according to our previous steady state model.

Recording of capnography during exploration of posterior fossa for eighth nerve tumour. Semi-sitting or lounging position.

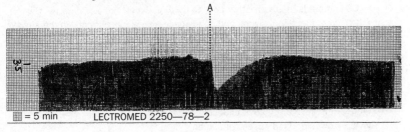

= 5 min   LECTROMED 2250—78—2

The $FE'CO_2$ remains fairly constant throughout the initial period of the operation. At A a precipitous fall in the $FE'CO_2$ occurs and subsequently recovers, and then overshoots the original value before subsiding to approximately the previous level. Most clinical records of capnography are much messier than this, with multiple emboli occurring. This one is so smooth that it looks like something 'pure' and we shall try to mimic its features with our model.

1.12.2 Characterizing the model

Alveolar dead space and hypoventilation

What are the effects upon gas exchange of the blockage of vessels by air? The fundamental effect is that the size of the alveolar dead space increases, since alveoli that have previously been optimally ventilated and perfused lose their perfusion. We shall assume that the subject is paralysed and mechanically ventilated and that total alveolar ventilation $\dot{V}A_{tot}$ is unchanged. This simple model predicts no change in oxygenation, since there is no mechanism for venous admixture in the model. This is of course an oversimplification, but moderate degrees of PAE can occur without discernible arterial desaturation.

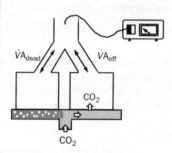

The alveolar compartment is now divided into two—a normal ventilated and perfused compartment and an alveolar dead-space compartment which is ventilated normally but no longer perfused.

The effect of this change of previously normally ventilated and perfused alveolar space to become alveolar dead space is two-fold:
- There is alveolar hypoventilation relative to the conditions prevailing prior to the embolus. Pa_{CO_2} will rise.
- There is dilution of alveolar gas from the perfused compartment by alveolar dead space, so that the end-tidal CO_2 concentration (FE'_{CO_2}) is appreciably less than that in the functional alveolar fraction. This is the basis for the use of capnography in detection of PAE.

Modelling assumptions

We summarize here the initial simplifying assumptions of the model (additional to those of the previous Pa_{CO_2} models):
- Air embolism is a single event that occurs instantaneously at time $t = 0$. Its magnitude is measured as the proportion of $\dot{V}A$ that is converted to alveolar dead space.
- At any instant an alveolus belongs to one of two mutually exclusive compartments—it is either ideally perfused and ventilated (functional alveolus) or normally ventilated and unperfused (alveolar dead space).
- Cardiac output $\dot{Q}$ remains constant. CO_2 production, $\dot{V}_{CO_2}$, is similarly constant.
- CO_2 output is in steady state prior to the PAE event.
- CO_2 from functional alveoli and dead-space alveoli mix perfectly in the airways and the resultant mixture is measured by capnography.

Of course, not all of these are justifiable, but they allow us to start.

Notation:
$\dot{V}A_{tot}$ Total alveolar ventilation
$\dot{V}A_{eff}$ Effective alveolar ventilation
$\dot{V}A_{dead}$ Alveolar dead space ventilation

1.12.3   Recovery

What do we expect to happen to the $PaCO_2$ and $FE'CO_2$ during and after PAE? The problem would actually only require a slight modification of the step change model but for one feature; air is cleared from the circulation and the $\dot{V}A$ recovers. Somehow, we are going to have to model recovery as well.

Recovery functions

Let us first see what happens if there is *no* recovery in $\dot{V}A$—at least within the early phase. We will track the $PaCO_2$ and $FE'CO_2$ after an embolus of magnitude 0.5—i.e. the PAE wipes out 50% of functioning alveolar ventilation—in a patient with $\dot{V}A = 4$ l/min and $\dot{V}CO_2 = 0.2$ l/min and hence a resting $PaCO_2$ of 5 kPa.

The 'no-recovery' air embolus is essentially a step change in $\dot{V}A$. We know that if we halve the $\dot{V}A$, then we will double the $PaCO_2$, so $PaCO_2$ will reach an equilibrium value of 10 kPa if total alveolar ventilation $\dot{V}A_{tot}$ remains constant. This will follow an exponential wash-in curve, as we have seen (1.11.4).

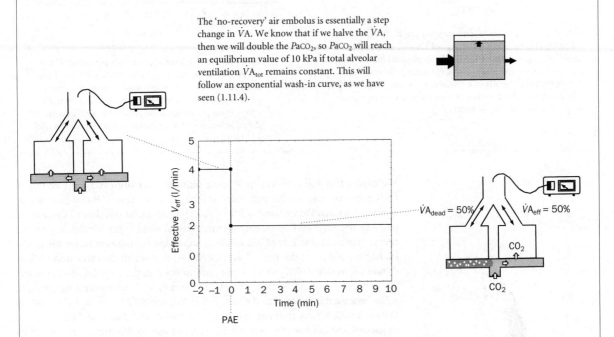

PAE

Since half of $\dot{V}A_{tot}$ is dead space, $\dot{V}A_{dead}$, then there is a 50 : 50 dilution of functioning alveolar gas CO_2 and the equilibrium $FE'CO_2$ is thus 5 kPa, as it was before the embolus—although this masks a large discrepancy in $PaCO_2$ and $FE'CO_2$. Since the dilution factor is constant, then the $FE'CO_2$ too will follow an exponential wash-in curve to reach equilibrium. The rate constant for the process is the same, although a superficial inspection of the graph may suggest that the $FE'CO_2$ is changing more slowly than $PaCO_2$: actually the proportional change in $FE'CO_2$ and $PaCO_2$ is the same at any time.

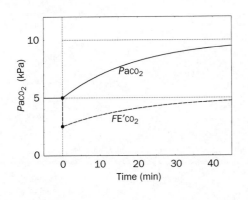

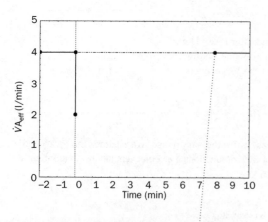

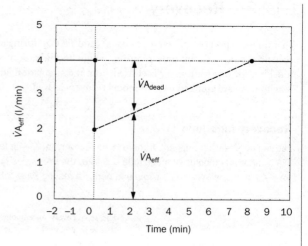

If the PAE recovers, then at some stage the graph of $\dot{V}A_{eff}$ with time will reach a plateau again at the original $\dot{V}A$—we have arbitrarily shown this occurring at $t = 8$ min. The shape of the line bridging the gap is not known—we shall call this the 'recovery function'. Even though we do not *know* how it behaves, we can simply *assume* that it is linear and see what happens. We cannot let ignorance stop our progress, so we just make something up.

Even with a simple linear recovery function, we shall still have to decide on its gradient—i.e. how quickly the $\dot{V}A$ is restored to function. For slow recovery rates, the pattern of $PaCO_2$ and $FE'CO_2$ will tend to the step change extreme above. For rapid recovery, the pattern will tend towards the equilibrium—i.e. a no-change picture. We shall model an 'in-between' solution.

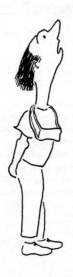

We expect that full recovery of $\dot{V}A$ will ultimately restore $PaCO_2$ and $FE'CO_2$ to their previous values, although there will be an initial rise in $PaCO_2$ (because of alveolar hypoventilation) and a fall in $FE'CO_2$ (because of dilution of dead-space gas). As the ratio of functioning alveoli/alveolar dead space increases with the recovery process, the rate of rise of $PaCO_2$ slows and the dilution factor diminishes. At a certain point the $PaCO_2$ has risen to a level at which the (now diminished) dilution results in $FE'CO_2$ which is the same as prior to the embolus. As the recovery process continues further, the $FE'CO_2$ 'overshoots' the starting equilibrium value because it is exposed to the elevated $PaCO_2$, and dilution further diminished. When the $\dot{V}A$ is fully restored, dilution is abolished, and $PaCO_2$ and $FE'CO_2$ move in parallel and fall purely exponentially back to their equilibrium values. We need to model this process quantitatively for any chosen rate of recovery.

1.12.4   The model

Modelling strategy

The model is built up in stages:

(1) The IOP is employed to produce an expression for the rate of change of $Paco_2$ as a function of time—a differential equation.

(2) This differential equation is solved to give values for the $Paco_2(t)$ at any time t after the occurrence of the embolus.

(3) The assumed recovery function—also a function of time—is used to calculate the prevailing factor by which the $Paco_2$ calculated in (2) is diluted by alveolar dead-space gas.

(4) A refinement is added to account for the fact that the embolized alveoli contain CO_2 at the outset which is washed out by the continuing alveolar ventilation in the alveolar dead-space compartment.

Input–output relations

input in $\delta t = \dot{V}co_2 \times \delta t$

output in $\delta t \approx \{FAco_2(t) \times \dot{V}A_{eff}(t)\}\delta t.$

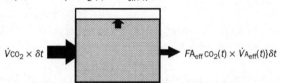

$\dot{V}co_2 \times \delta t$ → → $FA_{eff}co_2(t) \times \dot{V}A_{eff}(t)\}\delta t$

The only difference from the step change in ventilation example is that $\dot{V}A$ is no longer a constant during the equilibration period, but is now itself a time-dependent variable $\dot{V}A_{eff}(t)$. The routine derivation of the differential equation using the IOP is the same as before (1.11.2), but gives

$$[Paco_2(t)]' = \frac{1}{D^*}[P_i\dot{V}co_2 - \dot{V}A_{eff}(t) \times Paco_2(t)]$$

Unfortunately, there is no equation we can find of which this is the derivative; the differential equation is insoluble. However, this does not mean we cannot obtain an answer to our problem. We can employ a numerical method of solution that enables us to obtain a practically useful model. Numerical methods are briefly introduced in (2.16).

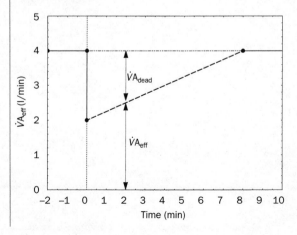

The CO_2 from functioning alveoli is diluted by gas from unperfused alveoli according to the proportion of the $\dot{V}A_{tot}$ which is $\dot{V}A_{eff}$. This diluted gas is the end-expired gas in which we measure FE'_{CO_2}. This, according to the model, will be

$$FE'_{CO_2}(t) = Pa_{CO_2}(t) \times \frac{\dot{V}A_{eff}(t)}{\dot{V}A_{tot}}\%.$$

The proportion ($\dot{V}A_{eff}/\dot{V}A_{tot}$) is obtained from the recovery function.

The final refinement is to add a term to account for the fact that the embolized alveoli contain CO_2 at the outset which is washed out by the continuing alveolar ventilation. The embolized, unperfused alveoli are modelled as having an unchanged ventilation and will thus have a proportional ventilation $\dot{V}A_{dead}$ to fraction of FRC (i.e. alveolar dead-space volume V_{dead}) which is constant. We know (1.10.1) that this will determine the rate constant of the washout process. This will add CO_2 to the expired gas and cause a 'slurring' of the otherwise abrupt fall in FE'_{CO_2}.

This term is

$$Pa_{CO_2}(0) \times e^{-kt} \times \frac{\dot{V}A_{dead}(t)}{\dot{V}A_{tot}}$$

where $k = \dot{V}A/V_{FRC}$.

This model formed the basis of a computer simulation of PAE, 'Embolus', developed by the author and Dr A. W. A. Crossley. The equation is solved using a numerical technique called the fourth-order Runge–Kutta method, which is a standard algorithm in science and engineering for the solution of ordinary differential equations. This generates a table of Pa_{CO_2} values at any time t after the PAE.

1.12.5 Computer simulation

Computer-based simulation of PAE

The computer program was developed to allow examination of the various factors affecting the pattern of Pa_{CO_2} and FE_{CO_2} after a PAE. A menu allows choice of

- $\dot{V}_{CO_2}$.
- $\dot{V}_A$ and hence with $\dot{V}_{CO_2}$ the steady-state Pa_{CO_2}.
- The extent of PAE as a proportion of $\dot{V}_A$.
- Rate and mode of recovery function. Three patterns of recovery are modelled; linear (choice of gradient) and both wash-in and tearaway type exponential functions (2.9.7) (choice of rate constant). All of these functions have a limit of the pre-existing $\dot{V}_A$.

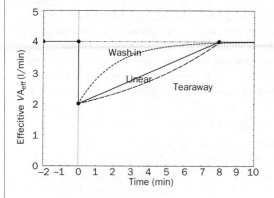

Output display is Pa_{CO_2}, FE'_{CO_2}, and the chosen recovery function.
An alveolar-end tidal P_{CO_2} difference of 0.5 kPa is incorporated.

FE'_{CO_2} continues to rise after the peak of Pa_{CO_2}. This is because the recruitment of embolized alveoli back into the functional compartment allows the dilution factor to diminish and expose more alveoli to the increased Pa_{CO_2}.

Once the recovery function has reached its completion and $\dot{V}_A$ is restored, the dilution factor is removed and Pa_{CO_2} and FE'_{CO_2} fall gently together (and now purely exponentially) back to the equilibrium value.

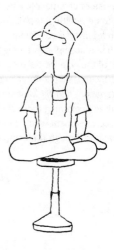

$\dot{V}_{CO_2} = 0.2$ l/min.
$V_t = 0.60$ l.
$f = 10$/min.
Effective embolus 50%
Recovery function: linear with gradient 0.1.
The computer output shows a five minute steady state period preceding the occurrence of PAE at $t = 5$.

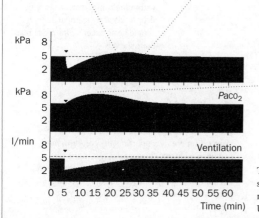

The Pa_{CO_2} reaches a peak before the full recovery of $\dot{V}_A$. This is because Pa_{CO_2} has risen to a point at which the (albeit still diminished) $\dot{V}_A$ produces a CO_2 elimination equal to production. Further recovery causes removal to exceed production and Pa_{CO_2} falls again.

The basic pattern of FE'_{CO_2} is similar to that of the clinical record in 1.12.1. Unfortunately, there is no clinical measurement of Pa_{CO_2} to compare.

This type of model enables one to examine the kinetics of a complex process in circumstances uncluttered by confounding factors. The model can be used to predict aspects of behaviour that might not be apparent in a qualitative description of the process; for instance, the initial return of FE'_{CO_2} to normal in slow-recovery embolus is actually masking a considerable rise in Pa_{CO_2}. The model will never be better than the modelling assumptions that underlie it, and these should always be kept under review when predicting from such models.

1.13.1   The one-compartment model

Pharmacokinetics is the study of the time course of drug disposition. Pharmacokinetics is dependent upon model-building and these models traditionally cause much anguish to students. Pharmacokinetic models are identical in principle to those we have been studying and the lessons we have learnt, for instance in modelling $PaCO_2$ or FAN_2 changes with time, should make coping with these models quite straightforward.

Single compartment kinetics

The purpose of pharmacokinetic models is to mimic the time course of plasma drug levels—nothing more. The models do not pretend to be a faithful representation of reality; the only criterion is how well they allow us to simulate measured plasma levels under diverse conditions.

     After bolus dosing, some drugs have a time course of action which seems to follow a simple exponential decline or washout of the type we have seen—warfarin, heparin, and insulin are examples. We know we can mimic a simple exponential washout by imagining a container washed through by a steady flow. This is what the step increase in $\dot{V}A$, circle system, pre-oxygenation, and N_2 washout examples all were in essence. In each case we needed a container or 'compartment' that represented something more complicated—a notional distribution volume D^* for CO_2, breathing circuit volume + FRC, and so on. This compartment was a modelling simplification or abstraction. In each case we also had a flow—$\dot{V}A$, FGF, or whatever—which washed through the compartment of fixed volume.

Initial drug concentration
$C(0) = M/V$

Drug concentration

0

Time

To reproduce a simple exponential washout, we need a compartment of volume V and a flow $\dot{Q}$ (in appropriate units) washing through it. To make the one-compartment model this is all that we do—we simply invent the compartment and the flow, assign suitable values to them, and we have a model. We do not need identifiable anatomical or physiological counterparts to these components. For a pharmacokinetic model, all we can say is that plasma must be contained within the compartment, since the drug levels in the compartment should be an accurate mimic of real plasma levels.

What is the flow in the pharmacokinetic model? We do not need a real visible flow such as we have had so far—$\dot{V}A$, cardiac output $\dot{Q}$, and so on—we simply need a notional flow analogous to the others. This flow is the *clearance*. Clearance is just an abstraction which enables us to make an analogy with similar models. Clearance has units of flow, e.g. l/min, l/hr.

$\dot{Q}$

Elimination of drug is merely viewed as overspill of the flow $\dot{Q}$ out of a single pathway. Drug is removed from the system at a rate governed by its prevailing concentration $C(t)$ and the clearance $\dot{Q}$. It is identical to the proportional removals that we have seen with CO_2, N_2, and isoflurane.

$\dot{Q}$

The volume of the compartment V will be measured in litres. This number can exceed the kilogram body weight of the subject, so V should be viewed simply as a proportionality constant, not real physical litres. This is analogous to the idea of tissue capacitance, except for our not being able to attribute the storage of a mass of substance to a particular tissue (1.7.2) This is body drug capacitance.

1.13.2 Distribution volume and clearance

The one-compartment model: assigning values to V and $\dot{Q}$.

We assume that the dose M of a drug is introduced into the single compartment at time $t = 0$, and instantaneously dispersed throughout the volume V. These are typical modelling assumptions. We know from previous models (1.10) that the rate constant for a simple washout process is the proportion of the container volume V filled in unit time by the flow $\dot{Q}$. This is $\dot{Q}/V$. The time constant τ is the reciprocal of this, $V/\dot{Q}$. We also know that a rate constant k for a simple exponential is the gradient of the log transformation straight line (2.9.10). (If the data are *not* from a single exponential, they will not lie on a straight line.) We can estimate this from real plasma data using techniques of linear regression (3.18). Hence we can obtain value for the ratio $k = \dot{Q}/V$, the rate constant—this tells us the relative size of V and $\dot{Q}$ but not the absolute value of either.

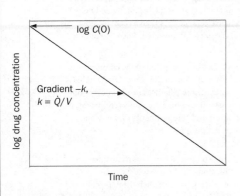
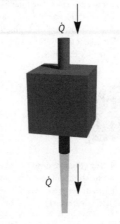

Extrapolation of the fitted line back to the log concentration axis gives a value for initial (log) concentration. This concentration (*not* the log concentration—we must antilog first) is M/V according to the model, where M is the (known) dose distributed throughout V. From this we extract a value for V, the distribution or compartment volume.

Since we can estimate the ratio $\dot{Q}/V$ from the gradient of the line, and V itself from knowing the intercept and dose M, we have completely characterized the model. This is all there is to the one-compartment pharmacokinetic model. The two-compartment model is only slightly more involved.

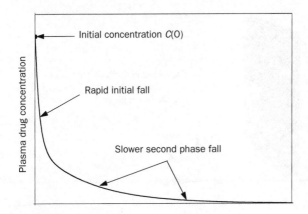

The IOP and the one-compartment model

The input–output interpretation of this model is that drug is introduced into a single homogeneous (i.e. 'well-mixed') compartment at time $t = 0$. The mass of drug (i.e. dose) M is distributed instantaneously through the volume of distribution V, leading to an initial concentration M/V. This is an initial condition and provided no further drug is introduced, the input is zero. Output is assumed to be proportional to prevailing drug concentration as the flow $\dot{Q}$ (i.e. clearance) through the constant volume compartment spills over, carrying drug with it. The derivation is identical to the N_2 washout example (1.9.3); $C(t)$ is equivalent to $F_{A}N_2$ and clearance $\dot{Q}$ is equivalent to $\dot{V}A$; Compartment volume V is equivalent to V_{FRC}.

$$\text{input in } \delta t = 0,$$
$$\text{output in } \delta t \approx \dot{Q}C(t)\delta t,$$
$$V\{C(t) - C(t + \delta t)\} \approx -\dot{Q}C(t)\delta t,$$
$$\frac{C(t) - C(t + \delta t)}{\delta t} \approx -\frac{\dot{Q}C(t)}{V}.$$

The rest of the derivation is identical to the N_2 washout example and the solution is

$$C(t) = A \exp\left[-\left\{\frac{\dot{Q}}{V}\right\}t\right]$$

where $A = \dfrac{M}{V} = C(0)$

There are unfortunately not many drugs whose time course is well modelled by the one compartment model. A much more typical pattern is an initial steep decline in plasma drug levels followed by a more leisurely fall. We need to improve our model to make the correspondence between its behaviour and the observed plasma levels better than we can achieve with the simple one-compartment model. We do this by adding a compartment. Two-compartment models are developed next.

1.13.3   **Clearance: infusion and steady state**

The notion of clearance seems to be poorly understood. Drug clearance is very simply the pharmacokinetic version of the 'obvious' flows that we have met in previous models, so that we can use these same models. It is sometimes called a 'virtual flow' because we cannot actually see it, although there is a real flow in that water is constantly passing through the body and drugs are eliminated with it in urine, bile, and so on. Creatinine or urea clearance are entirely analogous ideas.

Drug clearance

There are a number of different but equivalent ways of describing or viewing clearance.

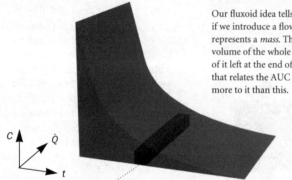

Our fluxoid idea tells us that if we have a concentration vs. time curve, then if we introduce a flow axis, the volume of any solid part of the figure represents a *mass*. The total mass of the drug M, the initial dose, must be the volume of the whole figure, since all of it is there at the beginning and none of it left at the end of elimination. The clearance $\dot{Q}$ is then a constant flow that relates the AUC to the mass of the drug administered. There is nothing more to it than this.

Clearance is the proportion of the compartment volume which flows in unit time: $\dot{Q} = kV$. This is just a statement of what we already know about rate constants and time constants (reciprocals of each other) and compartment volume V and flow $\dot{Q}$ relationships.

Another description of clearance is that it is the 'mass of drug eliminated/unit time/unit drug concentration'. This means that for a unit square on the front face of the figure (unit concentration and unit time) the depth along the flow axis is the mass removed. This just means the length of a fluxoid of unit area under the curve; if its front face has area unity, then the mass of drug contained in the fluxoid is the length of the fluxoid, the clearance $\dot{Q}$.

One-compartment pharmacokinetics is easy if one holds on to the ideas of clearance as a flow, the reciprocal relationship of time and rate constants, and that the time constant is the *time taken for the flow to fill the container*. The other ways of looking at clearance mentioned above are quite correct but do not necessarily do much to aid understanding. Standard notation denotes clearance by Cl; I have chosen $\dot{Q}$ to emphasize the flow nature of clearance and its equivalence to other flows we have met.

Infusion and steady state

The IOP, the fluxoid idea, and analogy with $\dot{V}A$ and Pa_{CO_2} enable us to deal quickly with the conditions which determine steady state plasma drug levels in continuous infusion; the rate of drug infusion (input: analogy $\dot{V}_{CO_2}$) must be exactly balanced by the output ($C_{equilibrium} \times \dot{Q}$) (analogy: $FA_{CO_2} \times \dot{V}A$), so that the only determinants are infusion rate and clearance.

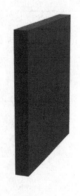

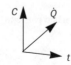

The volume of the fluxoid for unit time and for steady state conditions (flat top) must be the infusion rate of the drug.

1.13.4 Improving the fit: the two-compartment model

Adding a compartment

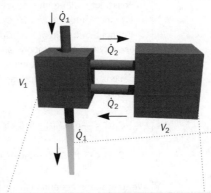

A typical pattern of decline in plasma drug concentration after bolus dosing shows a steep initial decline—the so-called *distribution phase*—followed by a slower fall in concentration—the *elimination phase*. It is impossible to mimic this with a simple exponential. One-compartment models cannot be persuaded to simulate this pattern.

We can simulate the bi-phasic pattern of decline by introducing a second compartment to the basic model. We distinguish a *central compartment* V_1, which is essentially the same as the single compartment of the simpler model. Drug concentrations in this compartment, $C_1(t)$, are the simulation of plasma levels. Elimination takes place only from V_1. Each compartment is assumed perfectly mixed and homogeneous.

The central compartment has a flow $\dot{Q}_1$ through it, the elimination clearance as before. This carries drug out with it through the elimination overspill pathway. This is in all respects identical to the single-compartment model.

The second constant-volume compartment is the *deep compartment* V_2 and is connected to V_1 by two pathways. A separate flow $\dot{Q}_2$—also somewhat confusingly called a clearance, although it does not clear anything—is envisaged as washing through the deep compartment. It enters V_2 through one pathway, carrying drug from V_1 in accordance with the prevailing concentration $C_1(t)$ into V_2. Since V_2 is a cul-de-sac of constant volume, all of this flow must return through the other pathway carrying drug back with it into V_1 according to the prevailing concentration $C_2(t)$ in V_2. $\dot{Q}_2$ is an intercompartmental clearance, although it might be better to think of it as an inner *circulation*.

Inputs and outputs in the two-compartment model

The presence of the extra compartment adds a little complication to the algebra, although the principle of balancing inputs and outputs is the same as in simpler IOP models. We will only deal with bolus dosing into the central compartment with no drug already present in the system.

The input into V_2 in δt is only from V_1:
$\dot{Q}_2 C_1(t)\delta t.$

The output from V_1 in δt is via two pathways:
- through the elimination pathway $\dot{Q}_1 C_1(t)\delta t.$
- from V_1 into V_2 $\dot{Q}_2 C_1(t)\delta t.$

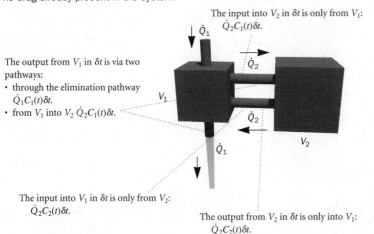

The input into V_1 in δt is only from V_2:
$\dot{Q}_2 C_2(t)\delta t.$

The output from V_2 in δt is only into V_1:
$\dot{Q}_2 C_2(t)\delta t.$

Constructing the equations for the two-compartment model

We have identified the inputs and outputs in δt in the two-compartment model. Note that one compartment's input can be the other's output. These can be used to construct a differential equation as before:

V_1: input–output in $\delta t \approx [\dot{Q}_2 C_2(t) - \dot{Q}_1 C_1(t) - \dot{Q}_2 C_1(t)]\delta t$,

V_2: input–output in $\delta t \approx [\dot{Q}_2 C_1(t) - \dot{Q}_2 C_2(t)]\delta t$.

These input–output relations are equated to concentration changes in the appropriate compartment in the usual fashion to produce *two* ordinary differential equations (ODEs)—one for each compartment—which are *simultaneously* true. We obtain

$$C_1'(t) = \frac{1}{V_1}[\dot{Q}_2 C_2(t) - \dot{Q}_1 C_1(t) - \dot{Q}_2 C_1(t)],$$

$$C_2'(t) = \frac{1}{V_2}[\dot{Q}_2 C_1(t) - \dot{Q}_2 C_2(t)].$$

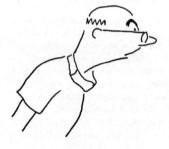

We treat these equations just like the simultaneous equations we did at school and after a large amount of tedious algebra and a little differentiation (details omitted), we obtain two second-order ODEs (2.15.3), one just in terms of $C_1(t)$ and its derivatives and the other in terms of $C_2(t)$ and its derivatives. These equations have the form

$aC_1''(t) + bC_1'(t) + cC_1(t) = 0$ for V_1,
$dC_2''(t) + fC_2'(t) + gC_2(t) = 0$ for V_2

which have solutions

$C_1(t) = Ae^{-\alpha t} + Be^{-\beta t}$
$C_2(t) = Ge^{-\beta t} - Fe^{-\alpha t}$

respectively. These solution functions are sums or differences of two exponential functions (2.9.11) of differing rate constant α and β.

1.13.5 The two-compartment model: solution functions

Examining the solutions

We have tried to see the pharmacokinetic models as just an extension of the IOP models which we developed earlier.

The purpose in defining values for V_1 and V_2 and the two clearances $\dot{Q}_1$ and $\dot{Q}_2$ (elimination and intercompartmental) is to predict the behaviour of the system—and hence if the model is a good one, of the real subject—to other doses, dosage regimes (e.g. infusion, or repeat dosing). Single-dose data and appropriate analysis of the model can do this. Whether or not the model predictions are fulfilled, even approximately, in reality is another matter. If they are not, this is not a fault of the model but of the modeller.

These are simulated curves for a hypothetical drug given to the model at $t = 0$ in bolus dose of 0.35 mg. The model is 'empty', i.e. there is no drug already present: $V_1 = 10\ \text{l}$, $V_2 = 12.96\ \text{l}$, $\alpha = 0.25/\text{min}$, $\beta = 0.025/\text{min}$.

At this point the concentration in V_2 has risen to equal that in V_1. This is a so-called pseudo-equilibrium. It lasts only instantaneously as continued elimination from V_1 ensures that $C_1(t)$ remains thereafter below $C_2(t)$, as can be seen in the graph.

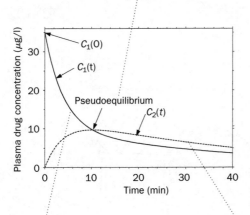

This function $C_1(t)$ models the time-dependent concentration in the central compartment V_1. Plasma is part of this compartment and this is essentially all we require of the model. We can fit the model optimally to experimental data of plasma drug concentrations (2.9.12, 3.18) and produce estimates of the values of α and β.

This function $C_2(t)$ has no meaning in reality whatsoever. It is merely the by-product of the model's ability to mimic values in V_1. Since the deep compartment has no counterpart in anatomy, we cannot measure $C_2(t)$. But we do need the deep compartment to be there to make the model work.

Model parameters

The various model parameters are obtainable from the experimental single-dose data. Values for A, B, α, and β are 'plugged in' to obtain the various parameters in sequence as follows. These are not to be memorized. They are only useful for actually examining model predictions under different circumstances from those of the single-dose data, i.e. for the working pharmacokineticist:

$$V_1 = \frac{M}{A+B},$$

$$k_{21} = \frac{A\beta + B\alpha}{A+B},$$

$$k_{10} = \frac{\alpha\beta}{k_{21}},$$

$$k_{12} = \alpha + \beta - k_{10} - k_{21}$$

$$\dot{Q}_1 = k_{10}V_1$$

$$\dot{Q}_2 = k_{12}V_1 = k_{21}V_2$$

$$V_2 = \frac{k_{12}}{k_{21}}V_1$$

We treat the starting concentration as an initial condition of the model rather than an input. The bolus dose M is treated as being instantaneously and uniformly distributed throughout V_1 at $t = 0$. These are typical modelling assumptions.

Drug is transferred by the inner circulation into the deep compartment V_2. The rate at which the concentration rises in V_2 will be governed by the rapidity of the flow $\dot{Q}_2$, how large is the space it is flowing into (magnitude of V_2) and how fast drug concentration is falling in V_1 as drug is removed from the model through the elimination pathway (the magnitude of k_{10} and V_1).

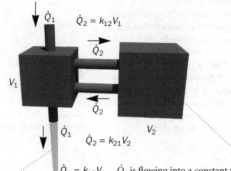

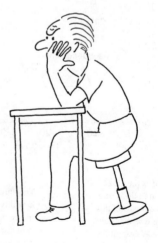

The elimination pathway has rate constant k_{10}, which is the ratio of elimination clearance $\dot{Q}_1$ to V_1. This is the usual flow/container volume ratio that we have seen in our other models.

$\dot{Q}_2$ is flowing into a constant volume container, V_2, and this same flow must return back to V_1: $\dot{Q}_{2in} = \dot{Q}_{2out}$. The same relationship of flow and container volume applies here, so that $\dot{Q}_{2in} = k_{12} V_1$ and $\dot{Q}_{2out} = k_{21} V_2$ and hence $k_{12} V_1 = k_{21} V_2$, where k_{12} denotes the rate constant for the flow from V_1 into V_2 and k_{21} denotes the rate constant for the flow from V_2 back into V_1.

1.13.6 Compartmental models and N_2 washout

Nitrogen washout

In considering N_2 washout in (1.9), we ignored the nitrogen in the tissues and treated the input of N_2 into the FRC as zero. Of the total N_2 stores in the body approximately 50% is in the FRC and the other 50% in the tissues, so the tissue N_2 cannot be ignored completely; tissue N_2 is of great importance in diving physiology, for example. The washout of N_2 from the FRC is rapid; we have calculated that it is practically complete in 2 min of effective pre-oxygenation in normal lungs. Removal of tissue N_2 takes about 2 h (i.e. 60 times more slowly), so that the effect of ignoring tissue N_2 on short-term prediction of FAO_2 is negligible—particularly compared with infelicities of pre-oxygenation techniques. This process can also be modelled by a two-compartment model, although here the model is rather more 'physiological' in that the superficial compartment V_1 can be identified confidently as the FRC, and the elimination clearance $\dot{Q}_1$ as the $\dot{V}A$. The deep compartment V_2 represents 'the tissues', which conceals a deal of lumping together of disparate components. $\dot{Q}_2$, the intercompartmental clearance or inner circulation, is largely represented by a composite tissue blood flow that carries the N_2 from tissues to the lung. This still involves considerable abstraction.

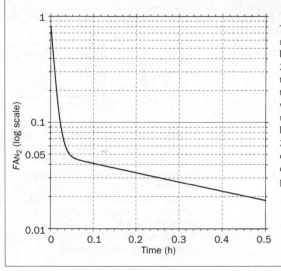

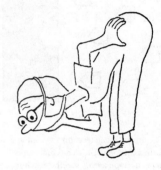

The rapid initial washout removes 50% of total body N_2 within about 2 min. The other 50% takes about 2 h. 50% of the volume of the N_2 washout fluxoid lies under the surface between $t = 0$ and $t = 2$ min. This is the curve of FAN_2 with time and is equivalent to $C_1(t)$ in the pharmacokinetic models.

Compartmental models are used for prediction. They may do this well or badly; if they do it badly in comparison with what actually happens, then we need a better model. This may need the addition of another compartment, or a new approach to the modelling altogether. Details are available in full treatments of what is a very involved topic. Whatever one may read about these models, it must be remembered what their purpose is: to predict from one circumstance what might happen in another. The fact that the models require imaginary flows through non-existent spaces should not disturb us too much. Somehow we feel that imagining millions of alveoli as a single or perhaps two 'spaces' is legitimate but the idea of a pharmacokinetic compartment is not so convincing. Actually, they are the same idea and both are ridiculous, but they do enable us to model, predict and explain patterns of change.

1.14.1   Receptors and agonists

We have studied the time course of drug action and how this may be modelled—pharmacokinetics. Now we turn to the effects of the drug at its site of action—pharmacodynamics. The concept of drug receptors was formulated by Clark in the 1920s and, despite refinements, the basic concept of a ligand interacting with a receptor in accordance with the Law of Mass Action remains valid. A ligand is a simply a molecule that binds to a receptor site. It may be a natural substance such as noradrenaline or a synthetic one such as isoprenaline. It may or may not produce some measurable effect. If an effect is produced, the ligand is an agonist at that receptor. We shall concentrate upon the mathematical models that the receptor concept predicts. Further details of receptor theory are available in any pharmacology text.

Drug–receptor interactions

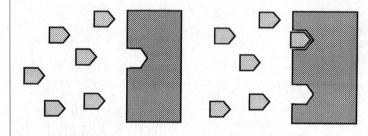

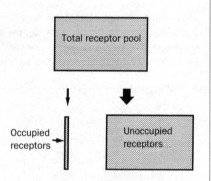

Total receptor pool

Occupied receptors

Unoccupied receptors

The drug [D] and receptor [R] combine to form a complex [DR]. The combination depends upon a fairly specific matching of drug to receptor. The formation of this complex may lead to a physiological response which is graded and dependent upon the concentration of agonist in the vicinity of the receptor.

The total receptors are viewed as a pool, with the individual receptors being disposed between two compartments according to whether or not they are occupied by ligand. Occupied receptors [DR] are in equilibrium with free drug [D] and unoccupied receptors [R]. The balance of the occupied and unoccupied receptors is determined by the equilibrium dissociation constant K_D. The proportion of the total receptor pool occupied by drug is the *occupancy y*:

In the simplest model, the drug combines reversibly with the receptor according to the Law of Mass Action, which states that at equilibrium the ratio $[D] \times [R]/[DR]$ is a constant:

$$\frac{[D][R]}{[DR]} = K_D.$$

$$y = \frac{[DR]}{\{[R]+[DR]\}}$$

Quite what [DR], i.e. the concentration of the drug–receptor complex means in the context of a membrane-bound macromolecule is unclear. This is another example of ruthless simplification in modelling. K_D has the units of concentration.

Receptors thus have the following properties:
- *Specificity*. The receptor is able to bind a rather narrow range of substances.
- *Affinity*. The receptor binds the drug more or less avidly. The more avid the binding, the smaller the value of K_D.
- *Stimulus–reaction coupling*. The occupation of the receptor may produce a measurable effect. This is the stimulus–reaction coupling (SRC). We are interested to establish the relationship between drug concentration and effect produced.

1.14.2 Occupancy and stimulus–reaction coupling

Receptor theory assumes that the effect produced by the combination of an agonist and a receptor is dependent upon the concentration of the drug–receptor complex [DR]. The combination of drug and receptor leads to some measurable response in the organism or isolated tissue in a tissue bath. The effect bears *some* sort of functional relationship to receptor occupation by agonist. The simplest model assumes a linear relationship between occupancy (proportional receptor occupation and hence [DR]) and the response. This is another example of a linear relationship as a default model.

Drug concentration and effect

We have three modelling equations to incorporate and we want to find a relationship between drug concentration [D] and effect E:

- $K_D = [D][R]/[DR]$ This is the Law of Mass Action equation. The equilibrium dissociation constant K_D is a measure of the specificity of the drug–receptor association. It is a dis-association constant and has a *high* value if the drug–receptor complex does not form easily—lots of free drug, small amount of drug–receptor complex.
- $y = [DR]/\{[R] + [DR]\}$. This is the occupancy or proportional occupation of receptors.
- Effect $= \alpha y$. We assume a linear relationship between the occupancy and the effect produced. This is the 'intrinsic activity' of classical receptor theory. It is a simple proportional response. α is the constant of proportionality and quantifies the change in response for any change in occupancy. The SRC is a 'black box'—we do not try to know *how* it achieves the response, but simply the relation between input and output. The proportional effect will be the same as the occupancy y.

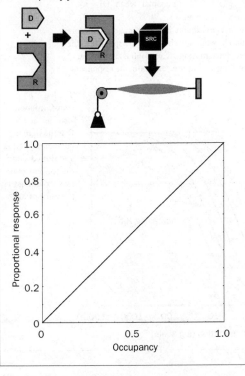

The occupancy function

We can express y in terms of only [D] and K_D by eliminating [R] and [DR].

Since $[DR] = \dfrac{[D][R]}{K_D}$,

$$y = \frac{\dfrac{[D][R]}{K_D}}{[R] + \dfrac{[D][R]}{K_D}}$$

$$= \frac{[D][R]}{K_D} \times \frac{1}{[R]\left\{1 + \dfrac{[D]}{K_D}\right\}}$$

$$= \frac{[D]}{[D] + K_D}.$$

This is an expression of the form

$$y = \frac{ax}{bx + c}.$$

This is a rectangular hyperbola (2.6.3) with a limiting value of 1 as x increases without limit. The occupancy y approaches 1 as the drug concentration increases.

1.14.3 **Dose–response curves**

Occupancy and effect

We have an expression relating drug concentration [D] and dissociation constant K_D to occupancy, $y = \dfrac{[D]}{\{[D] + K_D\}}$, and as occupancy is a proportion, this has a limiting value of 1. Since we further assume a proportional relationship between occupancy and effect $E = \alpha y$, we can draw a graph of drug concentration against proportional response, i.e. the proportion of maximum response.

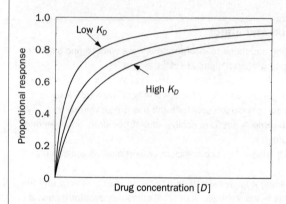

The gradient of the response curve at low concentration is very steep. We can expand the lower end of the scale by adopting a log transformation.

The graph is a rectangular hyperbola. All curves approach a limiting value of 1—i.e. the maximum attainable response—as the concentration is increased.

The value of the dissociation constant for any drug–receptor combination determines occupancy for any given concentration. The higher the value of K_D, the lower the response is. The occupancy is 0.5 (50% maximal) when $[D] = K_D$.

The effect of the log transformation is to expand the lower range of concentration scale where most of the action is, while still showing the approach to the maximum response at the higher concentrations. The graph is the familiar dose–response curve. In the mid-range of log concentration, the response is approximately linear.

The log transformation also has the effect that the sigmoid curves are parallel and shifted along the concentration axis according to the value of K_D.

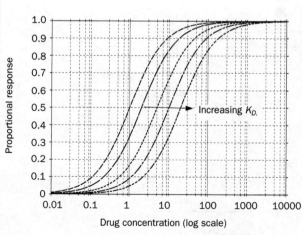

1.14.4 Linearization: the Hill plot

In order to characterize a drug–receptor interaction, we need to determine a value for K_D. If we look at the equation that we derived for response against occupancy, $y = \dfrac{[D]}{\{[D] + K_D\}}$, we can see that the response will be 0.5 when $[D] = K_D$. We would obtain a value for K_D by simply reading the value of [D] which produces a half-maximal response directly from the log-dose–response curve. It is difficult in practice to estimate this accurately from a dose–response curve. However, a simple manipulation of the occupancy equation enables us to produce a truly linear plot which allows a better estimate of K_D. Linear functions are so easy to manipulate that we often try very hard to find a linear transformation of a curvilinear function.

The Hill equation

We can rewrite the occupancy equation thus:

$$y = \frac{[D]}{[D] + K_D},$$
$$y\{[D] + K_D\} = [D],$$
$$y[D] + yK_D = [D],$$
$$yK_D = [D] - y[D]$$
$$= [D](1 - y),$$
$$\frac{y}{(1 - y)} = \frac{[D]}{K_D}.$$

The graphical method is due to A. V. Hill, and arose while investigating oxygen affinity for haemoglobin. Variation from a gradient of unity in the Hill plot implies a variable affinity of receptor for ligand, i.e. K_D is *not* constant. Variable affinity of haemoglobin for oxygen is well understood. A similar phenomenon may occur with drug–receptor interaction.

The Hill plot

Manipulation produces an equation $\dfrac{y}{(1 - y)} = \dfrac{[D]}{K_D}$. If we take logarithms (2.9) of both sides of our equation,

$$\log \frac{y}{(1 - y)} = \log[D] - \log K_D,$$

we obtain a linear plot. This method is the Hill plot.

When $\log[D] = \log K_D$, $\log \dfrac{y}{(1 - y)} = 0$. Since $\log(1) = 0$ for any base $\dfrac{y}{(1 - y)} = 1$, and $y = 0.5$, which we expect it to be. If we can fit a straight line to our dose–response data, the intercept on the log concentration axis is the estimate of K_D.

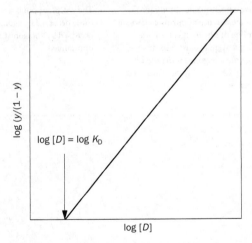

What about the gradient? The log[D] term is predicted by the model to have a coefficient of unity. The gradient of the line is therefore 1. If the experimental data suggest a non-linear relationship or even a linear plot, the gradient of which could not plausibly be unity, then the simple model based on the Law of Mass Action is inadequate and a more sophisticated model is required.

Experimental data can be plotted by this method and a line of best fit obtained by least squares. Linear regression techniques (3.18) can be employed to test for a linear relationship with a gradient of 1.

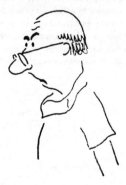

1.15.1   **Standardized concentrations**

Antagonists are classified as competitive or non-competitive. There are various ways in which the non-competitive antagonists may act but the most familiar—exemplified by phenoxybenzamine at the α-receptor—is the irreversible (or only very slowly reversible) reaction with a receptor site. The effect is essentially a depletion of the receptor pool [R] and hence a reduction in [DR] for any given agonist concentration. We concentrate on the more familiar competitive antagonism.

Competitive antagonism

Competitive antagonists are modelled as behaving in exactly the same way at the receptor site as do agonists. They obey the simple model based on the Law of Mass Action. The only difference is that they produce no effect. The intrinsic activity—the proportionality constant α in the SRC is zero.

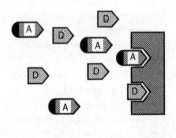 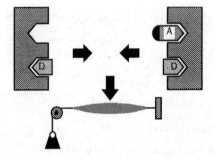 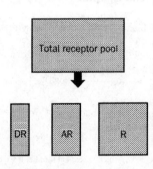

Agonist and antagonist compete for occupation of the receptor sites. A site occupied by agonist produces an effect as before. A site occupied by antagonist produces no effect and prevents access by the agonist. The balance is determined by the relative concentrations of agonist and antagonist, and the dissociation constants of each.

Antagonists have a quantifiable affinity for the receptor, but in the absence of intrinsic effect we can only determine this by its effects on the response produced by an agonist. The dissociation constant for the antagonist is denoted K_A. $K_A = [A][R]/[AR]$, where [A] is the concentration of antagonist A.

The receptor pool is now in three parts; those occupied by agonist, those occupied by antagonist and those still unoccupied.

Receptor occupancy in presence of antagonist

Since the value of K_D is the concentration at which the half-maximal effect (in the absence of antagonist) is achieved it can be useful to scale our prevailing concentration [D] relative to this K_D. We refer to the standardized drug concentration [D*], where [D*] = [D]/K_D. This relates our concentrations to the particular range of K_D. We can do the same for antagonist concentrations so that [A*] = [A]/K_A. The occupancy is still the proportional occupation of the total receptor pool by agonist, but there are now three possible states in which we may find any receptor—unoccupied, occupied by agonist, or occupied by antagonist.

$$y = \frac{[DR]}{[R] + [DR] + [AR]}.$$ Substituting for [DR] and [AR] and using standardized concentrations, we obtain a new occupancy function.

$$y = \frac{[D^*]}{\{1 + [D^*] + [A^*]\}}.$$

In the absence of antagonist [A*] = 0, and the equation becomes $y = [D^*]/\{1+[D^*]\}$. Since [D*] = 1 when [D] = K_D, we obtain a value $y = 0.5$ at this point as we require.

The presence of a non-zero concentration for [A*] increases the magnitude of the denominator for any given value of [D*] and hence the value of y—the response is diminished as expected.

Occupancy function in presence of antagonist

$$[AR] = \frac{[A][R]}{K_A} = [R][A^*],$$

$$[DR] = \frac{[D][R]}{K_D} = [R][D^*],$$

$$y = \frac{[DR]}{[R] + [DR] + [AR]}$$

$$= \frac{[D^*][R]}{[R]\{1 + [D^*] + [A^*]\}}$$

$$= \frac{[D^*]}{\{1 + [D^*] + [A^*]\}}.$$

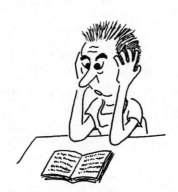

1.15.2 Dose–response curves and the dose ratio

Dose–response curves in the presence of antagonist

The familiar sigmoid log-dose–response curve is shown in the presence of various concentrations of antagonist. Each curve describes the response with a particular antagonist concentration. This shows a progressive rightward shift of the DRC as antagonist concentration is increased. The sigmoids remain parallel—there is no change in gradient or maximum response, merely a change in position along the log-dose axis.

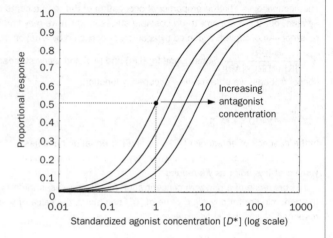

The parallel shift of the DRC by the presence of antagonist means that each point on the agonist-alone DRC is moved a constant distance along a horizontal (i.e. equal-response) line. Since the concentration is plotted on a log-scale axis—remember that this is a log-dose–response curve—this shift means that we need a constant *multiple* of the agonist concentration to achieve the same effect in the presence of antagonist.

In the presence of the particular antagonist concentration in this example, we require an agonist concentration tenfold greater in order to achieve the same effect as previously. Equal distances along a log scale means equal multiples. This multiple of agonist dose required is the dose ratio and is dependent upon the antagonist concentration $[A]$ and the value of its dissociation constant K_A. The dose ratio in this case is 10.

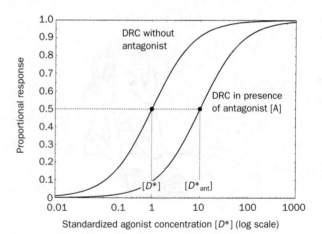

The dose ratio = $[D^*_{ant}]/[D]$, where $[D^*_{ant}]$ is the agonist concentration in the presence of antagonist at a particular fixed concentration $[A]$ which achieves the same response as $[D]$ with agonist alone.

When the log of agonist concentration is plotted against response, the antilog of the horizontal shift is the dose ratio. When we plot the *actual* standardized agonist concentration on a log scale as we have done, the dose ratio is read off the scale directly.

1.15.3 Extracting K_A: the Schild plot

Competitive antagonism: extracting K_A

We have established the idea of the dose ratio and we know that the value for any particular agonist–receptor interaction is dependent upon the antagonist concentration and the value of K_A. This is apparent in the occupancy equation

$$y = \frac{[D^*]}{\{1 + [D^*] + [A^*]\}}.$$

We now need to see how we can extract the value of K_A.

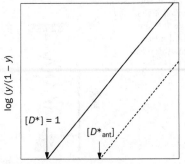

$[D^*] = 1$

$[D^*_{ant}]$

Standardized log agonist concentration $[D^*]$

The effect of the antagonist is to change the effective K_D of the agonist. This 'new' apparent K_D can be extracted from a Hill plot of the dose–response data in the presence of A. The DRC for drug with and without antagonist can be displayed as a Hill plot. The line and therefore the intercept shifts in parallel to the right as the dose of [A] is increased, provided that the simple mass action model is valid.

The Schild equation

We want to extract K_A. If, as before, we distinguish the concentration of agonist in the presence of antagonist, for the same response

$$y = \frac{[D^*_{ant}]}{\{1 + [D^*_{ant}] + [A^*]\}} = \frac{[D^*]}{\{1 + [D^*]\}},$$

$$[D^*_{ant}]\{1 + [D^*]\} = [D^*]\{1 + [D^*_{ant}] + [A^*]\},$$

$$[D^*_{ant}] + [D^*][D^*_{ant}] = [D^*]\{1 + [A^*]\} + [D^*][D^*_{ant}],$$

$$[D^*_{ant}] = [D^*]\{1 + [A^*]\},$$

$$\frac{[D^*_{ant}]}{[D^*]} = \{1 + [A^*]\},$$

$$\frac{[D^*_{ant}]}{[D^*]} - 1 = [A^*],$$

$$\{\text{dose ratio} - 1\} = [A^*] = \frac{[A]}{K_A}$$

The Schild plot

After some messy-looking algebra, we have arrived at a relatively simple equation relating the dose ratio to the antagonist concentration and the dissociation constant:

$$\{\text{dose ratio} - 1\} = [A^*] = \frac{[A]}{K_A}.$$

Taking logs of both sides, we obtain

$$\log\{\text{dose ratio} - 1\} = \log[A] - \log K_A$$

Like the Hill plot, this predicts a linear relationship between the variables with a gradient of unity and an intercept on the concentration axis of $\log K_A$.

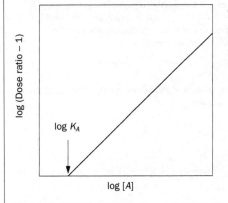

$\log K_A$

$\log [A]$

The gradient of the line from the simple mass action model is 1. Deviations from this indicate that the model does not adequately describe the receptor–agonist–antagonist relationship.

The horizontal axis is the log concentration of antagonist. The intercept is $\log K_A$.

Deviations from the predicted behaviour of the plots can be due to many factors. The receptor population may be non-homogeneous, the antagonist may not be purely competitive, or there may be inhibition of re-uptake by agonist or antagonist. Uptake processes may introduce non-linearity. These deviations from the linearity predicted by the simple model may help elucidation of the mechanism of action of the agonist or antagonist.

1.16.1   Masses and springs: Hooke's Law

Oscillating systems are seen everywhere. Anaesthetists are particularly interested in cyclical physiological processes such as the cardiac and respiratory cycles. As in previous modelling examples, we shall start quite simply and build up only such complexity as we need to describe the systems that concern us. We shall build a model of a typical arterial pressure waveform and see how this model relates to the physical behaviour of the clinical measurement systems that we use to display it. We start with the simplest ideal oscillating system, in which no frictional forces are involved.

The mass–spring system

Imagine a mass suspended from a spring. This will form the basis of our modelling of oscillations and waves. It is common experience that the spring will stretch when we attach the weight, and provided it is strong enough (does not break), the spring will support the weight of the mass acting downwards by an equal pull upwards. The tension in the spring acting upwards is a force equal and opposite to the force due to gravity acting downwards on the mass. If the mass is at rest, by Newton's Second Law, the forces are equal and opposite and no net force is acting.

There is no net force acting at the resting position and the force is negative when compressed and positive when extended. This is merely a convention to indicate direction of force i.e. to distinguish 'pull' from 'push'. Compression is a 'negative' displacement. The force of gravity acting on the mass downwards is balanced by the upward force due to the extension of the spring.

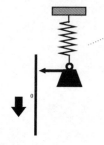

Hooke's Law: The force exerted by the spring when extended is proportional to the extension and is directed to restore the spring to its resting position—i.e. it pulls. Similarly, if we compress the spring, the force exerted is proportional to the compression and is again exerted in a direction to restore the spring to its resting length—i.e. it pushes. The proportionality constant (the gradient of the line) quantifies the force exerted for any given change in length and is the *stiffness*, of the spring, *k*; a bedspring has a higher value of *k* than an elastic band. This is, then, another simple linear relationship—at least until the spring is overstretched and undergoes an inelastic deformation, when it will not return to its original length. The law also breaks down with overcompression.

Newton's First Law: A body continues in a state of rest or uniform motion in a straight line unless acted upon by a net force.

Newton's Second Law

Force = Mass × Acceleration

$F = Ma$

Hooke's Law

Force = Stiffness × Extension

$F = -kx$

1.16.2   Simple harmonic motion: the sine wave

With our mass suspended at rest, we know from Newton's Laws that no net force is acting and that any forces involved must be equal and opposite. The force due to gravity acting downwards on the spring is mg, where g is the acceleration due to gravity. This downward force must be balanced by an equal and opposite force acting upwards due to extension in the spring. By Hooke's Law, this force must be of magnitude kx, where x is the extension of the spring from its resting length. If we consider extension is in the direction of positive x, i.e. downwards, then the direction of the force in the spring must be upwards in the direction of negative x:

$$mg - kx = 0$$

Since both m and g are constants, this initial stretching of the spring due to the weight of the mass will be a constant feature of the system and, when we look at the system after it has been set into motion, we are interested in how the mass oscillates about this resting position, at which the mass–spring system is in equilibrium at rest.

Oscillation of mass–spring

If we displace the mass from its resting position and release it, we set up a regular oscillation where the mass is constantly changing the direction and speed of its motion. The amplitude of the oscillation—how far the mass travels from its equilibrium position at maximum displacement—depends upon how far we displace it in the beginning. Experience tells us that if we attach a larger mass to the same spring, the oscillation will be slowed—the time taken to complete a cycle will be longer. Conversely, if we attach a spring of greater stiffness to any given mass, the system will oscillate more rapidly.

In any real system of this kind, the amplitude of the oscillations diminishes over time as the energy imparted to the system in the initial displacement is dissipated by frictional forces. However, we consider first an ideal system, in which the spring itself is of negligible mass and in which there are no frictional forces involved, so that the initial pattern of oscillation continues forever—this is typical of a first approach to modelling. The pattern of oscillation with time of such a system is called simple harmonic motion (SHM). It is described by the equation for a simple sinusoidal waveform:

$$A \cos \omega t + B \sin \omega t$$

Sinusoidal functions are considered in some detail in (2.10).

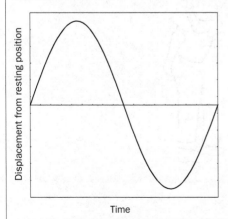

The vertical axis shows the displacement from the resting position with respect to time along the horizontal axis.

A larger mass for the same spring causes the oscillation to be slower. A stiffer spring for the same mass causes the oscillation to be faster. The relationship of the mass m to the stiffness k determines the rapidity of oscillation.

Potential and kinetic energy in the ideal mass–spring system

The ideal mass–spring system can be treated as a constant energy system, in which none is dissipated to the environment by frictional forces. The initial displacement and motion imparted to the system in setting it in motion determine the energy contained within it. The subsequent motion can be viewed as a continuous interchange of kinetic and potential energy. When the mass is at the maximum displacement from the resting position at either end of its excursion, it is momentarily at rest as it reverses direction of motion; the kinetic energy at this instant is zero, and the energy content is entirely potential; i.e. all of the energy is attributable to the stretching of the spring. As the mass whizzes past the resting position in either direction, it has maximal kinetic energy and the potential energy is zero; all of the energy is attributable to the motion of the mass.

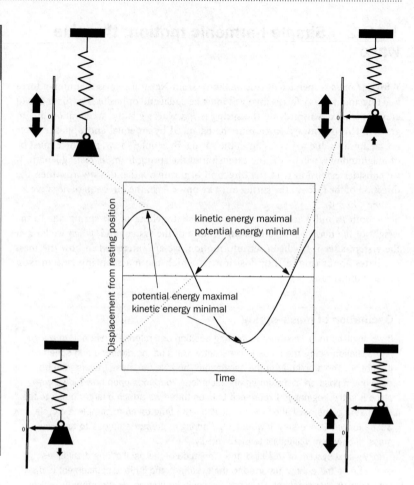

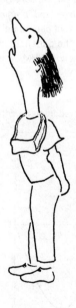

1.16.3 Simple harmonic motion: Newton meets Hooke

We have caused our mass–spring systems to oscillate and made some general observations about the influence of the size of the mass, the stiffness of the spring, and the resulting frequency of oscillation. We have decided to ignore for the moment the influence of frictional forces—we will incorporate these shortly as we build up a more general model. The total excursion of the oscillation depends upon the initial conditions—how far we displace the mass at the beginning, and how hard we push it in starting its motion. We will observe all of these factors in the modelling.

Modelling SHM using Hooke and Newton

Because the effects of gravity are constant, they have no influence on the oscillatory motion of the system, only upon the equilibrium position of the mass at rest; the mass would oscillate in the same way about its resting position if it were in the horizontal plane. We know from Newton's Second Law that the motion of the mass will be described by $F = ma$, where F is the force acting and a is the acceleration. The *position* of the mass changes with time and we will describe this position with respect to time as $x(t)$; $x(t)$ is the position function of time. We will identify the resting equilibrium position as $x = 0$, i.e. we measure displacement from this position—positive for extension and negative for compression. This is a convenient but otherwise arbitrary choice.

Velocity is the *rate of change of position* with time $x'(t)$—it is the first derivative (2.12.1) of the position function. The velocity of the mass is, however, not constant—it too is changing with time. The mass slows down as it approaches its peak displacement, and when it reaches this point it is instantaneously at rest before it reverses its direction. The *rate of change of velocity* $x''(t)$ is the acceleration and thus the second derivative of position with respect to time.

The force acting on the mass is thus $F = mx''(t)$ and this is determined by the tension in the spring, which from Hooke is $F = -kx(t)$:

$$mx''(t) = -kx(t)$$
$$x''(t) = \frac{-k}{m}x(t)$$

This is a second-order differential equation because of the appearance of $x''(t)$, the second derivative of the position $x(t)$. Second-order differential equations are described very briefly in (2.15.3).

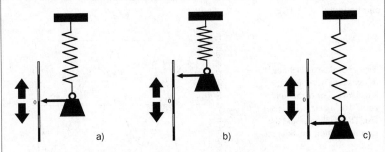

The mass oscillates about $x = 0$. The application of Hooke's and Newton's Laws gives us a differential equation which describes the motion of the mass with time. The solution to this equation is a sinusoidal wave.

1.16.4   Simple harmonic motion: solution function

The model system has given us a second-order differential equation to solve. A second-order equation arose from the two-compartment pharmacokinetic model in (1.13.4). The solution in this case, however, is different from the bi-exponential equation of that model:

$$x''(t) = -\frac{k}{m}x(t)$$

has the general solution $x(t) = A\cos\omega t + B\sin\omega t$, the general equation of a sine wave. (2.10.5)

Solving the equation

If we take the general solution and differentiate it twice to obtain the second derivative, i.e. the acceleration, we see that it only differs from the position function by a factor $-\omega^2$. Derivatives of sinusoidal functions are discussed in (2.10.4).

$x(t)$. This is the *position function*; it tells us *where* the mass is at any time t; how far away from the resting position it is (magnitude); and on which side of it (sign).

$$x(t) = A\cos\omega t + B\sin\omega t,$$
$$x'(t) = \omega A\sin\omega t + \omega B\cos\omega t,$$
$$x''(t) = \omega^2 A\cos\omega t - \omega^2 B\sin\omega t,$$
$$x''(t) = \omega^2[A\cos\omega t + B\sin\omega t]$$
$$x''(t) = \omega^2 x(t)$$

$x'(t)$. This is the *velocity function*; it tells us how fast the mass is moving (magnitude) and in which direction (sign) at any time t.

$x''(t)$. This is the *acceleration function*; it tells us how much the mass is changing its velocity (magnitude) and whether it is speeding up or slowing down (sign) at any time t.

Comparing this with our differential equation we see that $-\omega^2 = -k/m$ or $\omega = \sqrt{k/m}$. The quantity ω is the angular velocity of the oscillation—a measure of the frequency or rapidity of the cyclical motion. It is determined by the spring stiffness k (stiffer spring, more rapid oscillation) and by m (larger mass, slower oscillation.) This accords with our expectations of the behaviour of masses and springs.

But where does the amplitude of the oscillation come in? The arbitrary constants A and B determine this, and these are dependent only upon the initial conditions—where the mass is ($x(0)$) and how fast it is moving ($x'(0)$) at time $t = 0$.

Further details of the properties of sinusoidal functions and their derivatives can be found in (2.10).

Two sinusoidal oscillations. The dotted curve has double the angular velocity of the solid curve. It is oscillating twice as fast. The amplitudes and the starting position are different.

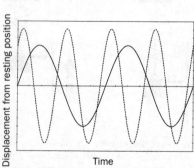

1.17.1 Modelling real oscillations: frictional forces and damping

We have studied the behaviour of a model system without considering frictional forces. The SHM oscillations continue undiminished for ever in such a model; the energy imparted to the system at the outset remains within the system. This is evidently quite unrealistic, since in reality we observe a progressive diminution in the amplitude of the excursion of the mass. If we suspended the mass–spring system in oil rather than air, we would expect the oscillations to be more sluggish (longer period of cycle) and to die away quickly (rapid diminution in amplitude.) We need to incorporate a frictional element into the model to account for this energy dissipation. The dissipation of energy from oscillating systems is damping.

Modelling damped oscillations

Energy is dissipated in real systems by frictional forces both within the materials and by resistance of the medium in which they move. The energy is released as heat. Frictional forces are generally proportional to the velocity of the moving parts with respect to the medium and act to oppose the direction of motion. We can quite easily adapt our simple mass–spring model to include a velocity-dependent frictional element called a dashpot.

By Newton's Second Law, the equation of motion of the system is now

$$mx''(t) = -kx(t) - rx'(t)$$

This can be rearranged into the form

- Elastic force due to spring, proportional to *position* $x(t)$.
- Resistive force due to dashpot, proportional to velocity $x'(t)$.

$$x''(t) + \frac{r}{m}x'(t) + \frac{k}{m}x(t) = 0$$

This looks a little unfriendly, but we can make educated guesses about the form of the solution. If $r = 0$, we recover the SHM equation and the solution is a pure sinusoid. If r is large, energy dissipation will be rapid; the period of oscillation will be prolonged and the amplitude will diminish quickly. But the energy to be dissipated will depend upon both the mass and the stiffness of the spring. We expect the ratio of r to k and m to play a role.

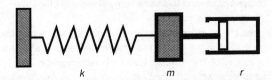

k m r

The dashpot is a component with a piston-like device within a cylinder. The piston moves within a fluid, the viscous characteristics of which determine the magnitude of the resistive force for any velocity. The frictional element is quantified by a dashpot constant r (for resistance).

The force now acting on the mass is the sum of:
- an elastic force due to the spring dependent upon position $-kx(t)$, and
- a resistive force dependent upon velocity $-rx'(t)$

Both forces oppose the motion of the mass and thus have negative sign.

This equation may be compared to that arising from the two-compartment pharmacokinetic model (1.13.4). The damped oscillation model has been constructed by an arrangement of three ideal elements—a mass element, an elastic element, and a resistive one. The premises upon which it has been made are very different from that of the pharmacokinetic model, but the equation to be solved looks very similar. But surely the solution function seems unlikely to be similar too? The answer is 'yes and no', as we shall see. Below the surface of the problem, there are similarities in that both systems have a resting state to which they 'wish' to return after a perturbation; for the oscillating system it is a state of rest with the mass motionless at $x = 0$; for the pharmacokinetic system after bolus dosing it is the complete elimination of drug from the system. Both are dynamic systems and under certain circumstances actually do behave very similarly.

1.17.2   The damping factor

Standardizing the damping

We developed a rather fearsome looking equation for our damped oscillation model:

$$x''(t) + \frac{r}{m}x'(t) + \frac{k}{m}x(t) = 0$$

This is another second-order equation. The details of how it is solved do not matter to us, but the solution function does. In fact, there are various solution functions depending upon the values r, k, and m.

We recognize the coefficient of $x(t)$, $k/m = \omega^2$, where ω is the natural angular velocity of the undamped oscillation. We shall call this natural velocity of oscillation ω_0, since we need to consider what happens to ω under various conditions of damping. We can quantify the effect of damping upon the system by a damping factor. We will omit details of derivation, but we need to introduce a term $\beta = r/2m$, which represents the balance between the magnitude of the mass and the resistive effect of the dashpot. The equation has now become

$$x''(t) + 2\beta x'(t) + \omega_0^2\, x(t) = 0$$

We describe a damping factor

$$\alpha = \frac{\beta}{\omega_0} = \frac{r}{2\sqrt{km}}.$$

$$\omega_0 = \sqrt{\frac{k}{m}}.$$

$$\beta = \frac{r}{2m},$$

This is not to be memorized, but we note that α is large for large values of r and becomes smaller for larger values of k and m. This is generally in accordance with our expectation—we expect a large resistive element to damp oscillations effectively, but for any given value of r, a stiffer spring and larger mass will be able to 'overpower' the resistive effect of the dashpot to a greater extent. Note that the creation of a damping factor is another example of standardization—we lump the defining factors of the model, r, k, and m, together to define a parameter to describe the particular system and to enable comparison with other systems with different values of r, k, and m.

We now have reorganized the equation enough to describe the various possible forms of behaviour of the system in the face of the different values of r, k, and m.

What do the solutions look like? The damping factor α is determined by the ratio β/ω_0. There are four different solution functions, two of which are very familiar:

- When $\beta = 0$, the damping factor $\alpha = 0$ also. The equation reduces to the ideal, undamped system of (1.16.4). and the solution is that of simple harmonic motion:

$$x(t) = A\cos \omega_0 t + B \sin \omega_0 t$$

where $\omega_0 = \sqrt{k/m}$ as before. The system oscillates at its natural frequency ω_0.

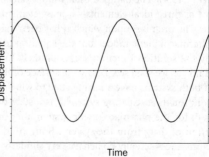

- In the case in which $\beta > \omega_0$, i.e. when $\alpha > 1$. The solution function is

  $x(t) = A \exp(-\phi t) + B \exp(-\gamma t)$

This solution is the familiar bi-exponential equation of the two-compartment pharmacokinetic model. The system is said to be overdamped, since the increase in the damping factor has removed any oscillation from the system—although there may be an initial overshoot of the starting value (dotted curve), the curve never crosses the horizontal axis. The rate constants are determined by a relation involving β and ω_0:

$$\phi = \beta + \sqrt{\beta^2 - \omega_0^2}, \qquad \gamma = \beta - \sqrt{\beta^2 - \omega_0^2}$$

We expect large values for the rate constants ϕ and γ—causing rapid diminution in the value of the function—when damping is high, i.e. when $\beta \gg \omega_0$ (2.9.8). This is all that we need note about these expressions.

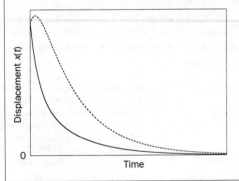

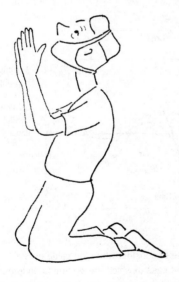

1.17.3   Intermediate damping solution functions

Partial and critical damping

We have described the solution functions for extreme values of α. The undamped case ($\alpha = 0$), and the overdamped ($\alpha > 1$). What about intermediate values of α?

- When $0 < \beta < \omega_0$, the damping factor $\alpha < 1$, the solution function is given by a rather complicated looking equation:

$$x(t) = [A \cos \Omega t + B \sin \Omega t]. \exp \{-\beta t\}$$

where $\Omega = \sqrt{\omega_0^2 - \beta^2}$. Although this looks daunting, we see that it is the product of an SHM sinusoid (inside the square brackets) and a negative exponential function. Let us look first at the sinusoid. A and B are the usual arbitrary constants that describe the initial conditions, but the natural angular velocity ω_0 of the system has been modified by the damping. Ω is always less than ω_0 if $\beta > 0$, i.e. if there is any damping at all. This means that the frequency of oscillation is diminished by the damping force; and, the larger the value of β the more pronounced is this effect. This is what we expect to happen.

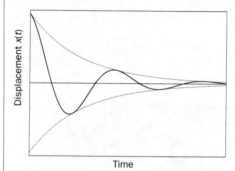

The effect of the exponential term is to cause the amplitude of the oscillations to die away with a rate constant β. The peak amplitudes of successive oscillations are points on an exponential decay curve, so that the sinusoid is contained within an exponential decay 'envelope'. Larger values of β cause a more rapid decay.

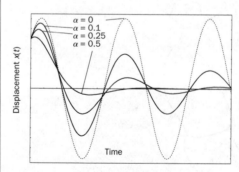

$\alpha = 0$
$\alpha = 0.1$
$\alpha = 0.25$
$\alpha = 0.5$

The effect of various levels of damping. Note that as the value of α increases, the decay of the oscillation is more rapid and the oscillation is slowed in accordance with our expectations.

- **Critical damping**

There is one last case to consider when the value of $\alpha = 1$. This represents the transition between the case in which the system is underdamped and when it is overdamped. This is critical damping, and is the minimum value of the damping factor that just prevents the decaying oscillation from crossing the horizontal axis, although there may still be an overshoot of the starting value.

When $\beta = \omega_0$, the damping factor $\alpha = 1$, the solution function is

$$x(t) = (At + B) \exp \{-\beta t\}$$

This is the product of a linear function and an exponential function. We see that the sinusoidal term has disappeared which means that the oscillatory behaviour of the system has been abolished by the damping.

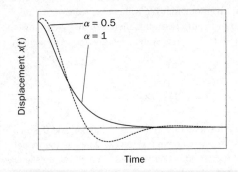

The underdamped system with $\alpha = 0.5$ still oscillates about the horizontal axis. The critically damped curve with $\alpha = 1$ subsides to the axis without crossing it. This is the minimum value of α that will abolish all oscillatory behaviour. Higher values of α cause decay with a bi-exponential curve, as we have seen.

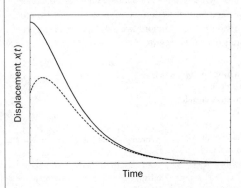

The condition of critical damping—or indeed over-damping—does not necessarily prevent an overshoot of the initial value but does abolish any oscillation. The presence or absence of an overshoot depends upon the initial conditions. These are both critically damped systems with different initial conditions only.

1.18.1   **Invasive blood pressure measurement**

We have spent some time modelling naturally oscillating systems, and we have seen how they respond to a displacement from their equilibrium position in the face of various levels of damping. We now need to look at how such systems respond to an applied vibration from outside. We will concentrate on the implications for invasive blood pressure measurement, but there are many circumstances in which we apply an oscillating force to a real system—high-frequency ventilation is another example.

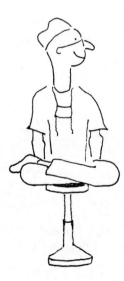

Forced vibrations

We need a model to incorporate the effects of a forcing oscillation and this is a simple extension of what we have already done for free oscillations. The model contains all of the elements of the previous one; a mass element, an elastic element, and a resistive one. We just add a forcing sinusoidal oscillation to cause the system to vibrate. A pressure transducer system can be considered to comprise these three elements and the applied pressure wave is the forcing oscillation. We wish to predict the behaviour of the system in the face of this forcing wave.

The motion of this plate is described by the output function and is the solution of the modelling equation $x(t)$. This is what is converted to an electronic signal in the transducer and displayed on the monitoring screen. This output function is still a sinusoidal one, but in principle will differ in both amplitude and phase from the input function. This leads to distortion: the output wave differs from the input wave.

A forcing sinusoidal oscillation ($F = A \cos \Omega t + B \sin \Omega t$) is applied to a plate connected to the mass, elastic, and resistive elements. The solution of the modelling equation describes the motion of the plate incorporating the mass element. The forcing oscillation is modified as it transmits through the system and we want our model to describe the output function. We may then compare the input function and output function.

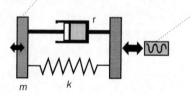

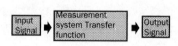

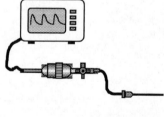

In order to be able to interpret the output, we need to understand how the input function (the blood pressure waveform—what we want to know) relates to the output function (what we see on the screen—what we do know).

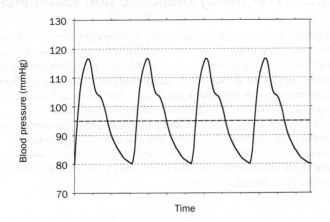

An arterial blood pressure wave is far more complex than a simple sinusoidal wave of the form $A \cos \Omega t + B \sin \Omega t$. We shall tackle this question too.

Forced oscillation modelling equation

The modelling equation has now become

$$x''(t) + 2\beta x'(t) + \omega_0^2 x(t) = F(t)$$
$$= A \cos \Omega t + B \sin \Omega t.$$

We have added a term $F(t) = A \cos \Omega t + B \sin \Omega t$ to represent the forcing sinusoid, which our system must now 'obey'. We are still interested to know what $x(t)$ is, since this is how the motion of the system is described. The method of solution is not explained here, but the solution itself and its implications are described.

Real pressure measurement systems have components which we can 'lump together' into the elements we have described—more modelling simplification. The mass of saline in the lines connecting artery to transducer is the main mass element and movement of this saline within the line is the chief contributor to the resistance element. The pressure sensitive diaphragm within the transducer is the main elastic component. We abstract the geometric and physical complexity of these real components into our idealized mass, resistance, and elastic elements.

1.18.2 **Frequency response and resonance**

The relationship of the input function—the forcing oscillation—to the output function is very important. Ideally, we should like the input wave to be exactly reproduced by the output waveform. In order for us to use our measuring systems intelligently, we must understand how the input signal is modified by the system, so that we can interpret the output signal and know how much reliance we can place upon it. We have so far only modelled the forcing oscillation as a simple sinusoidal function. Physiological waveforms are much more complex, and we will consider the modelling of these complex waves shortly. The input sinusoidal function is modified by the system so that the output function is still a sinusoid, but is in general different in both amplitude and phase from the input function. We will consider amplitude and phase separately.

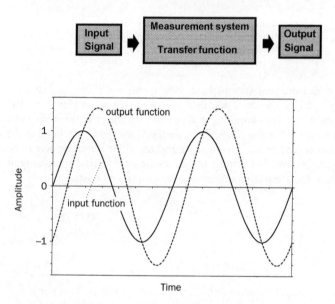

The output function differs from the input function in both amplitude—it is larger—and phase—the peaks of the input and output functions do not coincide. This means that what we see coming out is a *distortion* of what is going in. Relative amplitude is the ratio of output amplitude to input amplitude. If it is greater than unity there is amplification of the input.

Damping and relative frequency: ideal transfer function

The response of the damped mass–spring system to a forcing oscillation depends upon the natural oscillating frequency of the system, ω_0, and the frequency of the forcing function, Ω. We shall see that this relationship is critical in determining distortion by measuring systems of the input wave form in complex waves. We can standardize the input frequency as a fraction of the natural frequency of the mass–spring system as the relative frequency $\bar{\Omega} = \Omega/\omega_0$.

We expect that the degree of damping will also have effects upon the system response. In the face of high degrees of damping, we expect the output amplitude to be smaller than if damping is less. If damping is low and the forcing oscillation $\bar{\Omega}$ is close to the natural frequency , ω_0, i.e. $\bar{\Omega} \approx 1$, then the amplitude of the output is large compared to the input amplitude—there is amplification; relative amplitude >1. We can imagine the applied oscillation moving in synchrony with the natural oscillation of the system and reinforcing each swing to produce a large increase in amplitude. At forcing frequencies well away from the natural frequency, the system will wish to oscillate at a different rate and will 'co-operate' less. This phenomenon of increased amplitude when the applied wave is close to the natural frequency is *resonance*, and can be useful (tuning a radio receiver to a particular wavelength) or destructive (shattering of a wine glass by the cartoon opera singer). Resonance is a dramatic increase in output amplitude when the natural frequency of the system is approximated by the forcing function.

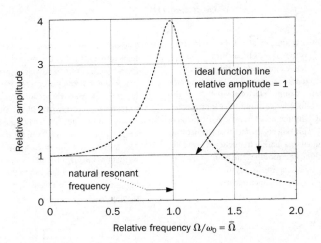

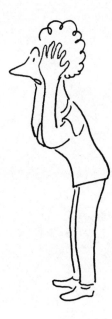

Relative amplitude increases greatly as the forcing frequency approaches the natural frequency. At higher forcing frequency, output amplitude diminishes until it falls below the input amplitude (relative amplitude < 1).

1.18.3 **Frequency response: amplification and phase shift**

Relative amplitude function

The solution equations look increasingly unpleasant, as the complexity of the model has increased. The output amplitude is a function of the system characteristics k and m—which determine ω_0—the damping factor α (dependent upon r), and the forcing amplitude and frequency Ω. This is for reference only:

relative amplitude =

$$\frac{1}{\sqrt{\{(1 - \overline{\Omega}^2)^2 + (2\alpha\overline{\Omega})^2\}}}.$$

Frequency response: amplitude

The relative amplitude—the ratio of the output wave amplitude and the input amplitude—should ideally be unity for a measuring system. This should be true for the whole range of frequencies of interest to us.

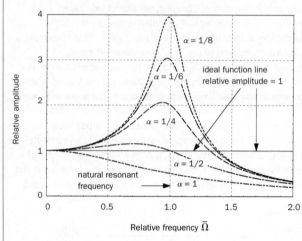

An ideal frequency response would lie along the line of relative amplitude = 1 for all frequencies. The output amplitude would always equal the input amplitude.

At a relative frequency $\overline{\Omega} = 1$ the forcing frequency Ω is the same as the natural frequency ω_0. The relative amplitude of the output is increased markedly around this value, especially when the damping factor is small. Note also that the peak relative amplitudes for higher levels of damping occur at relative frequencies below 1. This reflects the fact that the natural (undamped) oscillating frequency is lowered by damping and modifies the point at which the forcing oscillation and system are 'matched' and resonance occurs.

The aim of design of transducer systems is to ensure that the natural frequency ω_0 lies sufficiently far above the maximum frequency of interest in the input waveform so that relative amplitude stays acceptably near unity. The relative amplitude stays fairly close to unity (within about 1% even for $\alpha = 1/8$) for relative frequencies below 0.1, so that the resonant frequency needs to be about ten times higher than the highest frequency that we wish to display.

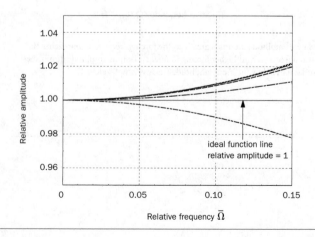

Frequency response: phase differences

Differences in amplitude are not the only source of distortion. Phase differences—the lagging of output wave behind input—may lead to infidelity of the output waveform. These are also dependent upon the relative frequency and damping. If all frequencies were treated equally, the phase difference would be of little consequence, since all frequencies would be shifted by the same amount.

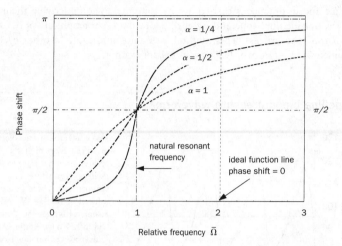

As we approach the resonant frequency of the system, $\overline{\Omega} \approx 1$, the phase difference approaches $\pi/2$ for all levels of damping. Higher input frequencies induce greater phase shifts.

Relative amplitude criteria lead us to design systems in which we keep relative frequencies below 0.1. Phase differences are greater for larger damping factors within this region.

Phase difference function

The frequency response for phase difference is given by

$$\text{phase difference} = \arctan\frac{2\alpha\overline{\Omega}}{(1 - \overline{\Omega}^2)}.$$

As the graph shows, this is a function of relative frequency and damping factor. Arctan is just the inverse function of the tangent of an angle ($\tan \phi = \sin \phi/\cos \phi$). It answers the question 'What angle ϕ has the tangent the value of which is z?'

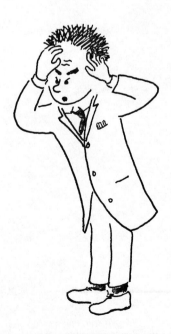

1.19.1   **Fourier analysis**

We have seen how a simple sinusoidal waveform arises from the modelling of a mass–spring system. Although this is cyclical, it does not otherwise much resemble the typical blood pressure waveform that we wish now to model. It is possible by the use of the technique of Fourier analysis to reproduce *any* repetitive waveform by a process of adding simple sinusoidal functions, and we shall use this technique to produce a replica of a typical arterial pressure wave. This process is simple in principle and in practice is carried out by computer. The underlying theory is, however, outside our scope and we shall adopt the usual graphical approach to demonstrate the process. This method is equally applicable to other cyclical phenomena—respiratory or ICP waveforms, for example.

Modelling blood pressure waveforms

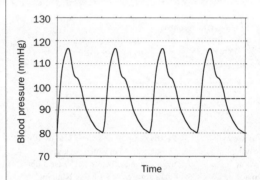

This is a typical arterial blood pressure waveform. It is a cyclical, repetitive wave which oscillates regularly, but not symmetrically, about a mean value of 95 mmHg. We will assume a heart rate of 60/min. Our task is to use simple sinusoidal waves as building blocks to construct a replica of this complicated waveform.

A very simple approach is to ignore the cyclical nature of blood pressure altogether and quote the mean value. Although this may seem ridiculous in our context, it is exactly what we do in clinical practice when we calculate such derived quantities as cerebral perfusion pressures or peripheral resistances.

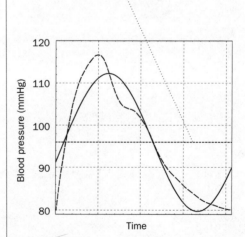

We can make a better approximation by taking a sine wave with the same mean value 95 mmHg and the same period of oscillation—i.e. 1 s—and we superimpose it on the wave that we are trying to replicate. We need to decide how large the amplitude should be and where to site it along the time axis to achieve the best fit.

We have chosen a sinusoidal wave of particular amplitude and phase. The fit is much better than the straight line of the mean value, but it is still not very satisfactory. The sinusoid is an expression of the general form $A \cos \omega t + B \sin \omega t$.

1.19.2   Refining the fit

Improving the model

The simple sinusoidal wave of the same period as the heart rate does not provide a very impressive fit. We can do much better than this. The frequency which is the same as that of the heart rate is called the fundamental frequency. If we now add a second sinusoid to the first, but this time with a frequency double that of the fundamental, we can improve the fit to our arterial waveform.

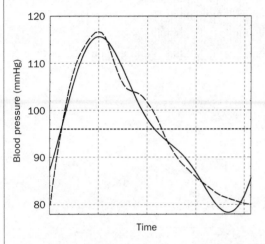

There is considerable improvement in the fit, but still some way to go to produce an acceptable replica of the waveform.

The pressure wave that we are attempting to replicate is the dashed line. We have now added a sinusoid, the frequency of which is double that of the fundamental. This is called a second harmonic. Again we must select an amplitude and a phase shift relative to the first wave. This wave has an equation $C \cos 2\omega t + D \sin 2\omega t$, where the choice of the constants C and D determine the amplitude and phase.

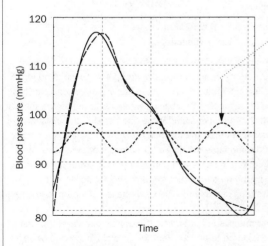

This wave is oscillating at three times the fundamental frequency—it has three cycles within the space of the whole pressure wave. We add this to the previous approximation, and the resulting wave is a better fit to the original. The shoulder of the dicrotic notch is beginning to appear. This new wave which we add has an equation of the form $E \cos 3\omega t + F \sin 3\omega t$. We must determine the correct values for E and F to improve the fit.

Note that the third harmonic starts near a minimum point in its cycle. The choice of values for E and F is sufficient to determine both magnitude and phase (2.10.5).

Digitized waveform

The process of Fourier analysis involves taking a pressure waveform and representing it as a digitized form, i.e. as a list of pressures and the times at which these are measured. These are subjected to a Fourier analysis algorithm by a computer that determines the coefficients *A, B, C, D* ... in the successive harmonics $A \cos \omega t + B \sin \omega t$, $C \cos 2\omega t + D \sin 2\omega t$, and $E \cos 3\omega t + F \sin 3\omega t + ...$ The sampling frequency determines how smooth a 'wave' is analysed. The Fourier-generated replica can never be better than the raw material wave that is trying to reproduce.

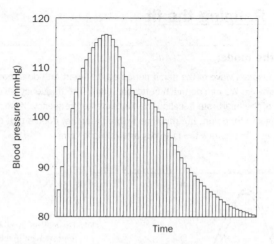

A digitized form of the same pressure waveform. The preservation of detail of the original wave depends upon the sampling frequency.

Fourier and invasive blood pressure measurement

The Fourier process tells us that we can construct any complex repetitive waveform to an arbitrarily close approximation by summing harmonics of the fundamental sinusoidal function. This involves only suitable selection of the coefficients in the expression

$A \cos \omega t + B \sin \omega t + C \cos 2\omega t + D \sin 2\omega t +$
$E \cos 3\omega t + F \sin 3\omega t + G \cos 4\omega t + H \sin 4\omega t...$

Our consideration of frequency response in invasive blood pressure measurement (1.18) shows us how the measurement system responds to variation in the input frequency of a pure forcing sinusoid. We can see now that the complexity of the wavefrom can only be reproduced with fidelity if we are able to record faithfully the higher frequencies which are responsible for the fine detail in the input waveform. The measurement system treats the incoming waveform as if it is a sum of the various harmonics of the fundamental as we have described. We have seen the origins of distortion in that amplitude and phase of the different harmonics will be treated differently by the measurement system. This is, however, predictable and electronic systems can use the theory we have outlined to correct for the predicted distortion.

We find that even five harmonics is not sufficient to mimic our waveform: ten harmonics is generally considered to be sufficient for physiological work. Changes in output amplitude and phase are fairly small for relative frequencies (with respect to the natural frequency of the measurement system) of less than 0.1, so our systems need resonant frequencies of about 100 times larger than the fundamental for good fidelity of output.

1.19.3   Higher harmonics: linear systems and static pressures

Mathematical sculpture

We continue the process of adding more harmonics and come closer to replicating our waveform each time we add a higher harmonic. The process is a 'mathematical sculpture'—we need to use finer and finer tools to reproduce the detail of the original. The higher harmonics are the fine tools. If we are sculpting from a fuzzy photograph, the likeness will not be very good—the digitized input waveform must have a reasonable sampling frequency.

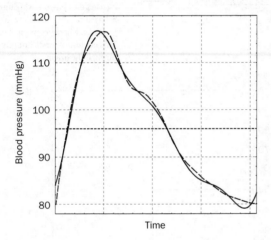

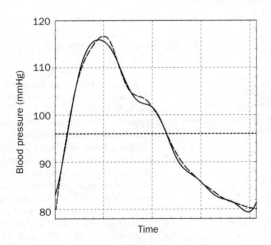

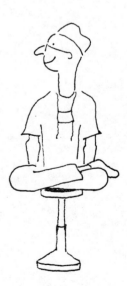

Adding higher harmonics improves the fit further. The result of adding the first five harmonics is quite a creditable replica of the original waveform, although there are still details to be refined. These would be ironed out if we continued in the same fashion for the next few harmonics. Computers are happy to do this for us, but humans get bored so we will move on.

Linear systems and BP measurement

In all of the complexity of Fourier analysis which is concerned with the fidelity of the waveform, we must not forget that the input and output of the system for *static* pressures must also be ensured. This is what we are doing with the calibration procedures. The transducer-display system must behave linearly (2.5) and is designed to do so, so that for any given change in input pressure, the display pressure will change proportionally. We can describe an input–output function for static pressure measurement, and this should be the function $y = x$, i.e. the line of identity.

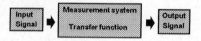

The display pressure for static pressures should be the same as the true input pressure. This means that we must instruct the system—which must behave linearly—to follow the function $y = x$; i.e. what goes in must come out. This is a line of gradient unity passing through the origin.

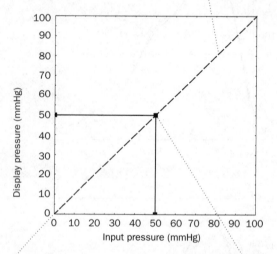

To fix the origin, the transducer is opened to atmosphere—our reference pressure—and the system instructed to call this pressure zero. This is 'zeroing' the system.

If all we do is fix the origin by zeroing, we have not established the necessary gradient of unity. We need a second point: this is usually done by means of a saline column of known height applied to the transducer and the calibration adjusted to ensure that the display reading matches this known pressure. A pressure of 50 mmHg is convenient, as this requires a saline column of 68 cm (13.6×50 mm), which can be applied using an ordinary 100 cm I.V. extension set. This is not a perfect solution since it involves an *extrapolation* to measure arterial pressures—i.e. outside the range of calibration. A better solution is to arrange a mercury column as reference. Measured values are then interpolated within the calibrated range; saline columns with say 250 mmHg to calibrate to arterial pressures would need a hole in the ceiling.

Part 2 **Mathematical background**

2.1.1 Numbers

This part on mathematical background should be viewed as a toolbox, from which the necessary implements are picked for a particular purpose; it is not meant to be read through from start to finish. There are certain patterns of relationship which occur frequently in modelling applications and we need a general familiarity with their behaviour. The emphasis is graphical and pictorial and relies heavily on the notion of the transformation which allows us to modify a basic pattern function to produce another related function. We also find composite functions arising by combining these basic pattern functions; for instance, a damped oscillation is a product of a sinusoid and an exponential function (1.17). This part is placed between those devoted to physiological and statistical modelling to emphasize the centrality of these patterns to solving problems in both of these areas. We open this part of the volume with a very brief consideration of numbers and notation. The classification of numbers need not detain us for too long, but we do need to define one or two classes before we can proceed.

The number line

The integers include the *natural* numbers—the ordinary counting numbers 1, 2, 3, 4, …—as well as zero and the negative integers 0, –1, –2, … An integer is a whole number. The integers can be displayed along a line in order of their magnitude—this device is the real number line. This forms the familiar picture of an axis of a graph.

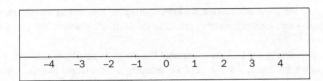

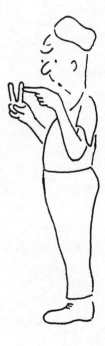

The spaces between the integers are occupied by the *real numbers*, which include the *rational numbers* that can be expressed as a ratio of integers (e.g. 3/29, 1/7, or 276/333) and the *irrational numbers*—such as π and e—which cannot be expressed exactly as a ratio of integers. All of these together (integers, rationals, and irrationals) form the real number system. There are extensions to this—for instance, the complex numbers which occur in more advanced applications—but we shall not need these.

We will also need the concept of an *interval*, which is a section of the real number line within which we may need to consider the behaviour or existence of a function. Why we look at particular intervals will usually be clear in the individual case. For instance, the concept of probability is only defined for the interval [0,1]. It may take any value within this interval, but a probability of –6 or 2.3 is nonsensical (3.8.1).

2.1.2   Notation

A good choice of notation can be an important aid to understanding; a poor choice can make even a simple subject seem incomprehensible. The notation and grammar of mathematics are closely bound together, and here we explore a few of the basic facts.

Mathematical notation

Mathematics is a language, and there are analogies with ordinary language which can help us understand what is going on. Notations are concerned with mathematical objects and operations carried out upon those objects. We will demonstrate this with a statistical example. Suppose that we have a set of nine data listed in order of size—in other words, in order of their position on the number line:

[1, 2, 2, 3, 3, 4, 5, 8, 8].

We might wish to refer to similar sets of data and identify individual members of the set. We can refer to any general member of the list x_i, so that in the above list

$x_1 = 1$, $x_2 = 2$, $x_3 = 2$, ..., $x_9 = 8$.

The x here refers to an *object*—a member of the list. Members of another data set might be identified by y to distinguish which set they belong to. Objects are the equivalent of nouns.

The subscript is essentially a description of *which* exact object we are referring to and performs the same function as an adjective in ordinary language: Which car? The *blue* one.

Operators are the mathematical equivalent of verbs: they tell us what to do to the objects—add, multiply, square, calculate the factorial, differentiate, integrate, and so on.

The expression $x_9 - \bar{x}$ tells us to subtract the mean of the above data set, $\bar{x} = 4$, from $x_9 = 8$ so that $x_9 - \bar{x} = 4$. $(x_9 - \bar{x})^2$ instructs us to multiply the result of this procedure by itself.

The summation notation, which is an instruction to add repeatedly in a specified manner, is a very important modifier; the operation of addition is the primary process, but the summation sign Σ tells us to do it repeatedly:

$$\sum_{i=1}^{i=9}(x_i - \bar{x})^2$$

tells us to take each member of the data set in turn (x_1, x_2, ..., x_9,) subtract the mean of the data set from it, square the result, and then add all of these squared values together. Note that the operation inside the bracket must be carried out first, followed by the squaring and *then* the summation. The order in which operations are carried out is often critical.

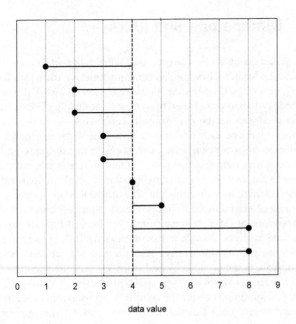

data value

The data points are shown along the number line. The vertical spread has no significance beyond separating the multiple points.

The distance from each point to $x = 4$ is calculated. This is the deviation from the mean ($x - \bar{x}$, which may be positive or negative. This deviation is squared: $(x_i - \bar{x})^2$. Each of these squares is summed for the whole data set:

$$\sum_{i=1}^{i=9}(x_i - \bar{x})^2$$ This example is studied in (3.10).

Further points of notation

$y > x$	y is greater than x
$y < x$	y is less than x
$y \geq x$	y is greater than or equal to x
$y \leq x$	y is less than or equal to x
$y \approx x$	y is approximately equal to x
$y \equiv x$	y is equivalent to x

$x! = x$-factorial $= x \times (x - 1) \times (x - 2) \times (x - 3) \ldots 3 \times 2 \times 1$

$|x|$ = the magnitude of x ie ignoring sign $x = 35$ and $x = -35$ have the same magnitude.

$x \sim N(0,1) = x$ follows a normal (N) distribution with mean $\mu = 0$ and variance $\sigma^2 = 1$.

$\exp(x) = e^x$. This enables complicated exponents to be made more legible.

Standard notations are established in many areas—respiratory physiology is an example. It aids understanding if the notation reflects the underlying concepts closely—it is easier if V is a volume and P a pressure. F represents a fraction, but is then unavailable for flow; since flow is a mass (Quantity transfer) in unit time, $\dot{Q}$ is a reasonable symbol. A dot above a quantity denotes the rate of that quantity in unit time. Thus $\dot{V}\text{CO}_2$ is the (volume) rate of production of CO_2 in unit time.

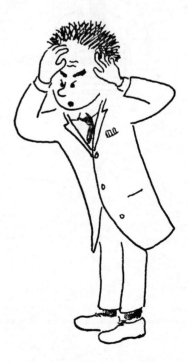

2.1.3   Dimensions and units

We define physical quantities by reference to certain fundamental quantities which cannot be reduced further. These fundamental quantities are mass [M], length [L] and time [T], as well as temperature [θ] and electrical charge [C]. A system of units, e.g. the SI system, is constructed from these basic building blocks. Any equations that we produce must be dimensionally consistent—the same dimensional quantities must appear on each side of the equation. In order to produce sensible numerical answers from our equations, we must ensure that the units used are also consistent throughout, but the actual system of units is largely arbitrary and is not fundamental. In the early stages of contemplating a problem, consideration of units can even interfere with clear thought. The idea of flux, for instance, is essentially one of rate of *mass* transfer from one region to another and must therefore have the dimensions of $[M][T]^{-1}$—mass/time. The *units* of flow are expressed as volume/time and might be thought to have dimensions $[L]^3[T]^{-1}$, but the essence of flow is not a transfer of volume but of mass; the mass of a substance is related to the volume of space that it occupies by its density. We may often describe the mass of a substance in terms of a volume—e.g. a CO_2 production, a $\dot{V}CO_2$ of 0.2 l/min—but this makes assumptions about the conditions in which this volume is measured. We need to keep these assumptions in mind, and if we get into difficulties, we need to refer back to the dimensions of the quantities involved.

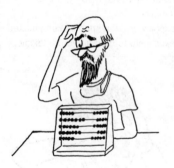

Rules for dimensions

1. Only quantities with the same dimensions may be added or subtracted. The resulting sum or difference has the same dimensions.
2. Equated quantities must have the same dimensions.
3. Quantities may be multiplied or divided regardless of dimensions.
4. Dimension is independent of magnitude. Units are the scaling factor to define magnitude.
5. Scaling by a dimensionless quantity ie a ratio or number leaves the dimensions unchanged.

Quantity	Dimensions	SI unit
Mass	[M]	kilogram
Length	[L]	metre
Time	[T]	second
Temperature	[θ]	degree K
Area	$[L]^2$	metres^2
Volume	$[L]^3$	litre
Velocity	$[L][T]^{-1}$	metres.sec^{-1}
Acceleration	$[L][T]^{-2}$	metres.sec^{-2}
Flux	$[M][T]^{-1}$	kilogram.sec^{-1}
Density	$[M][L]^{-3}$	kilogram.li^{-1}

2.2.1 What is a function?

Input, process and output

We use the idea of a function throughout this book, but what do we mean by a 'function'? We will treat a function as a *rule* that transforms one set of real numbers to another set of real numbers. The function is a process; we feed in a value at one end and the function rule generates an output value at the other end. We may need to be rather particular about defining the range of values that we may input into the function; for instance, the function $f(x) = 1/(x)$ is undefined at $x = 0$, and we must restrict the input range when defining the function to exclude $x = 0$, since it is impossible to divide by zero.

An important requirement for a function is that there must only be *one possible output* for any given input. The operation of taking the square root might be thought to be a function rule in its own right, but this is not so. The square root operation is only permissible with *positive* numbers, so the input range is restricted to $x \geq 0$. But if we take the square root of 9, there are two possible solutions: $y = 3$ and $y = -3$. A function must give a *unique* output, so for this example we need to specify that the function returns the positive root only *or* the negative root, but not both.

The function is a rule that processes real numbers from a defined range—the domain—and produces an output—the range, or co-domain. The output range may be restricted in the same way as the domain.

The function is frequently display graphically and we shall see plenty of examples of this. The input values are conventionally displayed along the horizontal axis. This is the independent variable. When the general aspects of functions are considered, this will usually be denoted the 'x' variable. We are often concerned with functions of time, with t as the input variable.

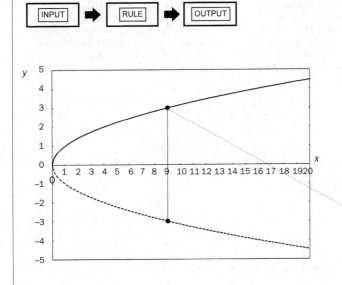

The output value is plotted on the vertical axis and is described as the dependent variable. We change the value of the input variable (independent variable) and the rule generates the value of the dependent variable. We vary the input and the rule determines the output, so that the dependent variable is *dependent* upon the rule and the input value. The dependent variable is often denoted by y.

The graph of $y = \sqrt{x}$ exists only for values $x \geq 0$. For any value of x, we obtain two possible values for y. This is *not* the graph of a function that must give a unique output. If we took the top half or the bottom half of the graph we would obtain a unique output, and we would have the graph of a function.

Points in the plane are defined by co-ordinates (x, y); e.g. this point has co-ordinates $(9,3)$. The first value is the position on the x-axis, and the second the position on the y-axis.

Distinctions between dependent and independent variables may depend upon the way in which we are looking at a problem. The dependence of $PaCO_2$ upon $\dot{V}A$ in the paralysed, ventilated patient has been examined in (1.3). However, if we consider the intact respiratory centre response to a rise in $PaCO_2$ effected by breathing CO_2 containing gas, this causes a reflex increase in $\dot{V}A$, so that $PaCO_2$ is now the independent variable and $\dot{V}A$ the dependent variable. Time is always an independent variable.

In statistical models, e.g. linear regression (3.18), the independent (input) variable may be called the *explanatory variable*, and the output variable the *response variable*. This is merely convention.

2.2.2 **Discrete and continuous**

Notation for functions:

There are two notational conventions for functions which we will encounter. Usually, we shall simply refer to the rule for a particular function as, for instance, $y = x^2 - 3$. However, there is often a need to talk about any *general* function of x without specifying the particular rule. This is described as $y = f(x)$ or $y = g(x)$ say, which allows us to talk about different functions of x in general terms. This notation is also used in a different sense, where $f(x)$ can mean the actual *value of the function* for the particular input x. We need this convention when discussing calculus (2.12). The distinction will usually be clear.

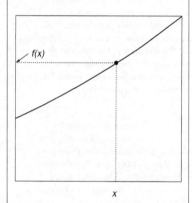

We are often interested in the gradient of a function at any point. The derivative of a function (the rate of change or gradient of the function) with these notations are described thus

$$\frac{dy}{dx} = f'(x) \text{ for the first}$$

derivative and

$$\frac{d^2y}{dx^2} = f''(x) \text{ for the}$$

second derivative (the rate of change of the rate of change) (2.12).

Steps and corners

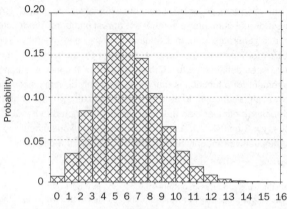

Graphs of functions do not have to be smooth curves. Probability distributions are functions. The Poisson distribution (3.2.2) $\mu = 5$ has an input range that is restricted to the non-negative integers 0, 1, 2, … (no negative or fractional events). The graph of this function has steps. It is discrete.

The output range is also restricted, since all probability values must lie in the interval [0,1]. The rule for the Poisson distribution takes the integer values 0, 1, 2, … and produces an output within the range [0,1] for each, which is the probability of that number of events in a Poisson process of $\mu = 5$.

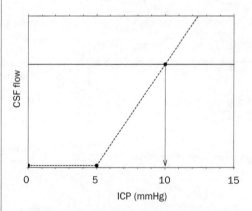

The function that we need to describe the uptake of CSF (1.2.2) is in two parts—the uptake below the threshold value is modelled as zero and above this level is linear. This means that two different rules are operating in different parts of the input range. As long as we define what they are, and there is only one output, we still have a respectable function. We have not so far specified what happens further up the ICP range—this function does not account for the reduction in CSF production when ICP reaches very high levels. We have restricted the function input range to an interval in which we expect this model to be a fair representation of reality. We have constructed for the CSF example a function out of bits of two pattern functions—the constant and the linear functions. (2.4), (2.5), This uptake function has a corner but is still continuous since there is a defined output value for all values along the ICP axis.

2.3.1 **Scaling**

We shall look at the properties of a number of important classes of function which are useful in modelling. In each case we shall emphasize that there is a 'basic pattern' function, which we may transform to other related functions by means of simple manoueuvres. These transformations will be demonstrated in general here graphically. This approach is intended to give a feel for how the mathematical solution to problems is found, rather than to give the ability actually to manipulate the functions.

Transformations in the plane: scaling

We shall look at some simple transformations in the plane—the usual two-dimensional axis system of graphs of functions of a single variable. To explore the general process, we examine transformations of a geometric figure—a square. We start by examining changing the size and shape by stretching.

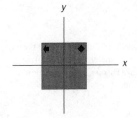

We take as a starting point the unit square sitting with its centre at the origin. A diamond in one corner and an arrow at another enable us to keep track of what has moved where.

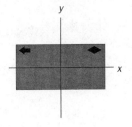

The square has been stretched along the direction of the x-axis. This distorts the shape into a rectangle. This is a *scaling* in the x-direction because we have effectively altered the scale along the horizontal axis. The y-direction is untransformed. We might equally compress the square in the x-direction.

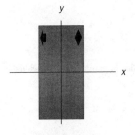

This is a scaling in the y-direction only, elongating the vertical scale but leaving the x-direction untransformed.

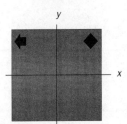

This is a symmetrical scaling in both the x- and y-directions simultaneously which leaves us with a larger square—the scale is different but the shape is unaltered. Note that in all of these transformations the position of the centre of the rectangle has not moved—it always sits symmetrically at the origin.

We shall use the term 'scaling' frequently for the process of stretching or squeezing a figure or graph. This is an example of a transformation in the plane (of the graph). It is termed a scaling because it is essentially a process of assigning a scale to the axes.

2.3.2 **Translation and rotation**

Translations

The next operation to consider is that of *translation*—moving the square to another position in the plane. The translation can be carried out in one direction or two. The translation might involve, say, moving one unit in the positive *x*-direction and one unit in the *y*-direction.

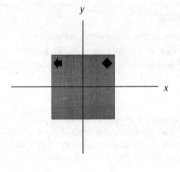

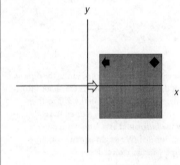

The square has been shifted bodily to the right. It has not experienced any deformation or scaling. This is a pure translation in the *x*-direction.

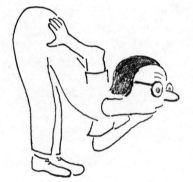

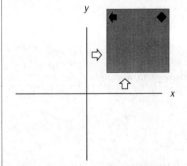

The square has been further translated in the *y*-direction.

Rotations

The next operation to consider is that of *rotation*—we pivot the square about the origin so that the figure occupies the same outline as before, but the relationship of the diamond and arrow to the axes has changed. We shall not need this transformation in our models, but the general consideration of transformations requires some mention of rotation.

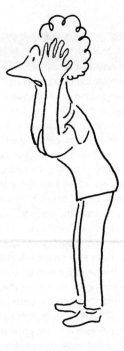

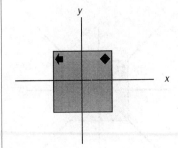

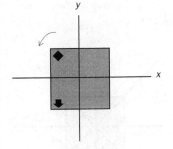

The square has been rotated about the origin three times through right-angles anti-clockwise. The rotation can be through any angle we choose, but if we rotate through a full circle we arrive back where we started—the identity transformation.

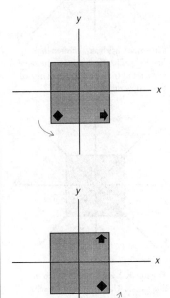

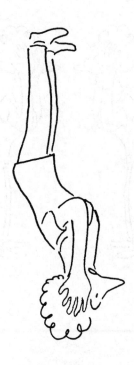

2.3.3 **Reflections and composition**

Transformations and functions

This simple idea of *operations* that we have performed on a square will be used to transform one *function* into another. It is apparent that we may perform combination operations by first performing a reflection (say) followed by a rotation. There are different ways in which we can obtain the same overall effect; for instance, reflection about the *x*-axis followed by a right-angle anti-clockwise rotation (composition of operations) gives the same result as a simple reflection in *y* = *x*. The *order* in which we perform these composite operations may be important. Changing the order of the composition of the reflection and the rotation gives a different position of diamond and arrow. The study of such operations and symmetries is the subject matter of group theory and abstract algebra.

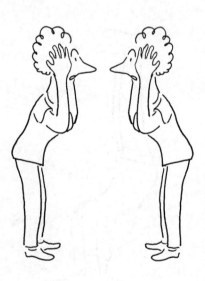

Reflections

The reflection of a graph or figure about a line in the plane is a simple idea which has important consequences. We shall be particularly interested in reflections about the axes and the line *y* = *x*.

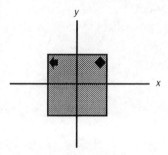

The square is in standard position.

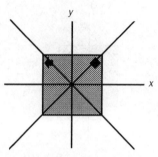

The square is in standard position and we have drawn lines for *y* = *x* and *y* = −*x*.

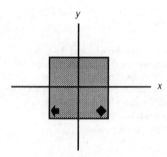

The square has been reflected in the line *y* = 0—the *x*-axis.

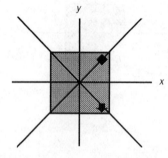

The square has been reflected in the line *y* = *x*. The diamond is in the same corner, but the arrow has been moved to the opposite corner.

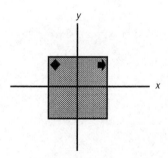

The square has been reflected in the line *x* = 0—the *y*-axis.

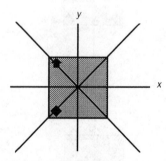

The square has been reflected in the line *y* = −*x*. The arrow is in the same corner, but this time the diamond been moved to the opposite corner.

2.4.1   Constants, parameters, and variables

The constant function

The simplest function that we can consider is the constant function. In fact, it is such a simple function that we might need convincing that it is a function at all. The example of CSF flow and ICP provides a good example.

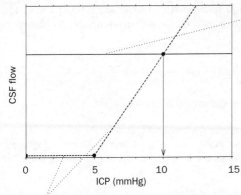

This is the graph of a function—whatever ICP we choose, the graph gives a (constant) unique value for the CSF production. The reality of control of CSF flow will, of course, be more complex. The rule for a constant function is $f(x) = a$, where a is the constant. We ask what the CSF production is for any value of ICP within the range and we always get the same answer—the constant, a.

A function may have different rules for different parts of its input. The CSF uptake is modelled as constant for part of its input and by a linear function for the rest. CSF uptake is a variable.

We shall see plenty of examples of the use of constants. Often, these will be constant functions of *time*. By definition modelling of steady states produces constant functions with respect to time. Other quantities are constant only under specified conditions: we know that SVP of an anaesthetic agent is dependent upon temperature, but if we control this variable, the SVP is a constant. There are other quantities such as R, the universal gas constant, or π or e, which are absolute constants that never vary under any circumstances.

We acknowledge others, such as the CO_2 production, $\dot{V}CO_2$, to be variables, but in order to model a system simply and gain understanding—particularly at the start of the modelling process—we may choose to treat them as constants.

We also need the concept of a *parameter*, which we shall use extensively; a parameter is a quantity which may in principle be varied but is held fixed for any particular set of calculation or runs of a model. The probability distributions form families of functions. There is a general rule that defines the function, but we need to specify one or more parameters to define which member of the family we are concerned with. For the Poisson distribution, the single parameter required is the mean of the distribution, μ. Substitution of this into the Poisson formula is sufficient to generate the whole distribution. The normal distribution needs two parameters to be specified—the mean and the variance—and these then define the particular normal distribution. The models for the distributions are general and 'picked off the shelf', the right parameters are inserted, and the requisite model for the problem in hand is produced. In modelling Poisson processes, for example, we assume a constant *mean* rate (i.e. unchanging with respect to time) for the random process, which, in turn, defines the parameter of the particular Poisson distribution that we use in the model (3.2).

2.5.1 **Straight-line relationships**

Linear functions are extremely familiar and are easy to handle; they are the mathematics of tea-making—'one spoon per person and one for the pot'. Linear functions are the simplest non-constant functions and are often used as a 'default' even when a more complex relationship is suspected, as we did in the air embolism modelling example (1.12). They are so easily manipulated that it is often worthwhile to search for a transformation that will convert non-linear relationships to linear ones. This is what we did with the Hill (1.14.4) and Schild plots, (1.15.3) and in estimating rate constants in exponential processes using log transformations (2.9.10).

Linear functions

The general formula for a linear relationship is

$y = a + bx.$

We will take our 'basic' function as $y = x$, where $b = 1$ and $a = 0$. b is the gradient of the line and a is the intercept on the vertical axis. Linear functions describe directly related variables.

This function returns the output as identical to the input. The gradient of the line is unity. The line intercepts the vertical axis at the origin.

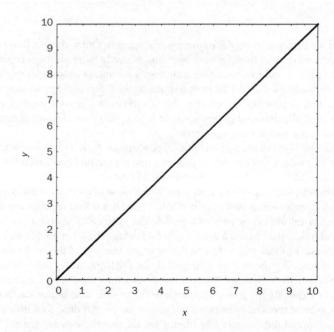

This is the function that we require, for instance, when we calibrate our invasive BP monitoring. We wish at all times to have the display pressure the same as the input (real) pressure (1.19.3). We are often interested in this function only for positive values of x. This function is also the defining relation of a completely useless diagnostic test. If post-test probability is identical to pre-test probability, the test is useless. (3.9.3).

2.5.2   **Transformations**

Transformations of $y = x$

We can take our basic function and apply some simple transformations. First, we apply a *scaling* by changing the value of b, the gradient.

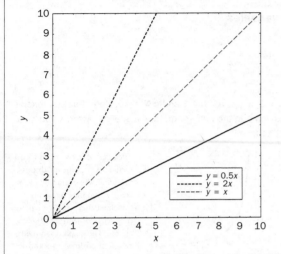

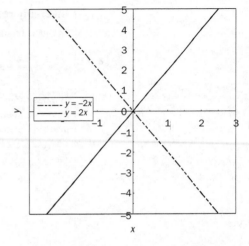

Scaling. This graph shows the functions $y = 2x$ and $y = 0.5x$. The gradient is altered by changes in the value of b: the larger the value of b, the steeper the gradient of the line—the smaller the value of b, the shallower the gradient. All pass through the origin.

Reflection. The graphs of $y = 2x$ and $y = -2x$. The effect of the minus sign is to 'reflect' the graph of $y = 2x$ around either axis as in a mirror. The value of the linear function is now decreasing as x increases. It is a decreasing function and the gradient is negative.

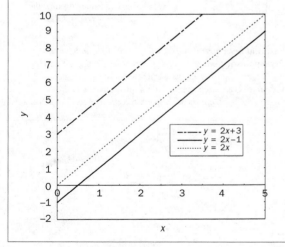

Translation. The effect of changing the value of the constant a in the function rule is to translate or shift the line so that it intercepts the y-axis (i.e. where $x = 0$) at a different point given by $y = a$. The gradient is unaffected by changing the value of a.

Note that the constant function $y = a$ is merely a linear function with gradient zero, i.e. $b = 0$. In linear regression we estimate a gradient for a line from linearly related data, and in order to demonstrate a linear relationship we have to be convinced that the gradient is significantly different from zero (3.18).

2.6.1 **Basic rectangular hyperbola**

The rectangular hyperbola is a function that very commonly arises in modelling. We shall again look at the basic function and then transform it to other related functions by simple manoeuvres. We shall concentrate our attention on transformations as they affect the graph in the first quadrant (x and y both positive).

Inversely related variables

The function rule is

$$y = \frac{a}{bx + c} + d.$$

The basic function is $y = 1/x$, i.e. $a = b = 1$ and $c = d = 0$. Note that the denominator is a linear expression and the numerator, a, is a scaling factor. y and x are inversely related quantities.

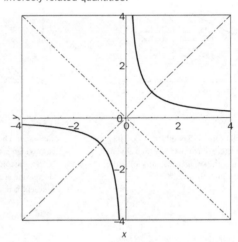

The graph is in two parts with a section in opposite quadrants of the graph. We cannot divide by zero, so that the function is undefined at $x = 0$, although we may get as close to zero as we choose. The graph is symmetrical about the lines $y = x$ and $y = -x$: if we reflect the graph in either of these lines, we obtain the same graph that we started from. As we approach $x = 0$, the gradient of the curve becomes steeper and steeper. As we move away from the origin along the x-axis in either direction, the gradient becomes shallower.

The curves approach the axes but never meet them: the axes are said to be *asymptotes*— these are lines which a curve approaches ever more closely, but never actually meets. The function is called a rectangular hyperbola because its asymptotes are at right-angles. Because the gradient of the curve is very steep near the origin, small changes in the x-value give us large changes in the y-value. This has important consequences in practice.

Quadrants

The standard graph plane is sectioned into quadrants. We may need to identify which quadrant we are in in describing the behaviour of functions.

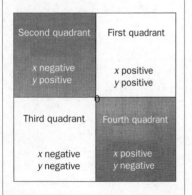

2.6.2   Transformations

Transformations of the basic hyperbola

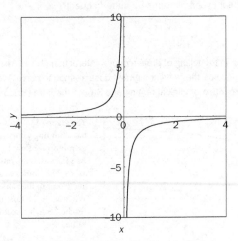

$y = -1/x$, $a = -1$. The minus sign has the effect of *reflection* about either of the axes.

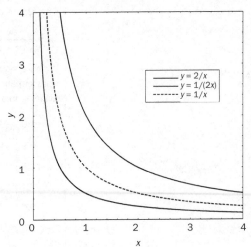

Scaling. Changing a and b.
$y = 2/x$, $a = 2$, $b = 1$, $c = d = 0$ and $y = 1/2x$, $a = 1$, $b = 2$, $c = d = 0$.
$y = 2/x$ simply doubles all the values of the basic function $y = 1/x$, a scaling by a factor of two. $y = 1/(2x)$ halves all the values of the basic function, a scaling by a factor of 0.5. Although the graphs have been shifted, this is *not* a translation.

$$y = \frac{a}{bx + c} + d.$$

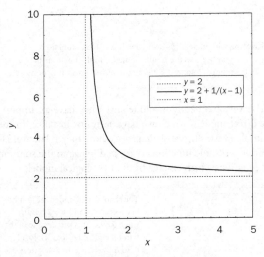

Adding a constant. Translation in y-direction. Changing d.

$$y = \frac{1}{x-1} + 2 \quad a = 1, b = 1, c = -1, d = 2.$$

The effect of adding a constant is to translate in the y-direction. Adding a constant of 2 to all values of the opposite function translates the whole curve 2 units in the positive y-direction (i.e. upwards).

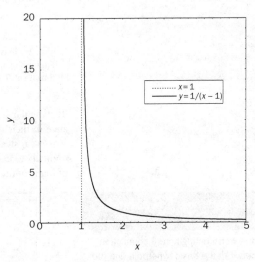

Translation in x-direction. Changing c.

$$y = \frac{1}{x-1} \quad a = 1, \quad b = 1, c = -1, d = 0.$$ The effect of $c = -1$ is to

translate the basic curve one unit to the right. Its vertical asymptote is now $x = 1$. When $x = 1$ the denominator has value zero, so this function is undefined at $x = 1$.

2.6.3   Rational functions

Another hyperbola

One variant of the rectangular hyperbola turns up quite frequently

$$y = \frac{ax}{bx + c} + d.$$

We have seen this equation in modelling of drug–receptor interaction (1.14). The log transformation of x-values gave us the familiar sigmoid dose–response curve. We also see this arising in the context of clinical testing and Bayes' theorem (3.9.3).

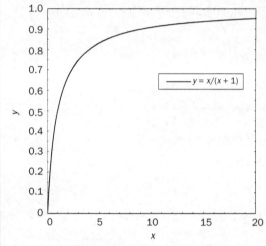

The graph of $y = x/(x+1)$ has a limiting value—an asymptote—of $y = 1$. As x increases, the ratio $x/(x + 1)$ becomes closer and closer to the value 1. When $x = 1$ the function reaches its half-maximal value.

We can see this function as a composite function, a product of two simpler functions:

$$y = x \times \frac{1}{x+1}.$$

$y = x$ is a linear function, increasing with increasing x, and $y = 1/(x + 1)$ is a function diminishing with increasing x. The graph shows the results of these simple functions battling it out. This is an example of a rational function—it is a ratio of two linear functions.

Rectangular hyperbolas arise very frequently in modelling. They have an importance in their own right as direct models, which we have seen, for instance, in the $\dot{V}A/P_{a}CO_2$ steady-state example (1.3). But we shall also see how they relate fundamentally to exponential and logarithmic functions (2.9), and hence to the solution of many of the differential equations which emerge from physiological models.

The hyperbola and natural log function

It is worth noting here a connection between the basic hyperbola and the tremendously important natural logarithm function which we meet in (2.9.5). The area under the curve of $y = 1/x$ between $x = 1$ and $x = t$ is $\log_e(t)$.

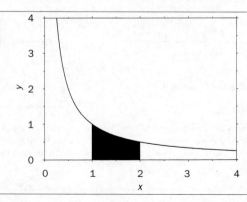

The shaded area under the graph between $x = 1$ and $x = 2$ has the value 0.693. This is the value of the natural $\log(2)$, i.e. $\log_e(2)$: $\log(1) = 0$, so the area is zero at $x = 1$. Areas under the curve below $x = 1$ have negative sign because the logarithms of numbers smaller than 1 are negative. The connection between this odd fact and the importance of the exponential and log functions should become apparent later (2.14.3).

2.7.1 Quadratics, cubics, and quartics

Polynomial functions are functions of the form

$$y = a + bx + cx^2 + dx^3 + \ldots,$$

where $a, b, c, d, \ldots$ are constants. They are sums of powers of x multiplied by constants—the coefficients of the powers of x. Polynomial functions are extremely important in modelling and statistical analysis. We shall not be concerned in any detail with any polynomials involving powers greater than x^2. Polynomial functions are classed according to the highest power of x in the equation. In fact, we have already met the two simplest; if all of the coefficients b, c, d, and so on are set at zero, we have $y = a$, the *constant function*. If a and b are non-zero, then we have $y = a + bx$, which is the equation of a *linear function*. Polynomials involving no higher power than x^2 are second-degree polynomials or *quadratic functions*; those involving x^3 are third-degree *cubic* functions; those with x^4 fourth-degree or *quartics*; and so on.

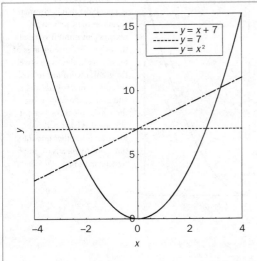

Polynomial functions

Examples of polynomial functions up to cubic functions are shown here.

Examples of constant (zero-degree polynomial), linear (first-degree), and quadratic functions. The quadratic function $y = a + bx + cx^2$ always has the same basic shape—a *parabola*. We examine parabolas in detail next. All quadratics can be obtained by transformations (scaling or translation) of the basic quadratic $y = x^2$.

The value of $y = x^2$ falls as it approaches $x = 0$ from the left (x negative). It is said to be decreasing for negative values of x ($x<0$). It is increasing in value for all positive values of x and is an increasing function for ($x>0$). At $x = 0$ the function is stationary, neither increasing nor decreasing.

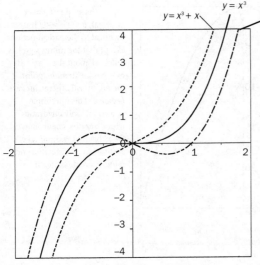

Cubics involve a term in x^3, so that when x is large and negative, the cubic term dominates, and y is negative ($-\times-\times-$); when x is large and positive ($+\times+\times+$), y is positive. All cubic functions can be obtained by transformation from one of these basic three pattern cubics.

The value of $y = x^3 + x$ is increasing at all points as x increases; it is an increasing function for all x-values. $y = x^3$ is increasing for all values of x except at $x = 0$ where it is stationary. $y = x^3 - x$ has a local peak at $x = -0.58$, and a local trough at $x = 0.58$. It is stationary at these points. Between these points, it is decreasing; it is a decreasing function on the interval $[-0.58, 0.58]$ and increasing elsewhere. These functions are further considered in (2.13.1).

2.7.2 Quadratic functions

Basic parabola and transformations

While quadratic functions do not arise very often as direct models in physiology, they are of immense importance in the solution of differential equations and in statistics. The laminar flow of liquid in a rigid pipe has a flow velocity profile which is a parabola. This can often be seen in a drip set with blood entering the saline column at the start of transfusion, where fluid at the axis of the drip tubing is moving more rapidly than that near the walls.

The general formula for a quadratic function is:

$$y = a + bx + cx^2$$

The basic quadratic function from which all others can be obtained by simple transformations is $y = x^2$.

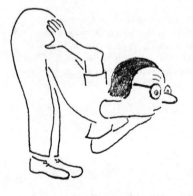

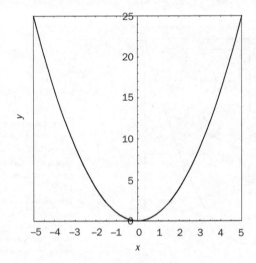

This is the graph of $y = x^2$. It is a parabola that is symmetrical about the y-axis and it reaches a minimum value at the origin. Because squares of numbers are always positive, the graph is confined to positive values of y (quadrants 1 and 2) i.e. it does not cross the x-axis. We will set about altering this basic parabolic function into other quadratic functions by means of simple transformations.

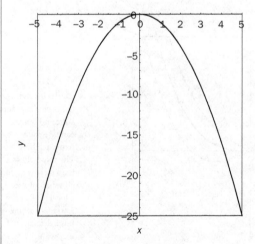

This is the graph of $y = -x^2$, i.e. $a = 0$, $b = 0$ $c = -1$. It is identical to the basic function except that the minus sign has reflected about the x-axis. It now has a *maximum* point at the origin. All other values are negative. This is a simple reflection. Only quadratics with a negative coefficient, c, for x^2 have a maximum, i.e. point upwards. Maxima and minima are discussed in (2.13).

2.7.3 Quadratic functions: further transformations

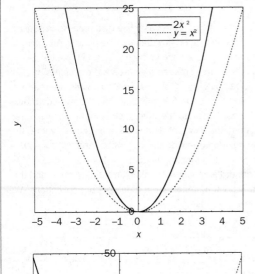

Scalings and translations

We apply some more transformations to the basic parabola and see how these relate to the quadratic function rule:

$$y = a + bx + cx^2$$

Scaling. The graph of $y = 2x^2$ is a straightforward scaling of the basic function—every value is simply doubled. The graph remains symmetrically disposed about the y-axis and has its minimum value at the origin—multiplying zero by 2 still gives zero.

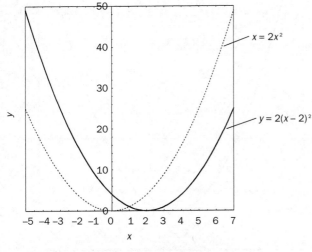

Translation: x-direction. The graph of $y = 2x^2$ has been moved two units to the right—a translation in the positive x-direction. The rule has now changed to $y = 2(x-2)^2$; this instructs us to subtract 2 from the input x-value, square, and scale by a factor of 2. Subtracting 2 from the input x-value gives us the same output as we obtain from the (unshifted) $y = 2x^2$, two units to the *left*. Note that the order of the operations is important: *first* subtract 2, *then* square, and *then* double. This may need some thought. This translates the basic curve to the right, and the minimum point is now at $x = 2$. The shape and size of the curve is exactly the same as $y = 2x^2$.

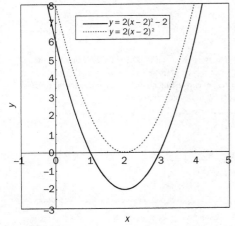

Translation: y-direction. A translation in the y-direction is easy—we just add or subtract a constant. This is the curve of $y = 2(x-2)^2 - 2$, i.e. the same curve as before, but we have merely subtracted 2 from every y-value calculated for the previous curve. This now has a minimum point that is still at $x = 2$, but the function value at this point is now -2. The curve now also crosses the x-axis, since it takes negative values between $x = 1$ and $x = 3$. We could, if we wished, express this same curve in standard form ($y = a + bx + cx^2$) by multiplying out, when we obtain $y = 2x^2 - 8x + 6$. The effect of the transformations is, however, more easily seen in $y = 2(x-2)^2 - 2$ form. This is the completed square form of the quadratic.

2.7.4   Quadratic functions: roots—maxima and minima

Quadratic root formula

The roots of quadratic equations $a + bx + cx^2 = 0$ cannot always be determined by factorization, but if they exist can be obtained from a formula simply by 'plugging in' the coefficients:

$$\frac{-b \pm \sqrt{b^2 - 4ac}}{2c}$$

- If $b^2 > 4ac$, then $b^2 - 4ac$ is positive and we can take the square root $\sqrt{b^2 - 4ac}$ and calculate the two roots of the equation from the formula.
- If $b^2 = 4ac$, then there is a single root—the parabola just touches the x-axis at one point.
- If $b^2 < 4ac$, then the quadratic has no real roots. Its roots are then *complex numbers*, which are interesting but beyond our scope. They will be mentioned in discussion of second-order differential equations (2.15.3), so we need to know of their existence at least.

Zeroes

Any quadratic function can be obtained from the basic one by a process of scaling, reflection, and translation, and we have seen how this may be done in principle. There are certain points of particular importance in the transformed quadratics:

1. The points (if any) at which the curve crosses the x-axis are the points at which the function value is zero: $a + bx + cx^2 = 0$. These x-values are the roots or zeroes of the function, and the need often arises to find the x-values that satisfy this equation. If the translation in the y-direction is in the positive direction, the graph does not cross the x-axis at all and there are no real roots. It may touch the axis at one point only—as do $y = x^2$, $y = 2x^2$, and $y = 2(x - 2)^2$—a single root. Or it may cross in two places, as does $y = 2(x - 2)^2 - 2$).

2. The x-value at which the quadratic reaches its minimum or maximum, and the value of the function at this point is important in a number of applications. We need this idea extensively in statistics.

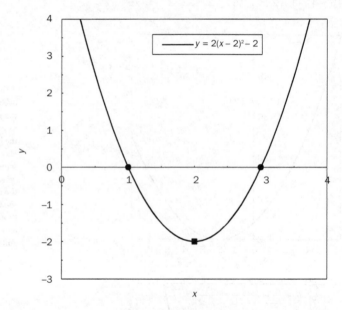

$y = 2(x - 2)^2 - 2$ can be rewritten as $y = 2(x - 1)(x - 3)$. When $x = 1$ or $x = 3$, the function value must be zero, since at each of these x-values one or other of the brackets will be zero. The process of converting quadratic equations to this form is *factorization*. This enables the roots to be determined.

Maxima and minima

A quadratic function always has a *minimum* value if the coefficient of x^2 is positive, since the parabola points downwards. If this coefficient is negative, the parabola points upwards and the function has a *maximum* value somewhere. The maximum or minimum is found where the gradient to the curve is zero. This point is found where $x = b/2c$; it is always midway between the roots if they exist. To see whether it is a maximum or minimum, simply look at the coefficient of x^2. We shall only need to deal with minima of quadratics. Maxima and minima are discussed in (2.13.1).

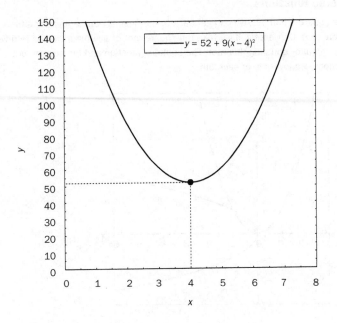

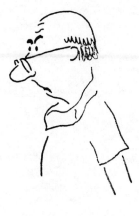

$y = 9x^2 - 72x + 196$. This parabola reaches a minimum value at

$$x = \frac{72}{2 \times 9} = 4.$$

The function value is then $y = 9 \times 4^2 - 72 \times 4 + 196 = 52$. We meet this function in (3.10.4), as an 'error function'.

2.8.1   Inversion of functions and reflection

A simple but important concept is that of an *inverse function*, which 'undoes' the work of another function. If we think of a function as a sausage machine—we put in the raw material (input range value), and out of the machine (rule) comes the sausage (function value)—an inverse function takes the sausage and gives us back the raw material. This is perhaps most easily seen with the quadratic and square root functions. It is not easily seen with a sausage machine.

Inverse functions

If we square a number, we can get back to the original number by taking the square root. Conversely, if we take the square root of a number we can retrieve the original by squaring this root. The squaring function and the square root functions are inverses of each other.

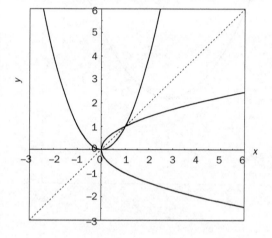

We can think of the inverse function idea as a *reversal of the axes*. We use the output of one function to read the graph 'backwards' to the original input. Essentially, we are reflecting the graph around the line $y = x$, so that the x- and y-axes are reversed. The square root graph is seen as the reflected image of the $y = x^2$ parabola.

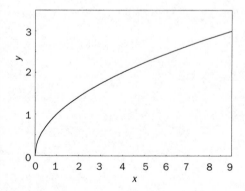

Each positive number has *two* square roots, as shown on the graph. We need to be careful to specify either the positive or the negative root to have a respectable function. This is the graph of the positive square root function. It is half of the $y = x^2$ parabola, reflected about the line $y = x$.

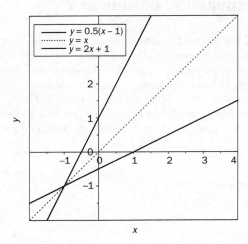

The inverse of the linear function $y = 2x + 1$ can be obtained by undoing the process that we apply to obtain it from the basic linear, $y = x$. The rule we use is first to double x and then add 1. To undo this we must first subtract 1 $(x - 1)$ and then halve the result, i.e. the inverse is $y = 0.5(x - 1)$. The graph of these two functions is shown; they are mirror images about the line $y = x$.

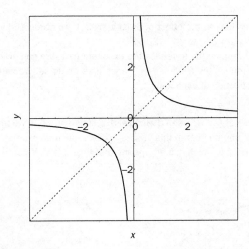

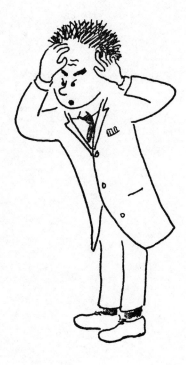

The idea of an inverse function will come into its own in the next topic—exponential and logarithmic functions (2.9). Another example is the rectangular hyperbola, which is its own inverse. If we take the reciprocal of a reciprocal we get back to where we started:

$$y = \frac{1}{x} \rightarrow \frac{1}{(1/x)} = x.$$

The graph of $y = 1/x$ is symmetrical around the line $y = x$, so that, reflection always gives us what we started with. The basic linear function $y = x$ is also its own inverse.

2.9.1 Exponents: powers of 2

The exponential function is of enormous importance in mathematical modelling. We have examined the properties of the polynomial functions $y = a + bx + cx^2 + dx^3 + \ldots$ (2.7); where the variable x appears in various powers—that is, multiplied by itself a number of times. We fix the coefficients and powers for our function rule and see how the function value varies with varying x. The exponential functions, on the other hand, describe the effects of *varying the power of a fixed number a, the base* $y = a^x$. The power to which a is raised is the *index* or *exponent* of a.

Exponents

Let us examine various powers of 2:

$$y = 2 \times 2 = 2^2 = 4,$$
$$y = 2 \times 2 \times 2 = 2^3 = 8,$$
$$y = 2 \times 2 \times 2 \times 2 = 2^4 = 16,$$
$$y = 2 \times 2 \times 2 \times 2 \times 2 = 2^5 = 32.$$

We have a collection of '2 raised to various powers'. Each time we multiply by another 2, we simply add one to the exponent. If we wish to multiply 8 by 4 we can arrange the calculation thus: $8 \times 4 = (2 \times 2 \times 2) \times (2 \times 2) = 2^3 \times 2^2 = 2^5 = 32$. It is evident that we can express a *multiplication* by *adding* the exponents. To achieve a consistent arithmetic, 2 itself must therefore be 2^1: $y = 2 = 2^1$.

It is a general rule that we can summarize as follows:

Rule 1: $a^m \times a^n = a^{m+n}$

Similarly, we can look at the effect of division by 2. If we divide 16 by 2 we obtain 8: $16 \div 2 = 2^4 \div 2 = 8 = (2 \times 2 \times 2) = 2^3$.

Division by 2 requires us to reduce the exponent by 1. We can divide by 2 more than once and reduce the exponent by 1 each time we do so. We can express *division* by *subtraction* of exponents:

Rule 2: $a^m \div a^n = a^{m-n}$

These rules work only if we keep the base, a, a constant, i.e. if we manipulate powers of the same number in this case $a = 2$. We can thus express fractions as *negative powers* of a, which actually means that Rule 1 is sufficient:

$$\frac{1}{2} = \frac{1}{2^1} = 2^{-1},$$

$$\frac{1}{4} = \frac{1}{2^2} = 2^{-2},$$

$$\frac{1}{8} = \frac{1}{2^3} = 2^{-3},$$

$$\frac{1}{16} = \frac{1}{2^4} = 2^{-4}.$$

This is a plot of some of the points that we have calculated where x along the horizontal axis is the exponent of 2. We have what appears to be a pattern that invites us to draw a smooth curve through the points—but this would demand giving a meaning to numbers such as $y = 2^{1.5}$.

We have not assigned a meaning to 2^0. The smooth curve joining negative and positive powers of 2 looks as though it should pass through the y-axis at $y = 1$. This would mean $2^0 = 1$. In fact, we do obtain a consistent arithmetic if we define *any* base to the power zero as 1: $a^0 = 1$.

2.9.2   **Fractional indices**

The exponential function $y = 2^x$

The square root of 2 if multiplied by itself gives us 2: $\sqrt{2} \times \sqrt{2} = 2^1$. We can define $\sqrt{2} = 2^{0.5}$, since if we use Rule 1 we can add the exponents and remain consistent: $2^{0.5} \times 2^{0.5} = 2^1$. In fact, we can continue like this; where, for instance, $y = 2^{1.5}$ means $2^1 \times 2^{0.5} = 2 \times \sqrt{2} = 2^{1.5} = 2.828\ldots$, which is the same as $4 \div \sqrt{2} = 2^2 \div 2^{0.5} = 2^{1.5} = 2.828\ldots$

It would follow from the rule that $2^{1.5} \times 2^{1.5} = 2^3 = 8$, i.e. that $\sqrt{8} = 2.828\ldots$, which it is.

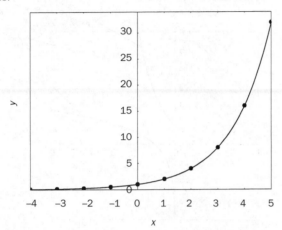

The smooth curve that we have drawn through the points is the graph of a function that allows fractional indices. We need to define for this function $2^0 = 1$. Since multiplication of a number by 1 leaves the number the same, then as we add indices to multiply, we must add zero to the index to multiply by 1. In fact, for *any a*, $a^0 = 1$. Any number raised to power zero = 1.

The function is always positive—it is confined to the upper two quadrants. It never meets or crosses the x-axis and hence never takes the value zero. It gets closer and closer to zero (i.e. asymptotically) as x becomes large and negative.

Filling in the gaps

We can produce a consistent arithmetic if we treat $a^{1/n} = \sqrt[n]{a}$, where $\sqrt[n]{a}$ is the *n*th root of *a*: if we multiply $\sqrt[n]{a}$ by itself *n* times, we obtain $(\sqrt[n]{a})^n = a$. For example, for $a = 27$ and $n = 3$, $\sqrt[3]{n} = \sqrt[3]{27} = 3$.

We can raise this n^{th} root of *a* to any power *m* so that:

$$a^{m/n} = \sqrt[n]{a^m}$$

For example with $a = 2$ $m = 3$ and $n = 2$, we have

$$2^{3/2} = \sqrt{2^3} = \sqrt{8} = 2.828\ldots$$

We can set *n* and *m* to any integers, and by a combination of raising to the *m*th power and taking the *n*th root, we can calculate a value for the function $y = a^{m/n}$ for any integers *m* and *n*, and hence for any fractional power *m/n*. So for any rational number (2.1.1) along the x-axis, we have a way of calculating $y = a^{m/n}$. We will assume that it is reasonable to extend this definition to include all real number powers of *a*—i.e. including irrational numbers.

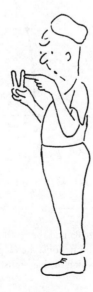

2.9.3 **Exponential and log as inverses**

We looked at the idea of an inverse function in (2.8). What about the inverse function of $y = 2^x$? This function would answer the question: If we input a number, what power of 2 is required to give that number? For instance, for the input 4, the power of 2 required = 2. If we input 2.8284 ... we would obtain output 1.5, since this is the power of 2 that gives the result 2.8284 ... This function is the logarithmic function for base 2.

Since the exponential function is confined to quadrants 1 and 2 (positive y), the inverse function, $\log_2 x$, is confined to quadrants 1 and 4 (positive x). Real logarithms of negative numbers do not exist.

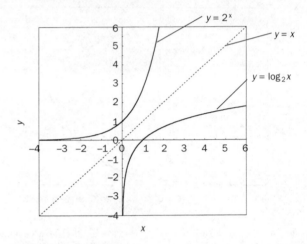

The logarithmic function $y = \log_2 x$

The log function with base 2 is shown. Comparison with (2.9.2) shows that this is the inverse function of $y = 2^x$. An inverse function is obtained by reflecting in the line $y = x$, which effectively transposes the axes.

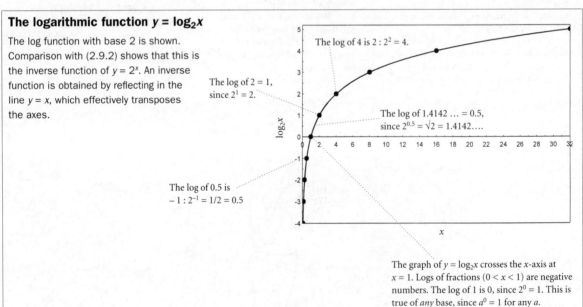

The log of 4 is 2 : $2^2 = 4$.

The log of 2 = 1, since $2^1 = 2$.

The log of 1.4142 ... = 0.5, since $2^{0.5} = \sqrt{2} = 1.4142....$

The log of 0.5 is $-1 : 2^{-1} = 1/2 = 0.5$

The graph of $y = \log_2 x$ crosses the x-axis at $x = 1$. Logs of fractions $(0 < x < 1)$ are negative numbers. The log of 1 is 0, since $2^0 = 1$. This is true of *any* base, since $a^0 = 1$ for any a.

We have explained the relation of the functions $y = 2^x$ and $y = \log_2 x$. Since these are inverse functions, then $\log_2 (2^x) = x$ and $2^{(\log_2 x)} = x$. The log of a number is the power to which the base must be raised to give the number.

2.9.4 Powers of 10: $\log_{10}x$

$y = 10^x$ and $y = \log_{10}x$

We have explored some of the properties of $y = 2^x$ and $y = \log_2x$. We now compare the exponential and log functions with different base, $a = 10$.

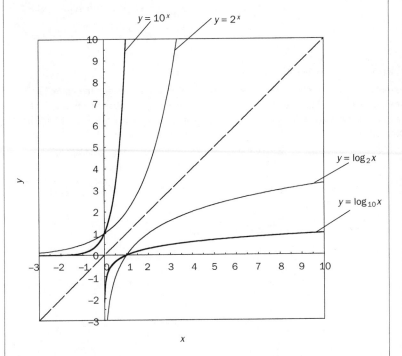

The curves for $y = 10^x$ and $y = \log_{10}x$ are again symmetrically disposed about the line $y = x$, since they are inverses of each other. They are just scaled versions of the curves of $y = 2^x$ and $y = \log_2x$ respectively. The curves of $y = 2^x$ and $y = \log_2x$ are shown for comparison. Because of the scaling involved, it becomes increasingly difficult with larger bases to display the features effectively on a single graph. As the base increases, the curves diverge more rapidly away from the fixed intercepts on the axes.

Note that both exponential functions cross the y-axis at $y = 1$. This is true of *any* exponential, since $a^0 = 1$ for any a. By the symmetry of the inverse function, it follows that $\log_a 1 = 0$ for any base a. These facts follow from the rules for indices (2.9.1).

Summary of properties of logarithmic functions

- The logarithm of a number $\log_a x$, is the power to which the base a must be raised to give that number: $\log_a x$ means $a^{(\log_a x)} = x$.
- Because the log is an exponent (index), addition of logs is equivalent to multiplication: $\log_a (mx) = \log_a (m) + \log_a(x)$.
- Similarly, subtraction in logs divides: $\log_a (x/m) = \log_a (x) - \log_a (m)$.
- Multiplication of a log by n raises to the nth power: $n\log_a (x) = \log_a (x^n)$.
- The log function is the inverse function of the exponential function to the same base: $\log_a (a^x) = x$ and $a^{(\log_a x)} = x$. The exponential function is the antilog function.
- One log function is obtained from another of different base by a simple scaling procedure. The rule is:

$$\log_a(x) = \frac{\log_b (x)}{\log_b (a)},$$

e.g. $\log_{10}(2) = \dfrac{\log_2(2)}{\log_2(10)}$

$$= \frac{1}{3.322} 0.3010.$$

2.9.5   The natural exponential function. Why *e*?

The numbers 2 and 10 are both familiar and we encounter them frequently. We have looked at the exponential and logarithmic functions based upon these numbers and found them not too difficult to comprehend, so why should we want to construct an exponential/logarithmic inverse function pair around the number $e = 2.718281828...$?

The exponential function $y = e^x$ and the natural logarithmic function $y = \log_e x$

These functions show exactly the same pattern as before, except that the scaling is intermediate between the base 2 and base 10 functions. The special feature of the exponential function $y = e^x$ is that *the gradient of the curve at any point is equal to the function value*; for example, when $e^x = 10$, the gradient to the curve at that point is also 10; when $e^x = 1000$, the gradient to the curve at that point is also 1000. We will see the important consequences of this fact shortly.

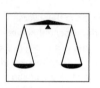

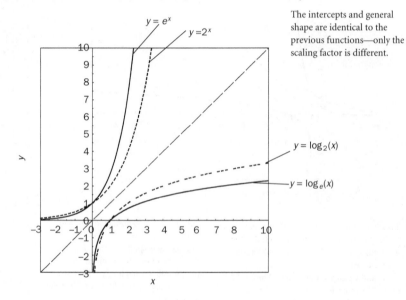

The intercepts and general shape are identical to the previous functions—only the scaling factor is different.

The gradient of the curve $y = e^x$ at any point is the same as the function value itself. At $x = 1$, the function value is $y = e^1 = e = 2.71828 ...$ The gradient of the curve at this point—the rate at which it is increasing—is also $2.71828 ...$; a tangent to the curve at this point has gradient $2.71828....$

The tangent and perpendicular make a triangle with the *x*-axis. Since the function value (the length of the perpendicular) is $2.71828 ...,$ the triangle must sit on a base on the *x*-axis which has a length of unity because the gradient is the ratio of the height to the base.

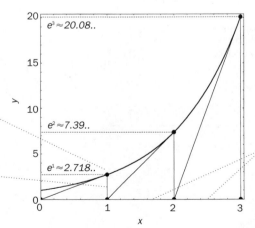

Because the gradient is always the same as the function value at any point, the base of the triangle formed by the tangent in this way is always of unity length.

Gradient of the natural log function

The natural log function, $y = \log_e x$, has a particularly simple derivative. The gradient at any point on the curve $y = \log_e x$ is $1/x$. Modelling equations frequently arise in which the rate of change of a quantity is given by $1/x$ (or a transformed version of it). We have explored the function $y = 1/x$ and its transformations in (2.6). These facts account for much of the importance of the exponential and logarithmic functions in modelling.

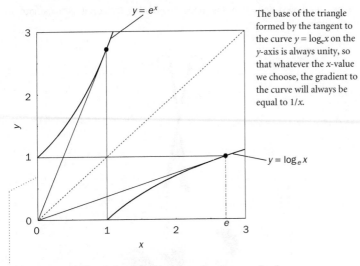

The base of the triangle formed by the tangent to the curve $y = \log_e x$ on the y-axis is always unity, so that whatever the x-value we choose, the gradient to the curve will always be equal to $1/x$.

By the symmetry of the relationship of the inverse functions $y = e^x$ and $y = \log_e x$ and the fact that the gradient of $y = e^x$ is always the same as the function value, the gradient of the tangent to the curve $y = \log_e x$ is $1/x$.

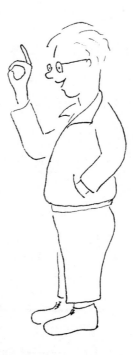

2.9.6 Exponential haircuts: Taylor series

Taylor series

There is another representation of the exponential function that may be encountered:

$$e^x = 1 + x + \frac{x^2}{2!} + \frac{x^3}{3!} + \frac{x^4}{4!} + \dots .$$

It is an infinite polynomial series and, if differentiated to obtain the gradient (2.12.3), it gives us exactly what we start with—all of the terms move along one, but since there is an infinite supply, nothing changes. This means the gradient is equal to the function value. If we evaluate the first few terms for $x = 1$, we obtain;

$$e^x = 1 + 1 + \frac{1}{2} + \frac{1}{6} + \frac{1}{24} + \dots .$$
$$= 2.708333\dot{}$$

Even with only five terms, we have a value quite close to $e = 2.71828 \dots$. This representation is called a Taylor series. Similar Taylor series can be used for a number of other functions; e.g. sin and cos. Calculations of series such as this are set in train when a function button is pressed on a pocket calculator.

Exponential processes: the exponential trichotome

Exponential processes are seen everywhere, and are not at all exotic. The characteristic feature is that a proportional change occurs: something doubled or halved, for instance—recollect how we calculated the N_2 washout discrete function (1.9.2). The hairdresser's pair of thinning scissors is an exponential machine; it removes half of the hair under the blades. If the hair is thick, lots of hair is removed; if thin, very little.

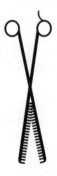

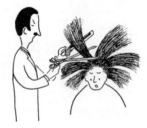

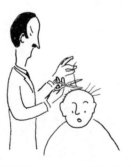

2.9.7   **Patterns of exponential change**

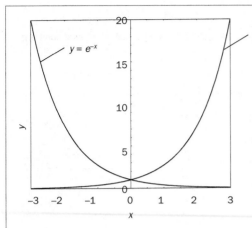

Transformations of the basic exponential function

There are three patterns of exponential change that we need to identify:

- the tear-away function
- the washout function
- the wash-in function

$y = e^x$

The basic exponential function $y = e^x$ that we have looked at so far is the *tear-away exponential function*. The exponent has positive sign. As x increases, the function value rapidly becomes larger—its gradient is identical with the function value and hence as the function increases, the rate of increase itself increases rapidly. The value of the function accelerates and 'tears away'. We shall not need this for modelling—although a truncated version appears as a candidate 'recovery function' in the computer simulation of pulmonary air embolism (1.12.5).

The tear-away curve reflected around the y-axis $y = e^{-x}$ is the negative exponential or *washout exponential function*. The exponent has negative sign. We will be particularly interested in this for positive values of x. (We will use t as the input variable when we are considering time-dependent functions. The use of x, t, or any other symbol is entirely arbitrary.)

This shows the detail of the washout function for positive values. The function value starts at 1 for $x = 0$ and diminishes in a smooth curve to approach the x-axis ever more closely. It never actually reaches the axis, but approaches it asymptotically. $y = e^{-x}$ is a decreasing function of x and approaches zero as x increases. The curve models the washing-out of a substance from a compartment or container by a flow.

If we subtract the washout function from 1, then instead of approaching the x-axis, it approaches a limiting value of 1. Since $y = e^{-x}$ approaches zero as x increases, then we subtract a smaller and smaller value from 1 as x increases. This is the *exponential wash-in function*, which is our third pattern. This is a reflection of the washout curve about the line $y = 0.5$. The curve models the wash-in of a substance into a container or compartment, carried in by a flow and mixing with the existing contents.

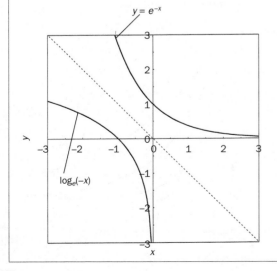

The inverse function of $y = e^{-x}$ is $\log_e(-x)$. Logs of negative numbers do not exist, but $\log(-x)$, when x is itself negative, is the log of a *positive* number ($- \times - = +$).

2.9.8 Exponential change: scalings and rates

Scalings in the vertical direction

Scalings in the vertical direction of the basic wash-in and washout functions are easily achieved by multiplying by a constant: $y = Ae^{-x}$ and $y = A(1 - e^{-x})$.

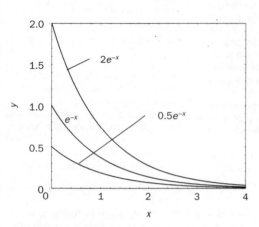
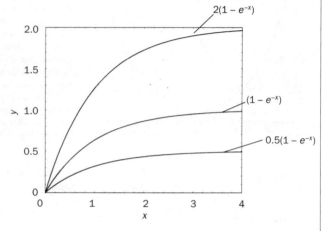

Multiplying by a constant A simply alters the vertical scale. The same *proportional function value*—i.e. as a proportion of *A*—occurs for any given *x*-value.

Scalings in the horizontal direction: rate constants

Stretching or compressing of the basic curves in a horizontal direction is achieved by manipulating the exponent. We will elsewhere change the variable from *x* to *t* since we shall mainly be interested in time-dependent processes. The choice of symbol is entirely arbitrary—*t* is just more familiar for time-dependent variables, which are of particular interest to us.

To achieve a horizontal scaling, we multiply the *exponent* by a constant α. This is the *rate constant*, since it scales in the horizontal (time) axis. The larger the value of α is, the more rapidly the exponential change occurs, since it amplifies the rate. Each wash-in curve is approaching the line $y = 1$ as its asymptote just the rate of approach is different.

The washout curves are each approaching the *x*-axis. The rate of the process is different. These are reflected versions of the equivalent wash-in curves about $y = 0.5$.

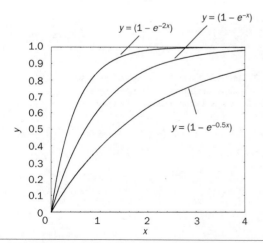
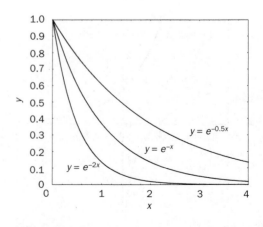

2.9.9 Rate constants, time constants, and half-times

Standardizing the change: the time constant

The rate constant α determines the rapidity with which a simple exponential process occurs. The basic time-dependent exponential process—whether wash-in or washout—has $\alpha = 1$. It is useful to be able to refer the value for any particular rate α to the standard basic exponential function by a standardizing procedure. This is the time constant τ, which we met in (1.10.1).

$$y = Ae^{-\alpha t}$$

$$\alpha t = 1 \quad \text{when } t = \frac{1}{\alpha} = \tau$$

$$\alpha t = 2 \quad \text{when } t = \frac{2}{\alpha} = 2\tau$$

$$\alpha t = 3 \quad \text{when } t = \frac{3}{\alpha} = 3\tau$$

$$\alpha t = 4 \quad \text{when } t = \frac{4}{\alpha} = 4\tau$$

Since, if we take the reciprocal of the rate constant, $\tau = 1/\alpha$, we obtain a time τ that is the time at which the exponential process will have reached 0.3679 of A—i.e. 36.79% of the starting value. Alternatively, we can say that $100 - 36.79\% = 63.21\%$ of the total change has taken place by time τ.

After time $t = 2\tau$, the function value has dropped to 13.53% of the starting value and at time $t = 3\tau$, the value is 4.98% of the initial value. The figure for $t = 4\tau$ is 1.83%. The time constant is a standardizing procedure; the proportions remain constant for any exponential function—all we need to do is to find a value for τ and we know the times at which these fixed proportional changes occur.

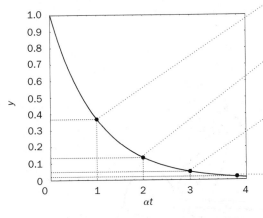

When $\alpha t = 1$, $y = Ae^{-\alpha t}$ has the value

$$y = Ae^{-1} = A \times \frac{1}{e} = A \times \frac{1}{2.7183} = 0.3679\,A \approx 37\% \text{ of } A.$$

When $\alpha t = 2$,

$$y = Ae^{-2} = A \times \frac{1}{e^2} = A \times \frac{1}{(2.7183)^2} = 0.1353A \approx 14\% \text{ of } A.$$

When $\alpha t = 3$,

$$y = Ae^{-3} = A \times \frac{1}{e^3} = A \times \frac{1}{(2.7183)^3} = 0.0498\,A \approx 5\% \text{ of } A.$$

When $\alpha t = 4$,

$$y = Ae^{-4} = A \times \frac{1}{e^4} = A \times \frac{1}{(2.7183)^4} = 0.0183\,A \approx 2\% \text{ of } A.$$

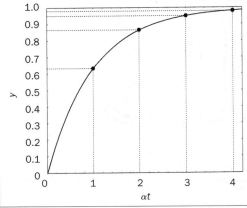

The same proportional changes occur in the wash-in curve. When $\alpha t = 1$, 63% of the change has taken place, 86% when $\alpha t = 2$, 95% when $\alpha t = 3$ and 98% when $\alpha t = 4$.

Half-time

The half-life, or half-time, of an exponential process is the time taken for the initial value to achieve 50% of its final value. Since the time constant is the time for a proportional change of 63% to occur, the half-time is less than τ. We need to find a value for t at which $Ae^{-\alpha t} = 0.5\,A$, i.e. the function value is 50% of A, the initial value. Cancelling A, we have $e^{-\alpha t} = 0.5$. Taking logs, we obtain $-\alpha t = -\log_e 2$, or

$$t = \frac{(\log_e 2)}{\alpha} = 0.693\tau.$$ The half-time is about 70% of the time constant.

Flows and compartments

There are some useful rules of thumb:

- The rate constant α and the time constant τ are reciprocals of each other: $\tau = 1/\alpha$, $\alpha = 1/\tau$.

- Dimensionally, α is a proportional rate and has dimension $[T]^{-1}$. The time constant is a time and must have dimension $[T]$: $\tau = 1/\alpha = [T]$, as required.

- When we have a flow $\dot{Q}$ washing through a container of volume V, we obtain a rate constant, $\alpha = \dot{Q}/V$. The time constant $\tau = V/\dot{Q}$ in these models is quite simply *the time taken for the flow to fill the container*. If we have a $\dot{V}A = 4$ l/min and FRC $= 2$ l, it takes 0.5 min for the flow to fill the container; $\tau = 0.5$ min. Thus 63% of nitrogen wash out will have occurred after 30 s (τ) of perfect pre-oxygenation, 86% after 1 min (2τ), 95% by 1.5 min (3τ), and 98% by 2 min (4τ).

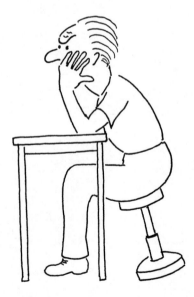

2.9.10 Making the curved straight: log transformations of exponential curves

Log transformations

It is very convenient to deal with linear functions, since they are very easy to manipulate and analyse. It is therefore often useful to be able to change a curved function to a linear one by a suitable transformation. The Hill plot (1.14.4) is one such. The log transformation of exponential data to linear form is extremely useful, and rests upon the inverse relationship between log and exponential functions. We consider linear regression in (3.18). If we take an example of the simple exponential washout curve, $y = Ae^{-\alpha t}$, we can take natural logs (2.9.4) of each side:

$$y = Ae^{-\alpha t},$$
$$\log y = \log(Ae^{-\alpha t})$$
$$= \log A + \log(e^{-\alpha t})$$
$$= \log A - \alpha t.$$

The natural log of a number is the power to which e must be raised to give the number. The log of $e^{-\alpha t}$ must therefore be $-\alpha t$. This follows from the inverse relation of the log and exponential functions (2.9.3).

In logs, multiplication means addition. A is a constant, so $\log A$ must also be a constant.

$\log y = \log A - \alpha t$ is the graph of a straight line—$\log y$ is a *linear function* of t. When $t = 0$, the function value is $\log A$. This is the intercept on the $\log y$-axis. The gradient of the line is $-\alpha$, the rate constant of the exponential process. If we can estimate the slope of this line by appropriate methods (3.18), we can estimate the rate constant α.

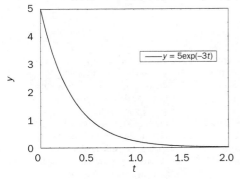

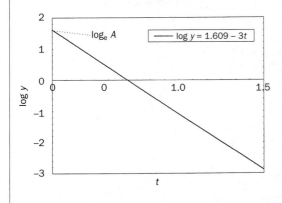

The curve of $y = 5e^{-3t}$. The rate constant is -3 and the vertical scaling factor is 5.

The curve of $\log y = \log 5 - 3t = 1.609 - 3t$. The intercept on the log y-axis is the log of the scaling factor A, in this case 5. The gradient of the line is the value of α, in this case -3. The part of the line below the horizontal axis is where the value of $\log y$ is negative. This means that the value of y is less than 1, since $\log 1 = 0$ for any base. The value of y then lies between zero and 1, where the line lies below the axis: $\log (0)$ does not exist.

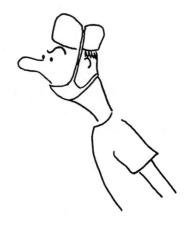

2.9.11   Sums and differences of exponentials

The two-compartment pharmacokinetic model and many other similar models in other contexts give rise to functions that are sums or differences of simple exponential functions. We may need to extract information about the contribution of the separate constituent exponential functions from the combination function.

Sum of two-exponential functions

The two-compartment model central compartment concentrations predict a sum bi-exponential pattern of the general form $y = Ae^{-\alpha t} + Be^{-\beta t}$. An example is shown $y = 5e^{-10t} + 3e^{-t}$.

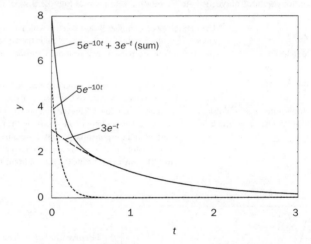

The two-component exponentials will in general have different scaling factors and rate constants. The more rapidly declining term causes the initial steep fall. It declines to a negligible value quite soon, leaving the slower term to dominate the latter portion of the curve. The component exponentials are shown.

This is a washout curve, with two simultaneous washout processes occurring. The principles for a wash-in curve involving two simultaneous exponential processes are analogous.

When $t = 0$, the y-value $= (5 \times 1) + (3 \times 1) = 8$. The difference in the rate constants ($\alpha = -10$, $\beta = -1$) means that the first term declines rapidly (exponent large and negative) to become negligible. Practically speaking, the latter part of the curve is almost entirely determined by the component with the slower rate constant. Where the rate constants of the two components are close, it becomes increasingly difficult to separate them.

Difference of two-exponential functions

The deep compartment equation in the two-compartment model is a function that is a *difference* of two exponential terms $y = Ge^{-\beta t} - Fe^{-\alpha t}$. We only dealt with the situation in which the deep compartment was empty (drug concentration zero at time $t = 0$) i.e. $C(0) = 0$. The scaling factors must therefore be equal for each of the two-component exponentials; i.e. $C = D$—only the rate constants α and β differ. The more rapidly declining term must be subtracted from the slower, so that nonsensical negative concentrations are not predicted.

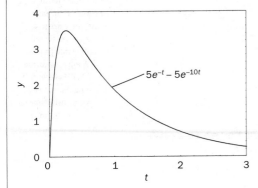

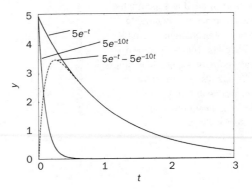

The graph shows a rising curve from the origin, although both terms are individually declining washout exponentials. This could be called a 'wash-through' curve, since it describes the wash into the deep compartment as well as the washout of it. As the rapidly declining component subtracted becomes negligibly small, the pattern becomes that of the single slower exponential. Early in the process, the pattern does not resemble a simple washout, since concentrations are increasing. The combination *difference* bi-exponential does have a maximum value, unlike the *sum* bi-exponential.

The deep compartment graph shows what happens in the deep compartment of the model. It has no counterpart in reality; it is merely the consequence of building a model to simulate the course of drug concentration in the plasma.

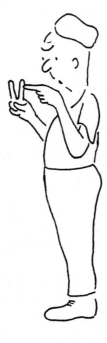

2.9.12   Sums and differences of exponentials: separating the components

Exponential stripping

When we have a model which involves two or more exponential terms, we may need to separate the individual components in order to determine rate constants and arbitrary constants. This is done by a process known as exponential 'stripping'. This is demonstrated for an ideal bi-exponential curve from a two-compartment drug model:
$C(t) = Ae^{-\alpha t} + Be^{-\beta t}$.

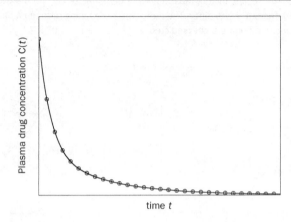

The more rapid process $Ae^{-\alpha t}$ declines and makes a progressively smaller contribution to the sum. If we look at the later points, these are practically governed by only the slower rate process $Be^{-\beta t}$. A log transformation (2.9.10) allows us to fit a straight line to these later points using linear regression techniques (3.18).

The line gradient is the estimated rate constant of the slower process β. By extrapolating back to the log concentration axis, we can determine log B and hence B itself.

The early points contain an important contribution from the more rapidly declining term, $Ae^{-\alpha t}$. Our regression line based on the later points predicts how much of the early concentration is attributable to the slower process. The deviation of the actual points from this regression line is attributed to the more rapid term. But these are deviations in *log* concentration—differences between one log curve and another—and hence represent multiples. These deviations must be calculated in absolute (antilog) form, since we need to add the contribution from $Ae^{-\alpha t}$ to $Be^{-\beta t}$. If we add in logs, we multiply.

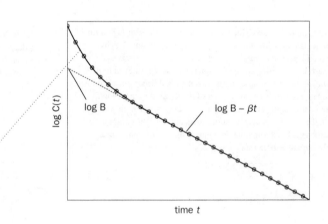

We replot the stripped slow exponential curve and calculate the deviations from the early points. These deviations are points on $Ae^{-\alpha t}$.

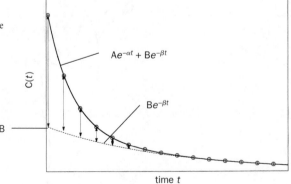

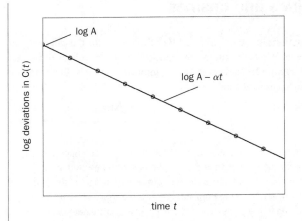

These *deviations* are plotted, and if only two exponentials are involved will lie on a single exponential decay curve. The *log* of these deviations can be fitted to a line of gradient α and intercept log A. We determine these in the same way, and have 'stripped' one exponential from the other. If these deviations do not fit a straight line convincingly, then we might need a model with another compartment added and hence a third exponential term.

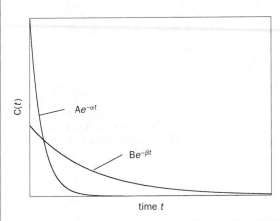

We can now plot the component functions and we have estimates of A, B, α and β.

In practice, the stripping of one exponential from another depends upon how different the rate constants are, how many points we have to fit our straight line to and the variability within the experimental data. Identifying any more than three exponential components is very difficult, or impossible, in practice.

Dye dilution again

Recirculation of dye in cardiac output determination (1.6.1) 'spoils' what is plausible exponential decay, but we can plot the 'middle' points between the wash-in of dye and the recirculation secondary peak. A log transformation of these should fit on a straight line, and the later deviations due to recirculation can be stripped off and discarded to reconstitute the 'pure' curve. This procedure is obsolete because the method is obsolete. However, the principle remains valid.

2.10.1   **Sines and cosines**

The sinusoidal functions are the building blocks for modelling oscillating and repetitive phenomena. We have studied the modelling of physiological pressure waves quite extensively in (1.19). This section summarizes some of the properties of the sinusoidal functions in general.

Sine and cosine

The definition of the sine (sin) and cosine (cos) functions is based upon a circle of unit radius. An arrow of unit length is fixed at the origin and rotated in the plane. The tip of this arrow traces out a circle if rotated through a full turn. For a rotation through an angle of θ to the horizontal axis, the arrow tip has an x co-ordinate (a projection on to the x-axis) which is $\cos\theta$ and a y co-ordinate (a projection on to the y-axis) which is $\sin\theta$. Both cos and sin are functions of angle θ.

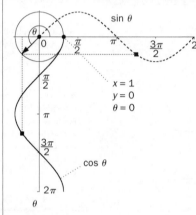

The circle is of unit radius. The values of $\sin\theta$ and $\cos\theta$ must lie between -1 and 1. When the arrow lies along the x-axis, $\theta = 0$: the x co-ordinate of the tip is 1 and the y co-ordinate is 0—$\sin 0 = 0$ and $\cos 0 = 1$.

The cos function

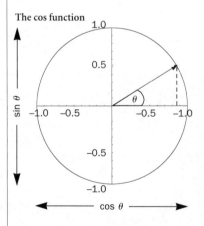

The cos curve is the x co-ordinate of the arrow tip as we rotate the arrow. It starts at 1 for $\theta = 0$, and then diminishes as θ approaches $\pi/2$. At $\theta = \pi/2$, the arrow lies along the y-axis and $\cos \pi/2 = 0$. The arrow tip enters the second quadrant and x is negative. The cos function is negative in this quadrant. It reaches a minimum value of -1 at $\theta = \pi$.

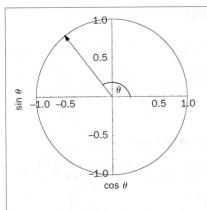

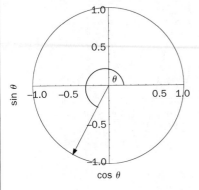

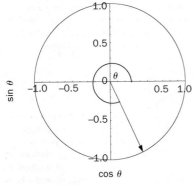

Radian measure

In proper mathematics, angles are measured in radians. A radian is the angle formed by an arc the length of the radius of the circle. Since there are 2π radii in the circumference of a circle, there are 2π radians in a full circle. 1 radian = $360°/2\pi \approx 57°$.

Degrees	Radians
0	0
45	$\pi/4$
60	$\pi/3$
90	$\pi/2$
180	π
270	$3\pi/2$
360	2π

As it enters the third quadrant, the tip of the arrow still has a negative x co-ordinate, but this approaches the y-axis at $\theta = 3\pi/2$, where it again has value 0. In the fourth quadrant, the cos again becomes positive and returns to the value 1 at $\theta = 2\pi = 0$. Because of the cyclical nature of the function, $\cos\theta = \cos 2\pi\theta = \cos 4\pi\theta = \cos 6\pi\theta$, and so on.

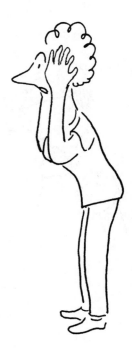

The sin function

The sin curve is the y co-ordinate of the arrow tip as we rotate the arrow. It traces out exactly the same curve as the cos function, except that it starts at $\sin 0 = 0$, increases to a maximum value of 1 at $\theta = \pi/2$, goes back to 0 at $\theta = 3\pi/2$, and so on. It is positive for θ in the first two quadrants; $0 < \theta < \pi$.

2.10.2   Transformations

We now take the basic functions of sin and cos and apply some of the usual transformations. We only explore these functions to the extent that we need for the modelling process; nor will we quote many of the standard trigonometric formulae.

Angular frequency

We treat θ as a function of time. We view the arrow as rotating at a particular constant angular frequency measured in ω radians per second (rad/s). If the oscillation has a frequency of 1 Hz, it completes one full cycle in 1 s. This is 2π radians, so the angular frequency ω is 2π rad/s. Hence frequency $f = \omega/2\pi$ cycles per second, or $\omega = 2\pi f$ rad/s.
Thus $\theta = \omega t = 2\pi ft$ and we obtain sinusoidal functions of time; $\sin \omega t$, $\cos \omega t$, and so on.

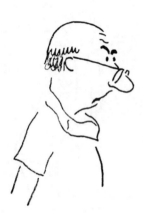

Translations: interconversion of sin and cos

The shape and size of the basic sin and cos functions are identical; the only difference is the starting point. We can transform sin into cos or vice versa by a simple horizontal translation.

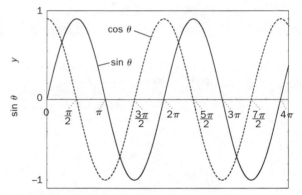

The curves of the functions $\sin \theta$ and $\cos \theta$ are identical except for their position along the axis. We can superimpose the curve of $\cos \theta$ on to that for $\sin \theta$ by shifting it along the axis to the right by $\pi/2$: $\sin \theta = \cos(\theta - \pi/2)$. Another way of looking at it is to shift sin to the left by $\pi/2$: $\cos \theta = \sin(\theta + \pi/2)$. Because of the cyclical repetitive pattern every 2π, these transformations are also true for any shifts of 2π (in either direction) in addition to these.

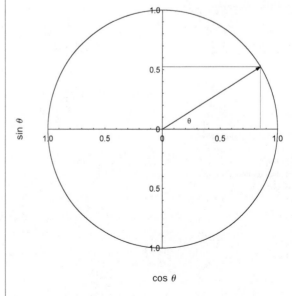

The horizontal axis and the rotating arrow make an angle θ. This is how the sin and cos functions are defined. In this book, we are only interested in time-dependent oscillations where the angle θ is itself a function of time.

2.10.3 Amplitude and phase

Transformations: scaling and translations

Translations of the basic function curves in the horizontal direction are termed *phase shifts*. The curve for cos can be obtained from the curve for sin by a phase shift of $\pi/2$ to the left; the curves are $\pi/2$ out of phase. Amplitude is the peak excursion of the oscillation from the central value. The basic functions have amplitude of unity.

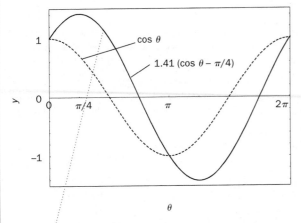

This sinusoid is shifted relative to the basic cos curve. It reaches a peak value at $\pi/4$ and so has a phase *lag* compared to the cos curve of $\pi/4$, since it reaches its peak later than cos. It is also a larger oscillation than the basic cos curve. Its peak displacement from the horizontal axis is about 1.4 instead of 1. The peak displacement of a sinusoid from its central value is the *amplitude* of the waveform.

The amplitude is a scaling in the vertical direction of the basic function. By incorporating the ideas of scaling and translation, we can describe any sinusoidal oscillation in terms of the basic cos function. We could equally well use the sin function as our building block.

General sinusoidal function

We have taken *two* basic functions—sin and cos, defined in terms of the x and y co-ordinates of the rotating arrow—and found another function, the general sinusoidal function that can be constructed from either of the originals by applying standard transformations e.g.:

$$y = A \cos(\omega t + \phi) + k$$

A is the vertical scaling factor for the amplitude. k is the vertical translation, which defines the mean value of the oscillation. ϕ ($-\pi < \phi < \pi$) is the phase shift (horizontal translation), which may be negative (phase lag) or positive (phase lead).

amplitude   angular frequency
(vertical scaling)   (horizontal scaling)

$$y = A \cos(\omega t + \phi) + k$$

phase shift   vertical shift
(horizontal shift)

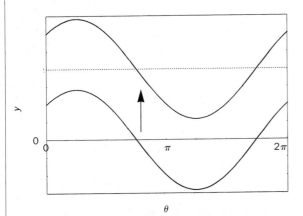

We may wish to describe a wave that oscillates about an axis other than $y = 0$. A blood pressure waveform oscillates about a mean value; say, 95 mmHg. This requires a simple translation in the vertical direction—the addition of a constant k.

2.10.4   Angular frequency

Transformations: horizontal scaling

The modelling examples of waveforms in this book are all functions of time. The frequency of the oscillation is measured as ω, the angular frequency in rad/s. The general sinusoidal function of time is given by $y = A\cos(\omega t + \phi) + k$. Increasing the value of ω increases the rapidity of oscillation; decreasing ω slows the oscillation. This is a horizontal scaling of the basic waveform—it expands or compresses the basic waveform along the time axis.

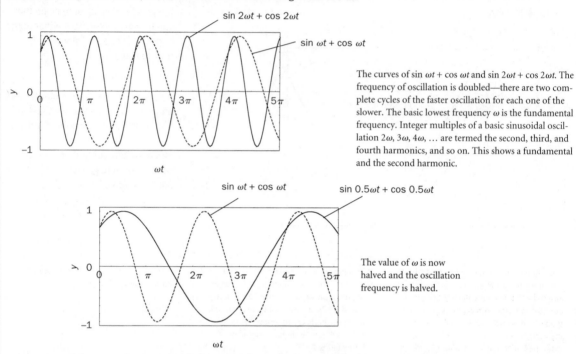

sin $2\omega t$ + cos $2\omega t$

sin ωt + cos ωt

The curves of sin ωt + cos ωt and sin $2\omega t$ + cos $2\omega t$. The frequency of oscillation is doubled—there are two complete cycles of the faster oscillation for each one of the slower. The basic lowest frequency ω is the fundamental frequency. Integer multiples of a basic sinusoidal oscillation 2ω, 3ω, 4ω, ... are termed the second, third, and fourth harmonics, and so on. This shows a fundamental and the second harmonic.

sin ωt + cos ωt

sin $0.5\omega t$ + cos $0.5\omega t$

The value of ω is now halved and the oscillation frequency is halved.

Derivatives of sin and cos

We shall need to know a little about the rates of change (2.12.1) of sinusoidal functions, the derivatives of sin θ and cos θ. These are particularly simple. The derivative of sin θ = cos θ.

The curves for sin θ and cos θ are shown: sin θ reaches a peak at $\pi/2$, at which point cos $\theta = 0$. The gradient at a maximum or minimum point must equal zero (2.13.1). Similarly, sin θ reaches a minimum at $3\pi/2$, at which point cos $\theta = 0$. Sin is *increasing* most rapidly at 0, 2π, 4π, ..., where cos has its maximum value 1, so the gradient at this point is unity: sin is *decreasing* most rapidly at π, 3π, 5π, ..., where cos = −1, so the gradient here is −1.

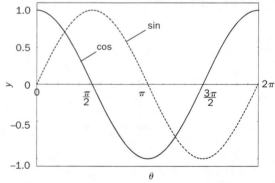

The curve for cos reaches a maximum value 1 at 0, 2π, 4π. ... Its gradient at a maximum must equal zero. Similarly, it reaches a minimum value at π, 3π, 5π ..., and the gradient at a minimum point is also zero. At these same points, the value of sin $\theta = 0$. So is sin θ the derivative of cos θ?

When cos θ is *decreasing* most rapidly—as it crosses the axis at $\pi/2$—the value of sin $\theta = 1$. Since the value of sin is positive and the gradient to cos is negative at this point, the derivative of cos θ cannot be sin θ. A similar argument applies at $3\pi/2$ when cos is increasing most rapidly and sin θ has the value −1. The derivative of cos θ is in fact − sin θ.

The main point to remember is that however many times we differentiate or integrate sin and cos functions, we will get sin and cos functions. Sinusoidal functions have incestuous derivatives like the exponential functions—it is all kept in the family.

2.10.5 **Sums of sinusoids**

Adding sin and cos: amplitude and phase

What happens when we add one sinusoid to another of the same frequency? Since sin and cos are out of phase with each other, the amplitudes do not simply add because the peaks and troughs are occurring at different times in the cycle.

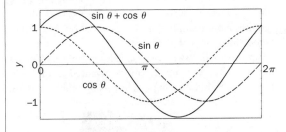

The basic cos and sin functions are shown together with the function that results when we add them together. The amplitude of the sum is greater than the amplitude (1) of the individual constituents, but less than the sum of the amplitudes (1 + 1). The amplitude is in fact $\sqrt{2} = 1.4142\ldots$

Not only is the amplitude increased, but the peak now occurs at a point intermediate between the peaks for the constituent curves—there is a phase shift relative to the constituent sinusoids. We have added two sinusoids of equal amplitude together. This curve can be described as either $1.4142 \cos(\theta - \pi/4)$ or $\sin\theta + \cos\theta$ the two descriptions are entirely equivalent.

Sums of sinusoids

Any arbitrary simple sinusoid can be described in terms of scaling and translation of the basic cos function $y = C\cos(\omega t + \phi) + k$, or as a sum of a sin and a cos function of the same angular frequency ω,
$A\cos\omega t + B\sin\omega t = C\cos(\omega t - \phi)$. They are two ways of expressing the same thing.
Where

$$C = \sqrt{A^2 + B^2} \text{ and } \phi = \text{arc}\cos\left(\frac{A}{\sqrt{A^2 + B^2}}\right)$$

arccos is the inverse function of cos and answers the question if the cos of an angle ϕ is z (i.e. $\cos\phi = z$), what is the angle ϕ?
   This looks very complicated, but is really just Pythagoras' theorem.
If we have $A = 3$ and $B = 4$, then
$y = 4\cos\omega t + 3\sin\omega t$ and we obtain $y = 5\cos(\omega t - 0.927)$, i.e.
$C = 5$. $\phi = 0.927 = 53.13°$.
   Because sin and cos are at right-angles to each other in their projections, they 'pull' in different directions, and we need to add them like we add forces in physics, using vector addition.

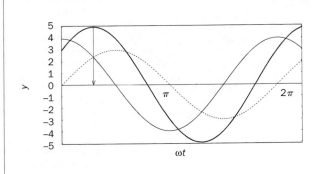

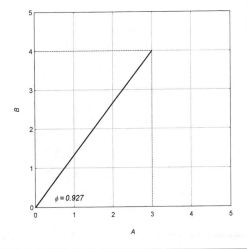

2.11.1   **Surfaces**

We have concentrated largely on situations in which the function value (the dependent variable) is determined by the value of a single independent variable. However, there are many circumstances in which we have functions that are dependent upon a number of variables. The first model that we constructed for the relationship of $PaCO_2$ and $\dot{V}A$ assumed a fixed value of CO_2 production, $\dot{V}CO_2$. We later allowed this to change and produced a 3-D graph, the surface of which showed all possible combinations of $\dot{V}ACO_2$, $\dot{V}CO_2$, and the resulting $PaCO_2$ according to the model. This was an example of a function of two variables. In fact, there was another variable, the atmospheric pressure P_I present in the equation, which we did not allow to vary. Evidently in reality this too varies, and altitude physiology requires close examination of this variation, but to keep things simple and comprehensible, we fixed it. This is the essence of modelling.

We can in principle treat functions of more than one variable in similar ways to those with a single independent variable—differentiation, determination of maxima and minima, integration, and so on, but these involve more advanced mathematical methods. We can deal with functions of more than two variables mathematically, but drawing graphs becomes impossible—we have only three dimensions to display on.

The surface that we used for the rebreathing example(1.5.2) can be used to describe the equilibrium ICP for different input values of CSF flow, $\dot{Q}_{CSF}$, and uptake pathway conductance (1.2.3). The threshold value for uptake is fixed and is indicated by the height of the platform. The rebreathing and CSF dynamics models are essentially the same. [Analogues: Output variables: ICP and $\dot{P}aCO_2$. Input variables: uptake conductance and $\dot{V}A$, $\dot{Q}_{CSF}$ and $\dot{V}CO_2$, uptake threshold and $PICO_2$].

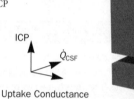

ICP

$\dot{Q}_{CSF}$

Uptake Conductance

Functions of two variables

A straight line is completely determined if we know its gradient and where it crosses the *y*-axis (or any other defined point that it goes through). If we are trying to decide a best-fit straight line to a data set (3.18), then the technique that we use must tell us the gradient and the intercept of the line. We use the least squares method, which minimizes the total of squared deviations from the line. The *RSS* is therefore a function of both the gradient and the intercept that we choose—i.e. a function of two variables. We select the gradient and the intercept to give us the minimum value of this function—the least squares that we can achieve by fitting a line.

The binormal joint distribution (3.19.1) is another example from statistics.

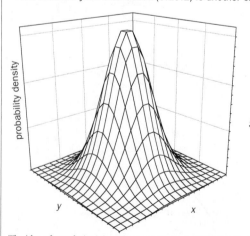

probability density

y   *x*

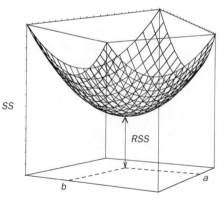

SS

RSS

b   *a*

The error function for the least squares method is a paraboloid—a 3-D version of a parabola. It has a minimum value *RSS* at certain values of gradient b and intercept a. These are the values that we choose to define our line. It is the same process as the error function for the mean, except that we now need to define two values to minimize the function.

The idea of correlation gives rise to a joint probability distribution, where the probability of a combination of values of the two constituent variables is determined. This probability is the output of a probability density function which requires the input of a value from each variable—a function of two variables.

2.12.1 Modelling, gradients, and rates of change: the derivative

Modelling processes frequently give rise to equations that describe the *rate of change* of a quantity. We saw this in the applications of the IOP to time-dependent variables such as step change in ventilation, nitrogen washout, pharmacokinetics, and simple harmonic motion. The simplest rate of change to deal with is when this is zero—the system is in steady state and the value of the quantity remains constant. We modelled steady-state conditions quite easily with $PaCO_2$ and $\dot{V}A$. We calculated steady-state $PaCO_2$ using modelling assumptions and simple arithmetic (1.3).

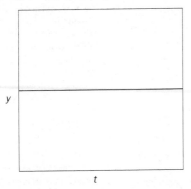

The next most easily modelled situation is that in which the value of the quantity of interest is changing, but is doing so at a constant rate. This is what we saw with the example of $PaCO_2$ and apnoeic oxygenation (1.8). We started with the empirical observation that the rate of rise of $PaCO_2$ in apnoea is approximately linear, and we modelled the problem with a single compartment. This problem was easily solved, with only elementary arithmetic, because we had a starting value for $PaCO_2$ and the assumption that its rate of rise was constant at 0.5 kPa/min. This enabled us to calculate the $PaCO_2$ predicted by the model at any time t thereafter.

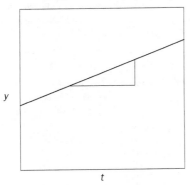

The mathematical problem became more difficult when we looked at nitrogen washout or the step change in ventilation problems since the rates of change of FAN_2 and $PaCO_2$ were no longer constant; they themselves were changing with time (1.9, 1.11). School arithmetic was no longer sufficient to solve the problem, although the principle of having an expression for the rate of change of a quantity with time and wishing to know the actual value of that quantity at any time was exactly the same. To solve these problems we needed knowledge of the behaviour of exponential functions (2.9). The basic exponential $y = e^x$ has a rate of change equal to the function value itself.

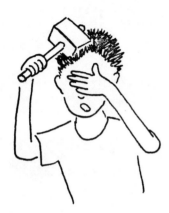

The derivative

The derivative is the gradient to a curve at any point. Its mathematical description is quite rigorous, but all we need to appreciate is that we can make a better and better approximation to the gradient of the curve at any point by making the interval between this point and an arbitrary adjacent one smaller and smaller. We can define a limiting value that this approximation approaches as we make the interval shrink towards zero.

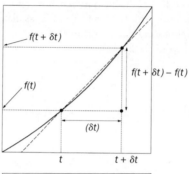

We have an arbitrary non-linear function, the value of which is here increasing as t increases. The gradient or rate of change is thus positive and changing with time. If we take any interval δt, we can make a straight-line approximation for the rate at which the function is increasing over the interval, by calculating the difference in the value of the function at the end of the interval and the value of the function at the beginning of the interval, $f(t + \delta t) - f(t)$, and dividing this by the time over which this change occurs, δt:

$$\frac{f(t + \delta t) - f(t)}{\delta t}.$$

If the interval is wide, the gradient at the beginning of the interval and the gradient at the end of the interval may be quite different, but the smaller we make δt, the smaller will be the change in gradient over the interval. We allow the size of the interval to shrink towards zero and the gradient approaches a limiting value; δt can never actually *become* zero, since we cannot divide by zero.

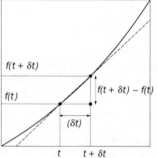

If we continue the process of making δt smaller and smaller, the gradient calculated becomes closer and closer to a limiting value. The limit that

$$\frac{f(t + \delta t) - f(t)}{\delta t}$$

approaches as we allow δt to shrink towards zero is the *derivative* of the function f at that point. This is denoted $f'(t)$.

$$\lim_{\delta t \to 0} \frac{f(t + \delta t) - f(t)}{\delta t} = f'(t).$$

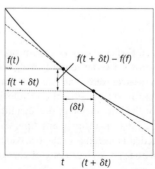

If a function is *declining* in value, then $f(t + \delta t) < f(t)$, so that $\frac{f(t + \delta t) - f(t)}{\delta t}$ is negative. If the gradient to the curve is negative at a point, the function is decreasing in value at that point.

If the gradient of a function is *zero* everywhere, then the function is the *constant function*, since $f(t + \delta t) - f(t) = 0$.

If the gradient of a function is a *non-zero constant* everywhere, then the function is a *linear function* since, $f(t + \delta t) - f(t)$ has the same non-zero value for any interval of width δt.

2.12.2 Limits

The idea of an approximation of one function to another is a common theme in this book. We encounter the idea of a limit in a number of contexts. This is actually a very subtle and important idea, but we need only to have a general graphical understanding of the concept. We met the idea in the alveolar ventilation example, in which $PaCO_2$ approached the horizontal axis as we increased the $\dot{V}A$. $PaCO_2$ can never cross the axis and become negative, but approaches it more and more closely as we increase $\dot{V}A$. In practice, there is of course a limit to how far we can increase $\dot{V}A$, but the *model* allows us to increase it without limit. There are plenty of other examples of asymptotic behaviour in the book—the power function (3.15.5), dose response curves (1.14.3), probability distributions, and so on.

Limiting behaviour: e

An important example of a limiting value is the function

$$y = \left(1 + \frac{1}{n}\right)^n.$$

This function approaches a limiting constant value as we increase the value of n. When $n = 1$, the function has value

$$y = \left(1 + \frac{1}{1}\right)^1 = 2$$

and when $n = 2$,

$$y = \left(1 + \frac{1}{2}\right)^2 = 1.5^2 = 2.25$$

and so on. The graph of the function is shown. As n increases, the expression inside the brackets becomes closer and closer to 1, but this is raised to a higher and higher power; 1 raised to any power is 1, but if we raise any number greater than one to a power greater than 1, it increases. The function approaches a limit which is the result of the 'battle' between these two tendencies. We do not prove it, but this limit is the number e = 2.718281828... .

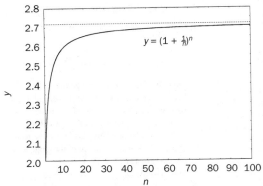

$y = (1 + \frac{1}{n})^n$

A limit for our purposes is a line or curve i.e. a function that we can approach (i.e. approximate to) as closely as we like without ever quite getting there.

By $n = 100$, the function value has reached 2.70481 .... . This is less than e, but we can see from the graph that it seems to be approaching some limiting value between 2.70 and 2.72. As we increase the value of n further, the graph approaches the dotted line more and more closely. The graph has an asymptote which is *e*. We can approach *e* arbitrarily closely with our function by increasing n, but never actually reach it. *However large we make n, our evaluation of e will always be an approximation.*

Notation for derivatives

There are two notational systems for derivatives in common use, and each has its advantages we use them interchangeably:

- *Functional notation.* The rate of change of a general function $f(x)$, its derivative, is denoted by $f'(x)$, said '*f* prime of *x*'. Higher-order derivatives are described by $f''(x)$, $f'''(x)$, and so on.
- *Leibnitz notation.* This is probably more familiar from scientific texts. The general function y, where y is some function of x (i.e. $y = f(x)$), has a first derivative denoted by dy/dx and higher derivatives d^2y/dx^2, d^3y/dx^3, and so on.

Thus:

$f(x) = y$,
$f'(x) = dy/dx$, $\quad f''(x) = d^2y/dx^2$,

and so forth.

There is an apparent paradox in our derivation of differential equations. On the one had, we seem to treat the change in the concentration, say, on one side of the equation as negligible over an arbitrary small time interval, δt, if this interval is 'small enough'; while at the same time, for the identical small time interval δt, we treat the change in concentration $[C(t + \delta t) - C(t)]$ as appreciable. When we divide this $[C(t + \delta t) - C(t)]$ by δt, we approximate this to the gradient to the function 'in the limit as $\delta t \to 0$'. This question caused great debate in mathematics in the early 19th century, and was only resolved by the refinement of the concept of the limit, which is a great deal more subtle than this brief glimpse might suggest. In essence, if the function is differentiable at a point, the derivative at that point is a limiting function that is approached as we shrink δt towards zero, just as the number e is a limiting value that is approached as we increase n towards infinity. This is the subject matter of real analysis.

2.12.3 Differentiation 1

Differentiation is the process of finding the derivative or rate of change of a function. If we differentiate a function, we obtain another function that describes the gradient at any point. This is generally quite a straightforward business once the rules have been learnt. We shall only describe some simple derivatives for reference, since we wish to concentrate on the modelling process rather than mathematical methods. Differentiation of even quite complicated expressions is not difficult with a little practice.

Differentiation of combinations of functions

There are a few rules that allow differentiation of complicated functions made up of basic functions. These are for reference only, but can be checked with the table of derivatives.

- *The sum rule.* The derivative of a sum is the sum of the individual derivatives:

$$\frac{d}{dx}[f(x) + g(x)] = f'(x) + g'(x);$$

for example,

$$\frac{d}{dx}[\sin x + x^2]$$

$$= \left[\frac{d}{dx}\sin x + \frac{d}{dx}x^2\right] = \cos x + 2x.$$

This extends to the case of 'adding' a negative function, i.e. the derivative of a difference is the difference of the individual derivatives:

$$\frac{d}{dx}[f(x) - g(x)] = f'(x) - g'(x).$$

- *The constant multiplier rule:*

$$\frac{d}{dx}k[f(x)] = kf'(x);$$

for example,

$$\frac{d}{dx}3[\sin x] = 3\cos x.$$

- *The product and quotient rule:*

$$\frac{d}{dx}[f(x) \times g(x)]$$

$$= f'(x)g(x) + f(x)g'(x)$$

and $\dfrac{d}{dx}\left[\dfrac{f(x)}{g(x)}\right]$

$$= \frac{1}{(g(x))^2}[f'(x)g(x) - f(x)g'(x)];$$

for example,

$$\frac{d}{dx}[\sin x \times x^2] = \frac{d}{dx}[\sin x] \times x^2$$

$$+ \frac{d}{dx}(x^2) \times \sin x$$

$$= x^2 \cos x + 2x \sin x,$$

$$\frac{d}{dx}\left[\frac{\sin x}{(x^2)}\right] = \frac{1}{((x^2))^2}$$

$$\left[\frac{d[\sin x]}{dx}g(x) - \sin x \frac{d(x^2)}{dx}\right]$$

$$= \frac{1}{x^4}[x^2 \cos x - 2x \sin x].$$

Limits and the derivative of $y = x^2$

We take another example of a limiting process in arriving at the derivative of $y = x^2$.

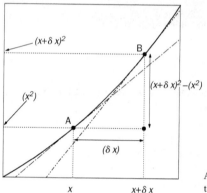

We consider a detail of the graph of $y = x^2$ and the usual arbitrary small interval δx. If the interval is wide, then the tangents to the graph at the beginning and end of the interval have appreciably different gradients. We wish to establish the limiting value of this gradient as the interval is allowed to shrink towards zero.

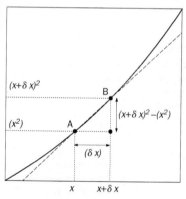

As we know, the addition of a constant term makes no difference to the gradient of a function, so this is also the gradient of $y = a + x^2$.

Scaling by any factor b, merely scales the gradient too, so that $y = a + bx^2$ has derivative

$$\frac{d}{dx}(a + bx^2) = 2bx.$$

At the start of the interval. The function value is $f(x) = x^2$ and at the end of the interval is $f(x + \delta x) = (x + \delta x)^2$. The change in value of the function over this interval is thus

$$f(x + \delta x) - f(x) = (x + \delta x)^2 - x^2$$

$$= (x^2 + 2x\delta x + \delta x^2) - x^2$$

$$= 2x\delta x + \delta x^2$$

This is the gradient of the chord between the points $A = (x, x^2)$ and $B = ((x + \delta x), (x + \delta x)^2)$.

We are interested in establishing the gradient of the function which is the limiting value of

$\dfrac{f(x + \delta x) - f(x)}{\delta x}$ as we shrink the interval towards zero, $\lim \delta x \to 0 \; \dfrac{2x\delta x + \delta x^2}{\delta x}$. As the points become closer together as δx becomes smaller (δx^2) becomes negligible and we can see that the value of the limit becomes $2x$. δx can approach zero arbitrarily closely, but cannot ever be zero (division by zero is meaningless). This is the gradient of the tangent to the curve at any point (x, x^2) and is the derivative of

$$y = x^2; \; \frac{d}{dx}(x^2) = 2x$$

Differentiation of simple functions

We have met some derivatives already; the rate of change of a constant function is evidently zero by definition. Similarly, a linear function has a constant gradient, so that the rate of change is constant.

The basic exponential function has a gradient that is equal to the function value itself, which makes it of very special importance. Transformed versions of the basic exponential function have derivatives that are proportional to the function value at any point. The gradient of the natural log function and how it relates to the exponential has been explained (2.9.5). Transformed versions of the log function will have derivatives that are just variants of the basic rectangular hyperbola.

The sinusoidal functions have derivatives that are also sinusoidal functions (2.10.4) like the exponential functions, the derivatives are kept within the family. We shall see that this fact makes these functions very important in solving differential equations.

- *The function of a function rule (chain rule).* This applies when one function of x, $g(x)$, is transformed by another function e.g. the sin function of x is squared $(\sin x)^2$:

$$\frac{\mathrm{d}}{\mathrm{d}x}\{f[g(x)]\} = \frac{\mathrm{d}}{\mathrm{d}x}[g(x)] \times g'(x)$$

$$\frac{\mathrm{d}}{\mathrm{d}x}\{\sin^2 x\} = \frac{\mathrm{d}}{\mathrm{d}x}\{\sin x\}^2$$

$$= 2\sin x \cdot \cos x$$

Table of derivatives

Function $f(x)$	Derivative $f'(x)$	
Constant k	0	
Ax^n	nAx^{n-1}	
Ae^x	Ae^x	
Ae^{nx}	nAe^{nx}	
$\log_e x$	$\dfrac{1}{x}$	k, a, A. constants.
$\dfrac{1}{a}\log_e(k-ax)$	$\dfrac{1}{(k-ax)}$	
$\sin ax$	$a\cos ax$	
$a\cos ax$	$-a\sin ax$	

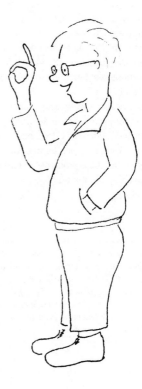

2.12.4 Differentiation 2

Derivatives of exponential functions

The general exponential function is $y = Ae^{\alpha t}$. We know that the basic exponential function $y = e^t$ has a derivative that is the same as the function itself: $dy/dt = e^t$. The scaled version $y = Ae^{\alpha t}$, where either A or α (or both) have values which are not unity—*neither* can be zero for an exponential function—has a derivative $dy/dt = \alpha Ae^{\alpha t}$.

This is in accordance with the rules: A is a constant multiple and just multiplies the basic derivative by A. On the other hand, α is a function within a function; the basic is $y = e^t$, and multiplying the exponent by α is not a simple multiple—it is a function of a function. The 'inner' function is αt, which then becomes the input into an exponential function, so we need the chain rule.

The negative exponential functions are merely forms of the equivalent positive function reflected about the y-axis. Symmetry tells us that the magnitude of the gradients will be equivalent, but the gradients will be negative.

The rate constant of the exponential process, α, is just that—a *rate* constant—and determines the horizontal scaling or speed at which the exponential process is occurring. Because this is a scaling of the *exponent*, this is not a simple multiple. For instance, if $\alpha = 2$ this means that $y = e^{2t} = e^t \times e^t$. The combination of these scalings should make the derivative seem sensible. If $y = Ae^{\alpha t}$, then $dy/dt = \alpha Ae^{\alpha t}$.

Derivative of linear functions

The linear function $y = a + bx$ has a constant rate of change, and this is determined by the value of the coefficient b, the gradient of the line, which may be positive (increasing function) or negative (decreasing function). The position of the intersection with the y-axis has no bearing upon the rate of change, but does determine the position of the line and hence the function value.

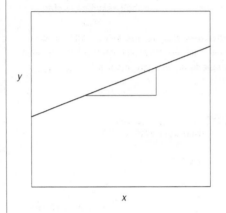

The derivative of $y = a + bx$ is $dy/dx = b$ (or alternatively, in function notation, $f(x) = a + bx$, $f'(x) = b$). The derivative does not depend upon the value of x, because the gradient is the same everywhere, b. In differentiating, any constant terms disappear because the rate of change of a constant is zero—obvious! This is differentiation of a sum, and the derivative is the sum of the derivatives of the constituents: $dy/dx = b + 0$.

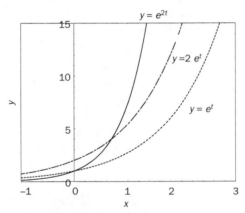

Since $y = Ae^t$ is just a vertically scaled version of $y = e^t$, the function value is changing A times as fast as the basic function. Its rate of change must therefore be $dy/dt = Ae^t$. This is a simple multiple of the rate of change of the basic function.

The rate of change of $y = 2e^t$ looks to be twice that of the basic function $y = e^t$, as we expect. Note that $y = 2e^t$ crosses the y-axis at $y = 2$. The graph of $y = e^{2t}$ crosses the y-axis at $y = 1$, but is increasing much more rapidly than either of the other two functions. The gradient at $t = 1$ is actually greater by a factor of $2e$—i.e. approximately 5.4—than the basic function. At $t = 2$ the gradient is greater by a factor $2e^2 \approx 14.8$.

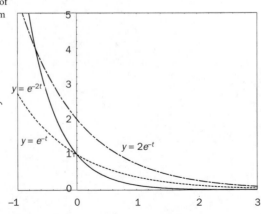

2.13.1   Local behaviour of functions

We often wish to know if a function has a maximum or a minimum value, and if so, where. Differentiation is the key to finding maxima and minima. To have a *maximum value*, the function must increase (+ve gradient) and then decrease (−ve gradient) as x increases. To have a *minimum value*, the function must decrease (−ve gradient) and then increase (+ve gradient) as x increases. In passing from +ve to −ve or vice versa, the gradient must be zero at the minimum or maximum point if the function is continuous. If we can determine where the gradient is zero, we have found a maximum or minimum point. Note that in more complicated functions the occurrence of a maximum or minimum is a feature of the *local* behaviour of the function. Many functions do not have maxima or minima; look at constant, linear, simple, and sum exponentials. The difference of two exponentials, however, may have a maximum or minimum (2.9.11).

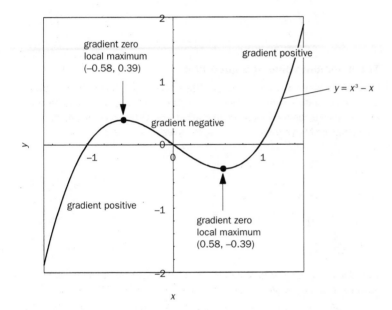

Any point where the derivative of a function and hence its gradient takes a value zero is called a stationary point. Not all stationary points are local maxima or minima. If we look at the graph of $y = x^3$ we can see that the gradient flattens out as it approaches zero. $\frac{d}{dx}\left(x^3\right) = 3x^2$, so that when $x = 0$, the gradient is also zero and we have a stationary point, but this is not a local maximum or minimum; the gradient is always positive except at $x = 0$ (because $3x^2$ is always positive or zero—what does the graph of $y = 3x^2$ look like? (2.7.3)).

The graph of $y = x^3 + x$ has no stationary points; we can see that it is increasing for all values of x. $\frac{d}{dx}\left(x^3 + x\right) = 3x^2 + 1$ which is always positive. There is no real solution to the equation $3x^2 + 1 = 0$; this is the same as saying that the graph of $y = 3x^2 + 1$ does not cross the x-axis (it is a vertical translation of $y = 3x^2$) and thus has no real roots (2.7.3, 2.7.4).

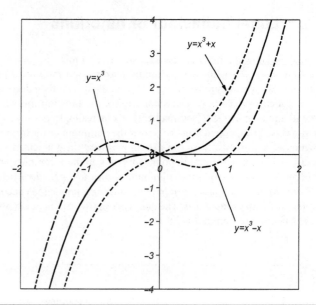

The minimum value of a quadratic

Error functions are described in (3.10). The squared deviation technique gives rise to a quadratic expression $TSS = 9x^2 + 72x + 196$, and we wish to minimize this to select a summary measure that minimizes dispersion of the data. Differentiation of this expression using the rules in (2.12.3) gives us

$$\frac{\mathrm{d}}{\mathrm{d}x}(9x^2 - 72x + 196) = 18x - 72.$$

Equating this derivative to zero,

$$18x - 72 = 0,$$
$$x = \frac{72}{18} = 4.$$

The minimum value indeed occurs at $x = 4$. The value here is $TSS = 52$. The minimum value of a quadratic $a + bx + cx^2$ occurs at $x = b/2c = 72/18 = 4$.

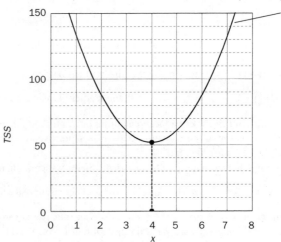

The function appears to have a minimum value $x = 4$.

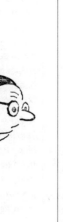

2.14.1   Anti-differentiation: integration

If we have a differentiable function, we can find its derivative and hence the gradient at any point on the graph. Our modelling equations are frequently expressed in terms of the rate of change or gradient of a quantity, and our task is to recover the original function. This process is integration, and is the reverse process of differentiation. The function the derivative of which we know is called a primitive. This is expressed in function notation as: $F(x)$ is a primitive of $f(x)$ which in turn has a derivative $f'(x)$. This also means that $F'(x) = f(x)$ and $F''(x) = f'(x)$.

A simple integration

The rate of change of a linear function is constant, because its graph is a straight line—i.e. of constant gradient. The derivative of $y = a + bx$ is b. Therefore if the rate of change of a quantity is constant, the function itself—the primitive—must be a linear function of the form $y = a + bx$. This is effectively the process that we used in solving the apnoeic oxygenation problem (1.8). Since any constant terms disappear on differentiation—because their rate of change is zero—we must re-introduce an arbitrary constant each time we perform an integration.

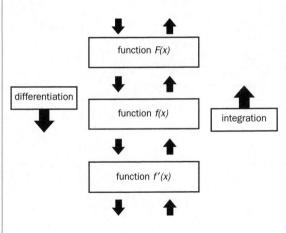

There is nothing sacred about a primitive or a derivative—each is a function in its own right. The terms refer only to the relationship between them. A derivative is obtained from a function by differentiation. If we integrate the derivative we can recover the original function (to within a constant). We have found a primitive.

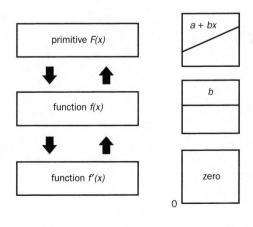

A function has only one derivative—it is unique, even if there is more than one way of expressing it. A function can, however, have an infinite number of primitives, because the constant term that we introduce can in principle take an infinite number of values. We always need some further information to select a particular function as the primitive we need.

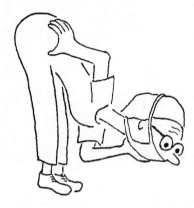

Standard integrals

Unlike differentiation, which is a straightforward application of rules, finding a primitive of a function is often difficult, or even impossible. Tables of known integrals are available, but many common functions have no primitive expressible in terms of known basic functions. This does not mean that these functions have no meaning or do not exist; they just have no simple integral. The normal distribution bell-curve function (3.11), for example, has no integral and other methods must be employed to evaluate the cumulative function numerically.

Table of integrals

$f'(x)$	$F(x)$
0	Constant k
Constant k	kx
Ax	$\dfrac{Ax^2}{2}$
Ax^n	$\dfrac{Ax^{n+1}}{n+1}$
Ae^{ax}	$\dfrac{A}{a}e^{ax}$
$\sin ax$	$-\dfrac{\cos ax}{a}$
$\cos ax$	$\dfrac{\sin ax}{a}$
$\dfrac{1}{x}$	$\log_e x$
$\dfrac{1}{(k-ax)}$	$\dfrac{1}{a}\log_e(k-ax)$

2.14.2 Integration and areas under curves

Integration arises naturally when we wish to find solutions to a differential equation, an equation which describes the rate of change of a quantity that interests us. Integration, if it can actually be performed, allows us to obtain the function for the quantity itself.

The other context in which integration frequently arises is the calculation of areas under curves; when we looked at step change in alveolar ventilation (1.11), we were able, from physiological argument, to predict the relationship of two areas bounded by curves. Integration allows us actually to evaluate those areas.

Areas under curves and integrals

What is the connection between finding a function the rate of change of which we know—solving a differential equation—and calculating areas under curves? The solution of the differential equation demands that we find a *function* and the calculation of an area under a curve requires us to find a *number*—the area. Let us look again at an arbitrary increasing function of time similar to the one which we looked at when considering the derivative.

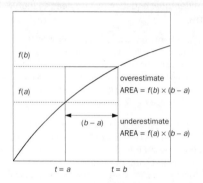

Suppose that we want to find the area under the curve between two points $t = a$ and $t = b$. We can make a crude overestimate by calculating the area of a rectangle $f(b) \times (b - a)$. We can similarly make a crude underestimate by calculating the area of a rectangle $f(a) \times (b - a)$. The true area will lie between these: $f(a) \times (b - a) < \text{AUC} < f(b) \times (b - a)$.

If we split the interval $[a,b]$ into two and perform the same process, we can make a better estimate of the area by adding the two lower rectangles (underestimate) or the two complete rectangles (overestimate). The true area will lie more closely between these. As we did with the derivative, we can split up the interval $[a, b]$ into smaller and smaller intervals δt. As the value of δt approaches zero, the upper and lower estimates get ever closer together—they approach a limit, the true area under the curve.

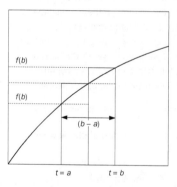

If we assume that there is function $I(t)$ which gives the true area under the curve, this will be a function of time, since the area under the curve depends upon how far along the axis we are. The true area under the curve in the interval $[t, t + \delta t]$ will therefore be $I(t + \delta t) - I(t)$: and will have a value between an underestimate and an overestimate calculated in this way.

$$f(t) \times \delta t < I(t + \delta t) - I(t) < f(t + \delta t) \times \delta t.$$
Dividing through by δt, we obtain

$$f(t) < \frac{I(t + \delta t) - I(t)}{\delta t} < f(t + \delta t).$$

As δt approaches zero and $f(t)$ and $f(t + \delta t)$ become more nearly identical, the expression in the middle of the sandwich becomes the derivative, of $I(t)$ and we have $I'(t) = f(t)$. This means that $f(t)$ is the derivative of $I(t)$, and hence $I(t)$ is the integral or primitive of $f(t)$. Thus, if we can integrate $f(t)$, we can find the area under the curve of $f(t)$.

If we wish to evaluate the area in a particular interval $[a,b]$, then we simply have to calculate the area below the interval $I(a)$ and subtract it from the total area $I(b)$, i.e. $I(b) - I(a)$.

2.14.3 Definite and indefinite integrals

Notation for integrals

The notation for integration is based upon the symbol '∫', which is a form of S signifying a summation procedure, since the evaluation of areas under curves is essentially a summing of areas of rectangles. If we have a definite integral such as that shown here, then $\int_1^3 (2x+1)\,dx$. The dx is an indicator that we are integrating the area under a curve which is a function of x. The sub- and superscript on the integral sign mark the lower and upper limits for our integral. The notation becomes important in more complicated integrals than we are concerned with here.

We have seen that the derivative of $\log_e x = 1/x$ and hence

$$\int \frac{1}{x}\,dx = \log_e x + c \ .$$ This was apparent from the symmetry of the inverse functions $y = e^x$ and $y = \log_e x$ (2.9.5). We have also seen the connection between definite integrals and areas under curves and in (2.6.3) we noted the connection between the natural log function and the basic hyperbola, $y = 1/x$. If we evaluate the definite

integral $\int_1^x \frac{1}{x}\,dx$, we obtain the area

under the basic hyperbola between $x = 1$ and x.

$$\int_1^x \frac{1}{x}\,dx = \log_e x - \log_e 1$$

$$= \log_e x - 0$$

$$= \log_e x$$

For $x = 2$ in the definite integral, this area has value $\log_e 2 = 0.693$

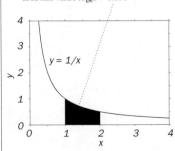

Evaluation of a simple integral

To demonstrate the technique, we will choose a straightforward example which can be checked with easy geometry. More involved integrals are evaluated in exactly the same way using the table of integrals in (2.14.1). We will evaluate the area under the graph of $y = 2x + 1$ between $x = 1$ and $x = 3$ by geometry and by using the integration tables.

The formula for this integral has an easily comprehensible geometric interpretation. We do not actually need the constant of integration here, because whatever constant we might introduce when we calculate the upper limit integral will be removed when we subtract the value evaluated at the lower limit of the integral. We are here calculating a *definite integral*—definite because the limits of the integral are defined ($x = 3$ and $x = 1$). Constants are not required for definite integrals. Note that the evaluation of a *definite integral* has given us a *number*—the area under the function curve. An *indefinite integral* gives us a *function*, which, when evaluated between defined limits, gives us the definite integral.

When we are integrating to solve a differential equation, we do need to introduce a constant, as we shall see (2.15).

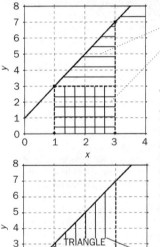

This is the area that we wish to calculate. It is bounded by the x-axis, the lines $x = 1$ and $x = 3$, and the line $y = 2x + 1$ above. Geometry suggests that we can calculate the area as the area of the rectangle $(2 \times 3) = 6$ + the area of the triangle $(4 \times 2)/2 = 4$. Area = 10.

The table of integrals tells us that the integral of $y = 2x + 1$, $\int (2x + 1)\,dx$, is $2x^2/2 + x +$ constant $= x^2 + x + c$. If we evaluate this for $x = 3$, we obtain $3^2 + 3 + C = 12 + C$. But this is the area under the curve between $x = 0$ and $x = 3$, and we need to subtract the area under the graph between 0 and 1, so we evaluate the integral at $x = 1$. We obtain $1 + 1 + C = 2 + C$. $12 + C - (2 + C) = 10$ as required. Note that the constant of integration disappears when we evaluate the integral.

What we have done is to apply the formula $\int (2x + 1)\,dx = x^2 + x$. x^2 is the area of the right-angled triangle with sides $2x$ and x. For $x = 3$, this has value 9. This is the triangle here. x is the area of a rectangle of unit height and length x.

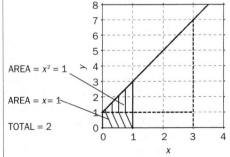

We need to subtract the area under the line between 0 and 1. This is evaluated from the integral in exactly the same way, by summing the area of the triangle and the rectangle.

AREA UNDER CURVE between $x = 1$ and $x = 3$ = $12 - 2 = 10$

2.14.4 Integration and areas: exponential models

Integrals and exponentials

The two-compartment model (1.13.5) gives us a solution equation:

$C_1(t) = Ae^{-\alpha t} + Be^{-\beta t}.$

Using the table of integrals (2.14.1), we obtain the integral of $C_1(t) = Ae^{-\alpha t} + Be^{-\beta t}$, as

$$\int C_1(t) = -\frac{A}{\alpha}e^{-\alpha t} - \frac{B}{\beta}e^{-\beta t}.$$

The integral of a sum function is the sum of the individual integrals.

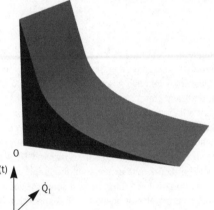

$C_1(t)$, $\dot{Q}_1$, t

The model requires that the AUC multiplied by the elimination clearance $\dot{Q}_1$ must give us the total dose M. This is the volume of the whole fluxoid.

$$\begin{aligned}
\text{AUC} &= \int_0^{\infty} C_1(t)\mathrm{d}t \\
&= \left[-\frac{A}{\alpha}e^{-\alpha t} - \frac{B}{\beta}e^{-\beta t} \right]_0^{\infty} \quad \cdots\cdots \text{ we evaluate at each of these limits} \\
&= [0] - \left[-\frac{A}{\alpha} - \frac{B}{\beta} \right] \quad \text{since } e^0 = 1 \text{ and } e^{-t} \to 0 \text{ as } t \to \infty \\
&= \left[\frac{A}{\alpha} + \frac{B}{\beta} \right] \\
&= \left[\frac{A\beta + B\alpha}{\alpha\beta} \right]
\end{aligned}$$

The elimination clearance $\dot{Q}_1 = V_1 k_{10}$

$$M = \left[\frac{A\beta + B\alpha}{\alpha\beta} \right]\dot{Q}_1 = \left[\frac{A\beta + B\alpha}{\alpha\beta} \right]k_{10}V_1$$

The quantity in the system at $t = 0$ is M. The quantity eliminated so far is 0.

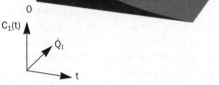

The quantity remaining in the system at $t = \infty$ is 0. The quantity eliminated is M. The solution function $C_1(t)$ has value 0 at $t = \infty$.

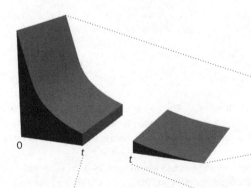

The quantity eliminated from the system at t is

$$\dot{Q}_1\left[\frac{A}{\alpha}e^{-\alpha t} + \frac{B}{\beta}e^{-\beta t} \right].$$

The quantity remaining in the system at t is

$$M - \dot{Q}_1\left[\frac{A}{\alpha}e^{-\alpha t} + \frac{B}{\beta}e^{-\beta t} \right].$$

Since $V_1 = \dfrac{M}{A + B}$, we have

$$M = \left[\frac{A}{\alpha} + \frac{B}{\beta} \right]k_{10}\frac{M}{A + B}$$ and solving for k_{10} we obtain

$$k_{10} = \frac{(A + B)\alpha\beta}{(A\beta + B\alpha)}$$

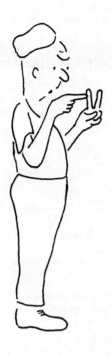

2.15.1 — Modelling with differential equations

We have seen plenty of examples in which our modelling has thrown up equations that describe the *rate of change* of the quantity that we are really interested in. These are examples of ordinary[*] differential equations (ODEs). Some of these—apnoeic oxygenation (1.8), for example—have been easy to solve; others—step change in V̇A (1.11), for example—have been soluble by other more technical methods;—and one ODE—air embolism (1.12)—has been insoluble except by using an appropriately programmed computer.

Most differential equations which arise in science and engineering are actually insoluble by other than numerical methods. General methods of solution to some classes of differential equation are available, but are beyond our scope; we shall be content to show how the differential equation and solution functions from some of our examples are related.

Direct integration

Sometimes we can use a technique of direct integration (i.e. using a table of integrals (2.14.1) to solve our differential equations, and this is what we do without even using any fancy mathematics when we have a rate of change $f'(x) = 0$ which must mean $f(x) = $ constant (i.e. a steady state); or a constant rate of change $f'(x) = $ constant, which must represent a linearly changing quantity $f(x) = a + bx$.

More mathematical sophistication is needed for dealing with second-order differential equations, but even some of these can be solved by direct integration. If $f(x) = a + bx + cx^2$, then $f'(x) = b + cx$ and $f''(x) = c$, so if we have a ODE with $f''(x) = c$, the solution function will be a quadratic expression, the graph of which will be a parabola. Acceleration due to gravity on Earth, g, is a constant quantity, and since acceleration is the second derivative of position with respect to time, we obtain a parabolic path predicted from Newton's Laws of Motion (1.16.3) for a particle moving under the influence of gravity. These applications of ODEs are in any text on elementary physics.

Our 'smooth' N_2 washout example, with V̇A modelled as a continuous flow, gave us an ODE

$$C'(t) = -\frac{V(A)}{V\text{FRC}} C(t)$$

This has the form $f'(x) = $ constant $\times f(x)$. The rate of change $f'(x)$ is proportional to the function value itself $f(x)$. We know that exponential functions have derivatives which are proportional to the function value (2.9.5), so the solution function must be exponential in form.

We can solve this by reference to tables of integrals (2.14.1). If $f(t) = Ae^{kt}$, then $f'(t) = kAe^{kt} = k \times f(t)$. Comparing with our ODE, $k = -V̇A/V_{\text{FRC}}$, so the solution is

$$C(t) = A \exp\left\{\frac{-V̇A}{V_{\text{FRC}}}t\right\}$$ where A is an arbitrary constant depending upon initial

conditions.

[*] These are ordinary because they have been functions of a *single* variable. Differentiation of a function of two or more variables is called *partial* differentiation; finding the minimum sum of squares—'least squares'—by choosing a slope and intercept of the regression line (3.18.2). involves partial differentiation. DEs involving partial derivatives are partial (i.e. not ordinary) DEs; these need advanced techniques.

2.15.2 First-order equations

Step change in $\dot{V}A$ ODE

In (1.11.2) we derived an ODE for the rate of change of $Paco_2$ following a step change in $\dot{V}A$:

$$(Paco_2(t))' = \frac{\dot{V}co_2 \times P_I}{D^*} - \frac{\dot{V}A}{D^*} \times Paco_2(t).$$

This is similar to the N_2 washout equation in that the rate of change is related to the function value itself, so we expect an exponential term in the solution. The difference is that this time we have a constant function

$$\frac{\dot{V}co_2 \times P_I}{D^*}$$

in the ODE as well, which makes a solution by 'guesswork' as we did for N_2 washout rather difficult.

We saw that the solution was

$$PaCO_2(t) = \frac{\dot{V}co_2 \times P_I}{\dot{V}A} + A \exp\left\{-\frac{\dot{V}A}{D^*}t\right\}$$

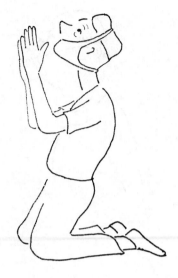

(where A is an arbitrary constant of integration), although we did not see where this solution came from. The solution is the sum of a constant term (the equilibrium solution) and a transient (time-dependent) term.

Note that this solution is not valid in apnoea ($\dot{V}A = 0$), since we may not divide by zero. The solution for apnoea is that $Paco_2$ is a linear function of time (which is what we started with).

$$Paco_2(t) = Paco_2(0) + at$$

where a is the rate of rise of $Paco_2$ in apnoea.

If we differentiate this solution function (2.12.3, 2.12.4), we obtain

$$(Paco_2(t))' = \left[-\frac{\dot{V}A}{D^*}\right] \times A \exp\left\{-\frac{\dot{V}A}{D^*}t\right\}.$$

Does this all fit together? Substituting for $Paco_2(t)$ into the ODE we get

$$(Paco_2(t))' = \frac{\dot{V}co_2 \times P_I}{D^*} - \frac{\dot{V}A}{D^*} \times PaCO_2(t)$$

$$(Paco_2(t))' = \frac{\dot{V}co_2 P_I}{D^*} - \frac{\dot{V}A}{D^*} \times \left[\frac{\dot{V}co_2.P_I}{\dot{V}A} + A \exp\left\{\frac{\dot{V}A}{D^*}t\right\}\right]$$

This expression in the brackets is just the solution function $Paco_2(t)$.

$$= \frac{\dot{V}co_2 P_I}{D^*} - \frac{\dot{V}A}{D^*}\left[\frac{\dot{V}co_2.P_I}{\dot{V}A}\right] - \frac{\dot{V}A}{D^*}\left[A \exp\left\{\frac{\dot{V}A}{D^*}t\right\}\right]$$

$$= 0 - \frac{\dot{V}A}{D^*} \times \left[A \exp\left\{-\frac{\dot{V}A}{D^*}t\right\}\right]$$

$$(Paco_2(t))' = -\frac{\dot{V}A}{D^*} A \exp\left\{-\frac{\dot{V}A}{D^*}t\right\}$$

So if we differentiate the solution function we get an expression which is equivalent to our modelling differential equation as required. Simple integration does not work here because we have the solution function itself and a constant in the ODE, and this solution required a standard technique for ODEs which we do not explore; details are available in texts listed in the bibliography.

2.15.3 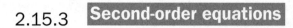 Second-order equations

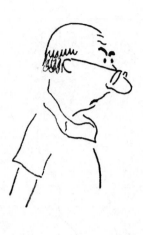

Second-order ODEs

Both the exponential functions and the sinusoidal functions have 'incestous' derivatives; all the derivatives of exponentials are exponentials; all derivatives of sinusoids are sinusoids. This makes the solution of some second-order equations possible.

The second-order ODE that we obtained from the two-compartment model (1.13.5) had the form:

$$aC''(t) + bC'(t) + cC(t) = 0$$

If we postulate a solution $C(t) = Ae^{\lambda t}$, then we obtain the following derivatives (2.12.3):

$$C(t) = Ae^{\lambda t},$$

$$C''(t) = \lambda A\, e^{\lambda t},$$

$$C''(t) = \lambda^2\, Ae^{\lambda t},$$

and the ODE can be arranged as

$$aC''(t) + bC'(t) + cC(t) = (a\lambda^2 + b\lambda + c)\, Ae^{\lambda t} = 0.$$

If we look at the form $(a\lambda^2 + b\lambda + c)\, Ae^{\lambda t} = 0$, we see that it is the product of two terms, an exponential and the term in brackets. A product can only be zero if one of its terms is zero. We know that the exponential term can never be zero (2.9) (unless A is zero, which is not very interesting), so the term in the brackets must be zero for a solution to the equation. But this is just a quadratic expression in λ, $(a\lambda^2 + b\lambda + c) = 0$ and *if* we can find roots—i.e. two values of λ that make the whole expression zero (2.7.4)—then both of these values λ_1 and λ_2 will satisfy our ODE as rate constants. This enables us to define a solution with *two* exponential terms—one for each root, since both satisfy the ODE—the familiar 'bi-exponential' equation:

$$C(t) = Ae^{\lambda_1 t} + Be^{\lambda_2 t}$$

We have solved a very important class of differential equation without actually doing an integration at all, but by solving a simple quadratic equation. However, the solution is fundamentally dependent upon the concept of differentiation/integration.

A similar approach with the basic sinusoidal function gives us a set of derivatives in which the second derivative is a simple multiple (ω^2) of the original function. This was how we solved the SHM second-order ODE (1.16.4):

$$f(t) = [A \sin \omega t + B \cos \omega t],$$

$$f'(t) = [\omega A \cos \omega t - \omega B \sin \omega t],$$

$$f''(t) = [-\omega^2 A \sin \omega t - \omega^2 B \cos \omega t] = -\omega^2 [A \sin \omega t + B \cos \omega t] = -\omega^2 f(t).$$

This gives a flavour of the approach to solution of second-order equations. Matters become mathematically more complex when damped and forced vibrations are modelled, and the mathematical techniques required are well beyond our remit. Further delving into this subject reveals some fascinating insights into the dynamic behaviour of systems—springs, respiratory systems, and pharmacological models—which have an equilibrium state to which they 'aspire' after any perturbation. Mathematical abstraction leads us to the conclusion that, under the surface, these apparently different models have much in common.

2.16.1 **An approximate method of solution**

We have studied some models which have given us ODEs that we have been able
to solve. 'Solve' here means we were able to find a *function* the rate of change of
which is given by the ODE. We cannot always find a function that satisfies the
ODE and the pulmonary air embolism (1.12) problem was an example of this; the
problem was real enough, and we would like to know the solution—but we cannot
find one. All is not lost, however; if we know the rate of change (from the ODE)
and a starting value (an initial condition), we can produce an *approximate* graph
of the function that we require. We demonstrate this with a known uncomplicated
function, so that we can compare the real and approximate solution.

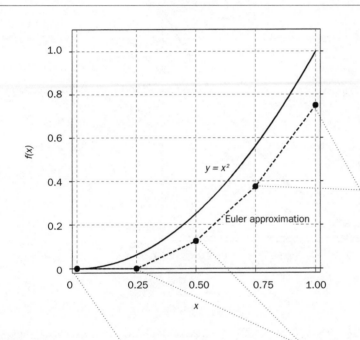

Euler's method

Consider the graph of $f(x) = x^2$, which
has derivative $f'(x) = 2x$. Let us start
at the origin, where $f(0) = 0$. We
choose an interval of size 0.25 to
demonstrate the principle.

We add on a line with gradient 1 for the next
point and we arrive at (0.75, 0.375), where the
gradient is $f'(x) = 2x = 1.5$.
Adding a line with gradient 1.5 for the next
interval gives us the point (1, 0.75).

The gradient here $f'(0)$ is zero, so we can draw a
horizontal line to represent its rate of change. As
soon as we leave the origin in the +ve x direction,
the gradient of the function is positive.

We choose $x = 0.25$ on the x-axis as our next point, the gradient here
is $f'(x) = 2x = 0.5$, and we draw a straight line from the point (0.25, 0) at a
gradient of 0.5 for another interval 0.25 wide, we reach the point (0.5, 0.125).
This is the point at which we calculate the next gradient $f'(x) = 2x = 1$.

Using only a starting value and the derivative, we have produced an *approximate* graph
of the function that we require; it is discrete and not smooth. The approximation is not
very good and gets worse the further we travel from the origin—the errors propagate.
We could improve the fit by taking smaller intervals, but this means more work. This is
Euler's method, and is the simplest numerical method for approximate solution to
ODEs.

Modified Euler's method

We can improve on Euler's method by taking a *mean* of the gradients at the beginning and the end of our iteration interval. The first line segment now has a gradient of $(0 + 0.5)/2 = 0.25$ and the second $(0.5 + 1)/2 = 0.75$. The approximation produced by this method is still discrete, but is much closer to the real solution than the simple Euler technique.

Much more sophisticated methods are available for use on computer—the air embolism problem was solved by a standard technique, the fourth-order Runge–Kutta method, and gave us a practical answer to our problem—but the fundamental idea is the same as demonstrated here. Instead of a *function* giving the solution value at any point, numerical methods produce a *table* of values. Tables of the normal distribution must be produced by a numerical method, since the normal probability density function is not integrable.

The numerical methods are iterative methods, in which the output from one cycle of the process is used to feed in to the next cycle. This is the idea we used in our discrete nitrogen washout function (1.9.2).

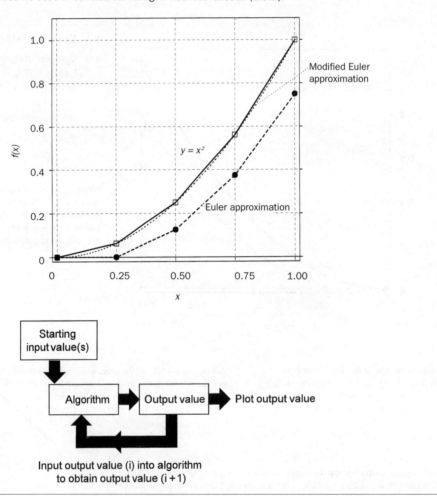

We have seen a method for numerical solution of ODEs. Similar techniques are available for the approximate solution of equations, finding roots, evaluation of areas under curves for non-integrable functions and so on. There are many pitfalls in the practical application of such techniques which can lead to propagation and amplification of errors. Numerical methods form an area of study in their own right, but this is as far as we go.

Part 3 **Probability and statistics**

3.1.1 **Probability and statistical modelling**

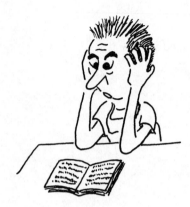

Probability distributions are functions and are used as models for problems involving random processes in exactly the same way as the other functions in the deterministic physiological models that we have developed. Just as we saw certain patterns arising in the physiological modelling, in probabilistic models certain patterns turn up frequently. Modelling assumptions are made which lead to probability models. These can then be used to make rational decisions about problems in which chance plays a part, or to make estimates of quantities with defined levels of certainty.

A technique which is of great importance in learning statistical ideas is that of *simulation*. Computers or statistical tables can be used to generate simulated samples from known distributions with known characteristics. Statistical inferential tests can be applied to these 'data' and we can see how the conclusions we would reach if these were real data compare with the known origin of the data. In real life, data are analysed in order to make *inferences* about populations of unknown characteristics; our purpose is learning, and it is useful to be able to know where our data have come from. This is a legitimate approach for instruction where it is clear that the data are simulated; but another word for 'simulated' is 'fake'.

I have placed a lot of emphasis on Poisson processes and the Poisson distribution for a number of reasons. The Poisson distribution is extremely important in describing all sorts of random situations and is particularly simple since it is defined by a single parameter. It is even easier to think of examples of Poisson processes than of normally distributed variables. Because such circumstances are so familiar, everyone has a 'visceral' feeling for how such random phenomena behave. It is possible to build upon this knowledge to introduce many of the basic ideas in statistical inference within a familiar context. The Poisson tends towards normality as the mean increases and hence provides a natural introduction to the supremely important normal distribution.

The scope of this part has been kept deliberately limited to concentrate on core ideas and hence much important material is left out; details of some standard, mainstream techniques—Fisher's test, the odds ratio and so on—have been omitted for reasons of space. The bibliography gives sources for further reading.

3.2.1 The Poisson process

Severe anaphylactoid reactions to general anaesthesia are rare. Let us suppose that reactions of a defined severity occur in about 1 in 5000 general anaesthetics. A city anaesthesia service administers 25 000 anaesthetics annually. How many such reactions might be expected annually? It does not require penetrating statistical insight to conclude that we *expect* there to be five. But what do we mean by the expectation of five reactions per annum? We know that such events tend to occur 'at random'—which means that such occurrences are largely unpredictable and unconnected with each other. This randomness means that we would actually be very surprised if our expectation of five events annually was fulfilled each year. We expect considerable variability around our expected value, but 'on average' there would be about five. How much variability do we expect and what number of reactions would lead us seriously to question the assumption that the average number of reactions was still five per year? Would we be surprised if there were ten reactions one year—or 14? In what proportion of years do we expect there actually to be five reactions? Just as we have modelled physiological and pharmacological systems by using simplifying assumptions, it is possible to model situations involving random processes in the same way. We shall first investigate a model which enables us to answer questions such as these quite precisely.

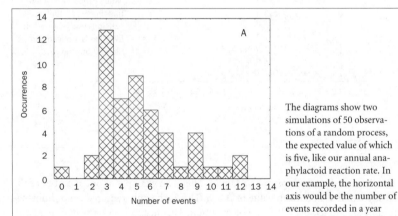

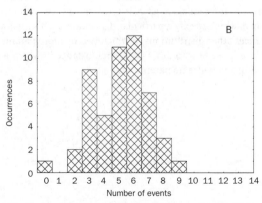

The diagrams show two simulations of 50 observations of a random process, the expected value of which is five, like our annual anaphylactoid reaction rate. In our example, the horizontal axis would be the number of events recorded in a year and the vertical axis the number of years in which that number of reactions occurred. Each diagram represents half a century of simulated observations.

Simulation of random events: Poisson processes

The essence of a random process is that although the events may be occurring at a certain underlying rate, the actual details of the occurrence remain mostly unpredictable—the factors causing the actual anaphylactoid reaction at a particular time in that place are complex. Although we may identify some factors in retrospect, they do not often help us to predict the next one. The occurrence of one reaction is generally unrelated to another one in another patient at another time—the reactions are independent of each other. Such random events, which are occurring at a constant underlying (i.e. mean or expected) rate but independently of each other, are examples of a Poisson process.

The summary measures show that the average is indeed close to 5:

mean	A = 5.38	B = 5.20
median	A = 5	B = 5
mode	A = 3	B = 6

The diagrams show a clustering around the central value of 5, but there is considerable spread—eight occurrences of nine or more events in one group and only one in this range in the other. There is no easily discernible pattern and random effects are prominent.

3.2.2 Counting events: the Poisson distribution

A discrete model of random events

Although there was little obvious pattern to be seen in the simulated examples, in fact the '*long run*' behaviour of such random processes can be modelled quite easily. The long-term relative frequency of the various possible outcomes—0, 1, 2, 3, 4, ... reactions annually—can be calculated from a simple formula. The only information that we require is the underlying mean rate μ at which the process is occurring: in our case $\mu = 5$. The long-term relative frequency of any particular outcome is the *probability* of that outcome. The way in which the probabilities are spread amongst the possible outcomes is the *probability distribution*. The probability distribution which describes the relative frequency of random events such as our anaphylaxis reactions is the Poisson distribution, named after its discoverer. The distribution is what we would obtain if we were to simulate an infinite number of samples in the same way.

The Poisson distribution is discrete—it only assigns a probability value to integer outcomes. We are *counting* events that can only come in whole number packages: 0, 1, 2, 3 ... . The distribution is therefore not smooth—there are steps between adjacent discrete probability values. We will later distinguish between counting (discrete) and measuring (continuous) variables and appropriate distributions.

The distribution is not symmetrical: there is a tail that extends further in the direction of higher values—the probabilities for large numbers of events are small, but they can happen. In the other direction, it is not possible to have fewer than zero events, so the distribution is necessarily skewed; that is, asymmetrical.

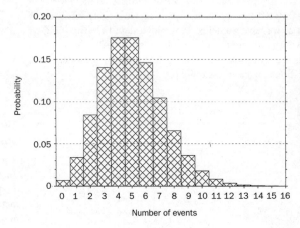

The probability of 14 reactions in a year is $p = 0.0005$. If the mean is truly $\mu = 5$, this outcome will occur in our example about once every two millennia. If we actually observed this number, we would probably conclude that the mean number of reactions was greater then five; that is, not compatible with our model.

The Poisson distributions form a family. This is an example of one member of the family—that with a mean value of $\mu = 5$. This is the only required bit of information needed to specify a Poisson distribution. The mean $\mu = 5$ is the defining *parameter* of the particular Poisson. Inferential statistics is often concerned with estimating parameters—numbers which specify a particular distribution. This is parametric statistics. We shall meet other distributions in which two or more parameters are required and also briefly see how to deal with a circumstance in which we have no candidate distribution and hence no parameter at all (3.20).

3.2.3 The Poisson distribution: general features

Poisson processes are at work everywhere—strokes after carotid endarterectomy, ruptured aortic aneurysms, subarachnoid haemorrhages, inadvertent dural puncture in epidural analgesia—each is occurring independently at random, and we expect a certain number to present depending upon the underlying rate in the population and the size of the population at risk. Many questions of clinical management are about minimizing complication rates—complications which occur sporadically—and are essentially questions about the mean of Poisson processes. We have looked at one particular Poisson distribution quite closely, and it enables us to give quantitative answers to some of the questions that arose in the anaphylactoid reactions problem. Let us look at the general features of the distribution by examining various members of the Poisson family.

The Poisson distribution: changing the mean

Poisson distributions of various means are shown. Certain general features can be seen. As the mean rate of the process increases, the *location* of the peak shifts along the horizontal axis. The peak probability always occurs at the mean value, although the probability of the value immediately below the mean is the same. (The equal peaks feature only with integer values of the mean and are not general to the distribution). The distribution remains stepped—that is, discrete—but becomes 'smoother' as the mean increases. The spread or *dispersion* of the distribution increases as the mean increases: the range of plausible values of the variable increases. The asymmetry or skewness which was prominent with $\mu = 5$ also becomes less obvious as the mean increases, although close inspection reveals that some asymmetry remains even at $\mu = 50$. Note that the scale of the vertical axis changes as the mean increases. Because the spread of the plausible values increases with the mean, the total probability of 1 must be distributed amongst a greater number of values, and hence the typical probability of any particular specified value must diminish.

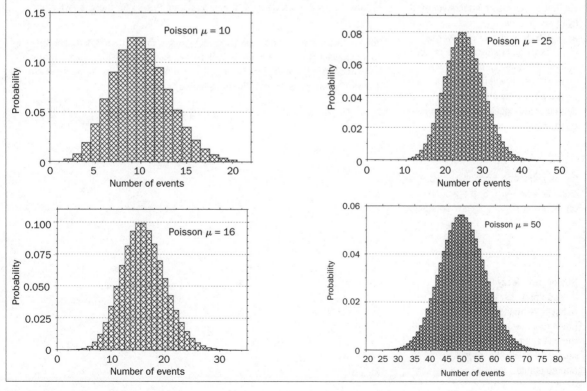

3.2.4   Poisson distribution: general features 2

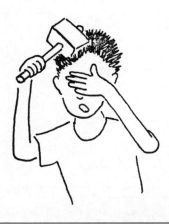

The Poisson distribution as a model of random processes

There is no space to derive the equation (below) which defines the Poisson distribution for any μ, but we can summarize the model upon which the mathematics is based. If the model is a good match to the real problem, then the Poisson will describe the long-term behaviour of the situation well. A classic study described the number of Prussian army cavalrymen killed annually by horse-kicks. The Poisson distribution was a good model—it has wide applicability as long as the modelling assumptions are fulfilled. Since these are very simple, Poisson processes are ubiquitous.

The number of anaphylactoid events annually or the number of cavalrymen killed by horse-kicks are examples of *random variables* (RV). We shall have more to say about RVs later.

Assumptions

1. The underlying process must be occurring at a constant rate over the period of observation. This determines the probability of an individual occurrence in any period. This is quantified as the mean rate or expected value. In the anaphylactoid example, this was $\mu = 5$. If we had asked how many reactions we expect to occur in 6 months, then the mean is $\mu = 2.5$.

2. Although taking place at a constant overall mean rate, the individual events occur at random—they happen independently of each other. The occurrence of one event is unrelated to the occurrence of any other—Poisson processes are said to be 'memoryless', because details of the history of the system are no guide to the future. We may of course be able to estimate the mean rate from past behaviour, as we did with the postulated $\mu = 5$ for the anaphylactoid example.

Poisson processes are not restricted to events in time. The same model arises in counting cells or bacteria in known volumes of fluids, or raisins in bars of fruit and nut chocolate, or defects in lengths of cable, for example. All we need are discrete occurrences in a continuum—time or space.

Calculating individual probabilities

The Poisson distribution for any mean μ is easily calculated, although the values for means up to $\mu = 50$ are commonly available in tables. For Poisson means higher than this, a normal approximation is usually more convenient (3.11). It seems paradoxical that the chaos and unpredictability of occurrence of a process such as anaphylaxis should be governed by an exact and rather simple mathematical relationship. It is a pity it does not tell us when.

The probability of observing the particular individual value x, where $x = 0,1,2,3,4, \ldots$, is

$$p(X = x) = \frac{e^{-\mu}\mu^x}{x!};$$

for instance, in our anaphylactoid example where $\mu = 5$, the probability of observing $x = 3$ reactions annually is

$$p(x = 3) = \frac{e^{-5}5^3}{3 \times 2 \times 1} = 0.1404.$$

Radioactive decay is an example of a Poisson process; the long-term behaviour—the half-life—is very predictable for any isotope, but the short-term behaviour—when the next β-particle will emerge—is unpredictable.

3.2.5 The cumulative Poisson distribution

Grouping probabilities

We might wish to ask a slightly different question about the anaphylactoid example. We might want to know the proportion of years in which there are more than six reactions, for example. This is not difficult to do, we simply add the probabilities for $x = 7,8,9,10, ...$ This can also be calculated as '1 – probability of six or fewer reactions'. We need to take care to include the right values to answer the exact question; more than six is seven or more.

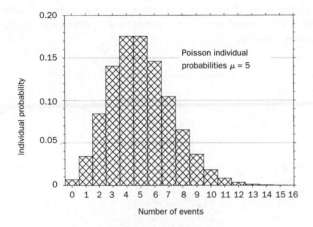

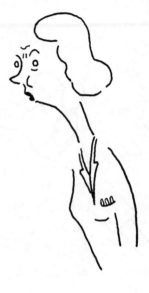

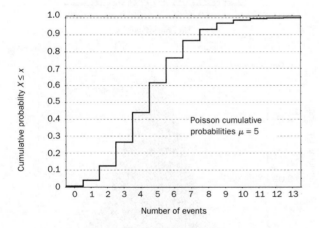

This is the graph that tells us the probability that there will be 'x or fewer reactions annually', where x is any number that we specify. There will be six or fewer reactions in about $p = 0.76$ of years—about once every four years ($p = 0.24$) we expect there to be seven or more. This is the *cumulative Poisson distribution* for $\mu = 5$, and is easily obtained by stacking all the individual probabilities of Poisson $\mu = 5$ progressively. For example, the probability of three or fewer reactions is the sum of the individual probabilities for 0, 1, 2, and 3 reactions = $0.0067 + 0.0337 + 0.0842 + 0.1404 = 0.265$. We meet other cumulative distributions later.

Parameters and the Poisson

When we examined the Poisson process, we noticed that as the mean rate μ increases, so does the spread of plausible values. We did not feel the need for separate information on how spread out were the likely outcomes; the randomness somehow already contains this information, and we were not surprised that the variability is higher for higher values of μ.

The Poisson is specified uniquely by one parameter; the mean rate μ. The degree of dispersion is already 'built in'. The dispersion of a distribution is measured by its variance (3.10), and the Poisson has the very convenient property that *the mean and the variance are equal*. We shall examine the significance of this later. When we study the normal distribution, we shall discover that the mean and the variance of that distribution need to be specified separately, since they are independent. In fact, all of the distributions that we meet, except the normal, have a 'built-in' variance.

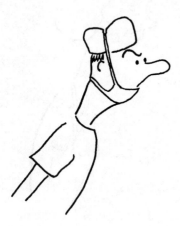

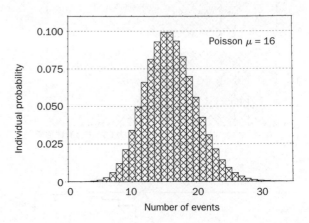

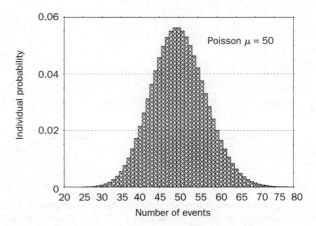

The greater dispersion of the Poisson $\mu = 50$ compared with that with $\mu = 16$ is apparent.

3.2.6   Plausible and implausible outcomes

We constructed our model of anaphylactoid reactions on the assumption that the mean rate was five reactions annually. This was based upon an assumed incidence (1 : 5000) and the size of the population at risk (25 000); we have prior information. The Poisson distribution with $\mu = 5$ gave us the individual or cumulative probabilities. If we observed, say, 14 reactions one year, we would find from the cumulative distribution that this (or a more extreme number) is going to occur only once every 2000 years or so on average, if the mean is truly 5. This is such a small probability that we would reject the assumption that the mean is 5. The event is simply not very plausible for $\mu = 5$. We may wish to decide a range of values that we will accept as being compatible with the assumed distribution. Any occurrences outside this range will cause us to question or reject the assumptions upon which the model was based—this may mean the distribution itself (*is* it a Poisson process after all?) or the parameter that we have assumed (it *is* Poisson but the *mean* is different). The threshold level of probability at which we reject our assumed model is essentially arbitrary—it is up to us to decide.

Is it likely?

The assumed distribution (form and parameter) is termed the *null distribution*. It is based upon the hypothesized model—the 'null' hypothesis that the data are from a Poisson distribution with mean $\mu = 5$. The word 'null' is conventional but otherwise not very helpful.

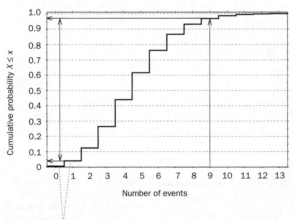

The probability of there being no reactions in one year on the null hypothesis is $p = 0.0067$—less than 1%. The probability of either one ($x = 1$) *or* no reactions ($x = 0$) is $p = 0.0404$—about 4%.

We might look for a range of values along the horizontal axis that causes the cumulative distribution to occupy, say, 95% of the vertical axis. Because the distribution is discrete, we cannot find an exact answer.

The upper end probabilities show that more than ten reactions occur with a probability $p = 0.0136$—just over 1%. More than nine (i.e. ten or more) has a probability $p = 0.0317$—in other words, 96.83% of the distribution lies below 10 (i.e. nine or fewer).

If we want to determine a range of acceptable values—that is, counts of reactions annually—which would be compatible with our model, we must decide a probability level which we feel is inconsistent with the model. Let us take a level of $p = 0.05$: we will reject our model if we observe a value which will occur in only 1 in 20 occasions (or even more infrequently) by chance. We have a problem, because the null distribution is discrete—it has jumps—and it is asymmetrical or skewed. With this discrete distribution, we are unable to choose a middle range which will give us *exactly* 95% of observations of the null distribution. If we choose an acceptable range 2–9 (inclusive), we encompass 92.8% of the null distribution. If we choose 1–10 (inclusive), we encompass about 98%. The range 1–9 gives us 96.2%, so this might be the range we would choose. We shall look again at this idea in more detail later (3.12).

3.3.1   The exponential distribution

From Poisson to exponential

The probability distribution has a simple and familiar form; it is a wash-in exponential function. The probability of waiting less than $T = t$ between events is

$$p(T \leq t) = 1 - e^{-\mu t},$$

where μ is the mean of the associated Poisson process. The mean waiting time is $1/\mu$. The Poisson formula can explain this.

The Poisson rule is

$$p(X = x) = \frac{e^{-\mu} \mu^x}{x!}.$$

For $x = 0$ ie no events—we are still waiting, $\mu^0 = 1$ and $x! = 0! = 1$, so we have $p(X = 0) = e^{-\mu}$. If we consider observing the same process for 6 months, our expected number is now $\mu/2 = 2.5$. The probability of waiting longer than 6 months is thus $p(T > t) = e^{-\mu t} = e^{-5/2} = 0.082$. The probability of waiting a shorter time than 6 months is thus $p(T < t) = 1 - e^{-\mu t} = 1 - e^{-5/2} = 1 - 0.082 = 0.918$.

We are beginning to feel more familiar with Poisson processes, so let us stay with them a little longer but look now at a different aspect. If we return yet again to the anaphylaxis example, we might ask how long we would expect to wait between one reaction and the next. Again it is simple to state that, since the expected number annually is five, then we expect to wait 0.2 years—about 73 days on average. Since the process is random, however, we know that there will be a spread of waiting times. We have exactly the same circumstance, but we are asking a different question about the situation. Whereas previously we were *counting* events in a given time, now we are *measuring* times between those same events. The distinction between counting and measuring is an important one.

A continuous distribution

The appearance of 'e' in the Poisson formula means that we may not be surprised to discover that waiting times between events in a Poisson process are distributed exponentially. The negative exponential distribution answers the question 'What is the probability of waiting less than time t since the previous event in a Poisson process with mean rate μ?' Evidently, the more rapid the process (the greater the Poisson mean, μ) the shorter will be the mean waiting time.

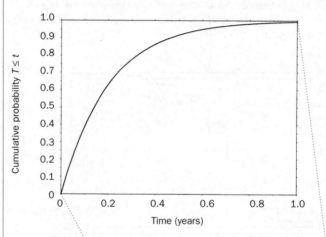

The probability of waiting less than zero years is obviously zero.

The probability that there were *no* events in the Poisson $\mu = 5$ was $p = 0.0067$. This must be the same as the probability of waiting longer than one year for a reaction in our anaphylaxis example. This point must therefore have a value $p = 1 - 0.0067 = 0.9933$.

The distribution of waiting times is smooth—it has no steps, since we can wait for any length of time. This is an example of a continuous distribution. Continuous distributions are used to model processes in which we are measuring rather than counting. We are observing the same process as before, but the question is different and the model is also different, although intimately connected to the Poisson.

3.4.1 **The binomial distribution**

Suppose that we have eight candidates taking the fellowship exam and there is a published pass rate of about 30%. Each individual's exam is a 'trial' and passing the test is a 'success'. 'Success' and 'trial' are technical terms in probability theory and are obviously very appropriate here. We suppose that one candidate's success is independent of another's—no cheating. We *expect* 2.4 candidates to pass, but obviously the *realization* will be different—only a whole number can pass. We would probably say that two was the most likely number, since this is the integer closest to 2.4. We would not be surprised if three or even four passed, but what about five or none at all? We can be certain that we will observe an outcome that lies in the range 0, 1, 2, 3, …, 8. The Poisson distribution was unrestricted at the upper end: a Poisson with $\mu = 2.4$ specifies probabilities for 9, 10, 11, … events which are impossible outcomes in our exam problem, so the Poisson will not do—we need a different model.

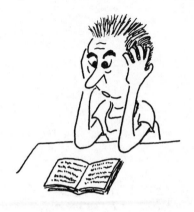

Simulating the examination:

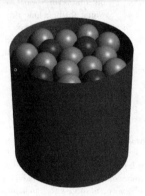

Suppose that we have a bin filled with a large number of well mixed beads: 30% of the beads are black and the rest white. We select samples of beads eight at a time and record the number of black beads in each sample. We return the beads, mix them well between samples, and repeat the process a large number of times. What proportion of the samples contain 0, 1, 2, 3, … 8, black beads? This is the distribution of a simulation of 500 samples.

The modal—most common—value is indeed 2, although three and four black beads out of eight are not uncommon. This is a simulation and open to random effects, but the pattern is clear. The mean of all 500 samples $\bar{x} = 2.352$, quite close to the expected value $\mu = 2.4$.

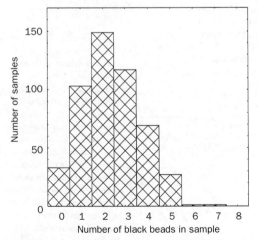

This is a physical simulation model of the examination problem. Each bead in the samples represents a candidate, and the selection of a black bead signifies a pass. The distribution of the number of black beads in the samples should mimic the number of candidates passing, if the model is a good one.

Actually, we do not need to mess about with beads and bins, since there is a mathematical model which gives us the probabilities directly—this is the binomial distribution. As with the Poisson, there is a simple expression that enables us to calculate probabilities of each of the possible outcomes. It depends upon the value of two parameters, n, the number in the sample, and p, the probability of a success at any one trial. The values for our examination problem are $n = 8$, $p = 0.3$. Tables are available that give the probabilities for various values of n and p.

The model depends upon a mathematical formulation of the bead selection process, and requires certain assumptions which can be summarized as follows:

- Random selection: each time we select a bead, there is a constant probability of success. This means that the proportion of beads is always the same, and the beads are always well mixed.
- Each bead selection is independent of the other selections: this implies a large number of beads, so that removal of a bead does not materially alter the proportion of those remaining.
- A fixed number, n, is drawn to form the samples.

3.4.2 The binomial distribution: general features

Individual and cumulative probabilities

The binomial distribution arises when we have a fixed number of trials with a fixed probability of success in any individual trial. There were eight trials in the exam example, with a fixed probability of success of 30% or $p = 0.3$. This is the null distribution based upon the published pass rate and the knowledge that we have eight candidates entered. The binomial distribution $B(8, 0.3)$ describes the pattern of variability that we expect on these assumptions. We might question whether our candidates are better (or worse) than the average. $p = 0.3$ is the probability of any randomly selected candidate—not just our own—passing. If ours are better prepared than most, then p for them will be larger.

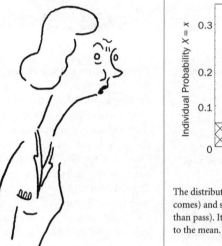

The binomial distribution gives us the theoretical probabilities of the various outcomes. This is what we would obtain in long-run relative frequencies for repeated simulations such as the previous one with the beads.

The distribution is discrete (only integer outcomes) and skewed to lower values (more fail than pass). Its modal value is the integer closest to the mean.

Since anybody who does not pass fails—it is a binary process, win or lose—this distribution must be the complement of binomial $(8, 0.7)$. The probability of three passes, for instance, must be the same as the probability of five failures. All we need to do is reverse the scale of the horizontal axis to obtain the distribution $B(8, 0.7)$.

The distribution needs two parameters to define it—unlike the Poisson, which needs only one. We need to know the number of trials n ($n = 8$ here) and the probability p of success at an individual trial ($p = 0.3$). The expected value or mean $\mu = np$.

This is only a good model in so far as the assumptions of the model are matched by the real circumstances. For example, examiners with favourite questions in a poorly-structured oral examination, which are passed on to later candidates, could affect the independence of the trials. A number of other circumstances can be envisaged that might violate the assumptions upon which the distribution is constructed. Try to think of some. The comparison of real life with the model is an essential component of the modelling process.

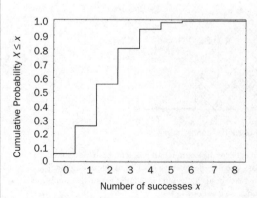

We can construct a cumulative distribution in the same way as we did with the Poisson, by stacking up all the preceding probabilities cumulatively to produce a distribution that answers the question 'What is the probability of x or fewer passing the exam?' We see that just over 80% of the time three or fewer will pass on the null assumption of $p = 0.3$. In all discrete distributions, it is easy to make mistakes in reading the cumulative distribution: 'three or fewer' includes three—'less than three does not'.

3.4.3 **Parameters, symmetry, and skewness**

A symmetrical binomial

The fixed number of trials determines how the probabilities are distributed: we would not expect as many to pass the exam if there were only seven candidates, even with the same pass rate. We might expect the degree of asymmetry to depend upon the value of p, and this is true. For $p = 0.5$, the distribution is entirely symmetrical whatever the value of n. The distribution for $n = 10$, $p = 0.5$ is shown. We shall find a use for this distribution later. (3.15.1)

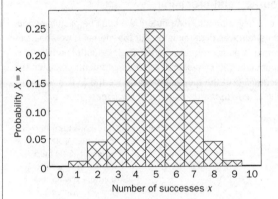

The distribution is discrete but now is also symmetrical.

Like the Poisson, the binomial distribution has a built-in variance. Under conditions when n is large and p small, the binomial and the Poisson probabilities (with $\mu = np$) are very similar, and the Poisson may be more convenient to calculate.

Binomial probabilities

As in the case of the Poisson, we omit derivation of the model, which is a mathematical formulation of the bead selection process. The binomial probabilities are easily obtained from a formula, but the results are more conveniently available from tables—which saves tedious calculation:

$$p(X = x) = \frac{n!}{x!(n - x)!} p^x (1 - p)^{n-x},$$

the probability that the variable takes the value x when the probability of success is p and the number of trials is n.

The mean of a binomial distribution is $\mu = np$ and the variance = $np(1 - p)$. For the distribution shown here, $\mu = 5$ and the variance is 2.5.

For large n and small p, the binomial and Poisson distributions of the same mean ($\mu = np$) are very similar, and we can often use the Poisson, making calculation much easier. The now familiar Poisson $\mu = 5$ and B (20, 0.25)—in other words, also with $\mu = 5$—are shown. They are not identical, but they are quite similar. This approximation of one exact distribution to another of a different family is seen quite frequently in studying probability. We shall see other examples.

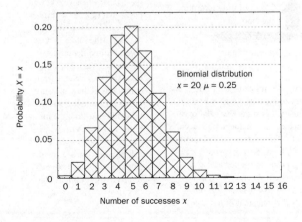

Binomial distribution
$x = 20$ $\mu = 0.25$

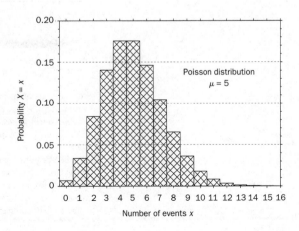

Poisson distribution
$\mu = 5$

3.5.1   **Estimation and measurement error**

A pharmaceutical manufacturer has produced a new volatile anaesthetic agent and, in order to deliver it by vaporizer, needs to establish a value for the saturated vapour pressure (SVP) at 20°C. The SVP of a substance at any fixed temperature is a physical constant—it has no inherent variability. Unfortunately, the measurement method itself is subject to error, and even though the laboratory might control the experimental conditions as well as possible, there is always some variability in the measurement. The manufacturer has been using the same method for a long while, and knows that on average 95% of the SVP measurements fall within 8 mmHg to either side of the mean value.

Measurement: accuracy and precision

Measurement errors are usually normally distributed. We shall be examining the normal distribution and its relatives in detail later. For the moment, we shall simply assume that the normal is an appropriate model. The amount of variability in measuring the same quantity is the *precision* of the measurement: precision is concerned with the *repeatability* of the measurement. Since the SVP is a constant, all of the variability is due to the measurement technique.

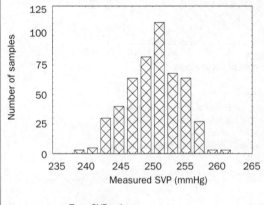

This shows the results of a simulation of 500 measurements from the SVP-ometer. We can see that there are very few examples of measurements outside the range 242–258 mmHg. The spread is roughly symmetrical around a central value of about 250 mmHg. The way in which we choose to group the data to form the histogram has some bearing upon the exact shape of the display, but the general picture remains the same.

The variability of the method means that when we take samples—that is, make a number of repeated measurements of the SVP—the values that we obtain from different determinations will vary. The mean value that we calculate from collections of these measurements (i.e. samples) will usually be different from the mean μ of the *method* itself—which should not vary or 'drift'. This will become clearer as we discuss the sampling process. We return to this example later (3.13).

The accuracy of the method is quite distinct from its precision. Accuracy is a measure of how close the mean μ of the *measurement method* itself is to the *true value* of the SVP. Errors in determination can be due to poor accuracy or poor precision, or both. An accurate method homes in on the true value even if it is erratic or imprecise: it just takes larger samples to get close to the correct value. Statistics can say nothing about accuracy here, but has plenty to say about precision. We shall assume our method to be completely accurate; that is, μ = true SVP.

3.6.1 The uniform distribution

We have seen examples of a number of situations in which random factors are operating and we have introduced four different patterns of variability—the Poisson, exponential, binomial, and normal distributions. These distributions are expressions of the behaviour of probability models. The real-life examples have all been typical *random variables*. A random variable (RV) is simply any quantity that varies according to some random process, and our first task is to choose an appropriate probability model to parallel the real situation, if we can. Sometimes this is easy—the result of the throw of a fair die calls for a very simple model—but sometimes it is impossible to produce a plausible probability model. There are a number of standard models such as those we have seen, which can be used in a wide variety of situations. The important point is that the assumptions upon which the model is based and the real-life situation should be closely matched and, if necessary, modifications made to the model, or appropriate caution used in interpreting the results. Part of the art of statistics is finding a good model.

There *are* ways of dealing with problems in which no direct probability model suggests itself, although the analysis of such situations does still demand the use of probability models. This is the distribution-free (or non-parametric) approach, which we shall meet briefly (3.20.).

Equally probable outcomes

No book on probability can avoid the throwing of dice. The throw of a fair die has an equal probability of showing a 1, 2, ..., 6. This is a feature of the physical construction of the die. The number appearing on the upper face after a single throw is a RV, and the associated probability model is an example of a uniform distribution. Even this is a simplification of reality: How do we deal with the die falling against something and resting on an edge? This is easy—we ignore it and throw it again, but the probability model does not account for this outcome.

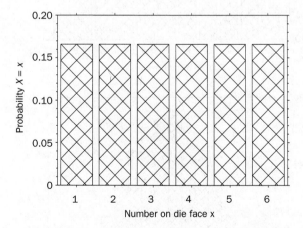

All outcomes are equally likely, with $p = 1/6$. The distribution is discrete and uniform. It has an expected or mean value of $\mu = 3.5$. We can never observe this expected value in a single throw of the die. What we mean is that 'on average, in the long run', 3.5 is the score that we obtain.

Simulation of a binomial variable using random numbers

Random numbers from the uniform distribution are available in tables or on pocket calculators. They can be useful for simulation techniques and random allocation procedures. Each digit 0, 1, 2, 3, ..., 9 has an equal probability of occupying any slot in a table of random numbers: the tables are, in essence, results of rolling a ten-sided die. If we wished to simulate samples from $B(8, 0.3)$, as in the examination example, all we need to do is start anywhere in the table and take the digits in groups of eight at a time ($n = 8$). We merely count, for each group of eight, how many occurrences of the digits 0, 1, 2 (say) there are. One of (0, 1, 2) will occur on 30% of occasions; that is, $p = 0.3$ (three of ten possible digits with an equal probability of occurrence in any slot in the table). We can thus use one distribution to simulate another by adopting an appropriate selection method.

If we start here* and take these eight digits, the simulation gives the result $x = 3$: three candidates pass the exam, since 0 occurs twice and 1 once, and 0, 1, or 2 signifies a success.

Table of random numbers from uniform distribution

94384	64989	74446
42298	48320	87255
32938	57234	73482
71337	*77050	197*48
98123	36655	93261

3.7.1   **Adding RVs**

Sums of throws of a die

The die is an example of the uniform distribution which is almost as simple as a distribution can get. But if our RV is the *sum of two throws of a die*, what distribution do we get then? The range of outcomes is now 2, 3, …, 12, but is the distribution still uniform? Each throw of the die is independent and each possible combination—six for the first throw and six for the second—occur with equal probability; 36 possibilities in all. The *sum* of the two throws, however, does not give an equal probability for each of the possible outcomes 2, 3, 4, …, 12. This fact has profound implications.

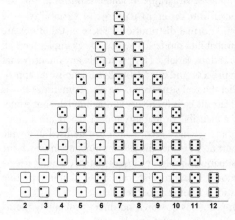

There are more ways in which we can obtain values in the centre of the range than values at the extremes. We only get an extreme value when we add values from the same end of the single throw distribution: (1 + 1) or (6 + 6). Values in the middle of the distribution of the sum can arise either by obtaining two middle values or by extreme values from opposite ends of the single throw distribution: (1 + 6) or (6 + 1).

The simple process of adding two independent observations from one RV has given us another RV of very different shape. The mean value is now $\mu = 7 = (3.5 + 3.5)$, and the range of possible outcomes has increased.

This is the distribution of the sum of three throws of the die. The mean is now $\mu = 10.5$ and the range of possible values has increased further. The scaling of the probability axis (now measured in 1/216ths, since there are 6^3 = 216 possible combinations) is such that the jumps between one probability value and the next are smaller—the distribution is becoming smoother. It is symmetrical and is beginning to look like a crude version of the normal distribution.

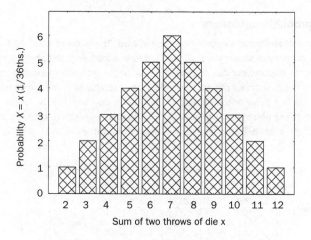

Sum of two throws of die x

Note that the mean $\mu = 10.5$ is just 3×3.5, three times the mean of the individual throw—*the mean of the sum is the sum of the means*. However, the range has increased even further, and it is true that for sums of *independent* variables (as these ones are), the *variance of the distribution of the sum is the sum of the variances* of the component variables. We will learn more about the variance as a measure of variability or dispersion soon (3.10).

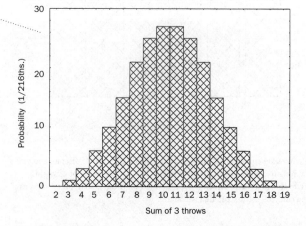

Sum of 3 throws

3.7.2 The centralizing tendency

What we have seen with the die example is of profound importance in understanding random processes. The sum of independent observations from a random variable has given us a distribution which has very different features from the the original, and this is *due to the summing procedure itself*. The data are independent observations from a uniform distribution and remain uniformly distributed until we add them together, when their sum follows a different distribution. What about the distribution of the *difference* of two throws of a die: say we subtract the second throw score from the first? We expect the distribution to be centred around zero (since the mean score for each throw will be the same) and the range will be –5 (1 – 6) to + 5 (6 – 1). The distribution has exactly the same shape and probability values as the sum, but is relocated around a central value of zero. These can be seen as horizontally translated versions of the same function.

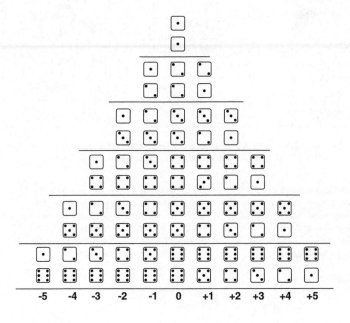

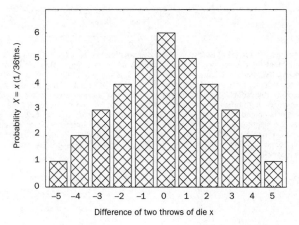

Difference of two throws of die x

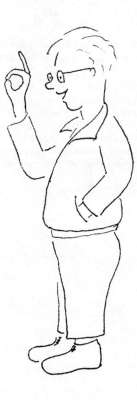

Sums and differences of random variables

We shall meet circumstances in which we need to know what happens when we add or subtract RVs. The important points to note at the moment are as follows:

- When we add or subtract RVs, we obtain another RV which may have a different form compared to the variables that we sample from. The shape becomes more like a normal distribution as we add more observations, even if we are sampling from a non-normal distribution. Observations tend to 'clump' in the middle: there is a centralizing process or tendency at work. The posh name for this phenomenon is the Central Limit Theorem; but we shall call it the centralizing tendency
- The mean of the sum is the sum of the means: the mean of adding two throws of the die is 3.5 + 3.5 = 7. The mean of a difference is the difference in means: the mean difference of two throws of a die is 3.5 − 3.5 = 0.
- The variability or range of values increases.

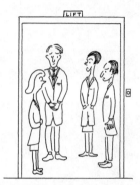 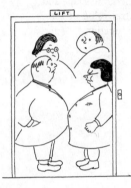 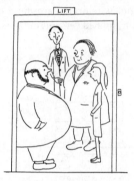 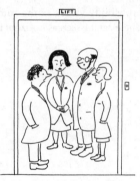

Extremes of the sum RV arise when observations from the same end of the underlying distribution occur together.

Middle values occur either by summing central values or by summing values from opposite ends of the underlying distribution.

The total mass of people in a lift is an example of a sum random variable. Lift manufacturers need to know the probable extreme values of the sum distribution so that the cable does not break and the motor will be adequate to the task. However, it is easy to see how the independence criterion may be violated; if a weightwatchers' convention is held in the building, the model of a sum of independent observations from the whole population mean weight will need modification.

The difference of two RVs can be imagined as the net force on the rope in a tug-of-war; the teams form sum RVs of strength. These two sum RVs are applied in opposite directions to the rope. The net force is dependent upon the difference in the two teams' strengths.

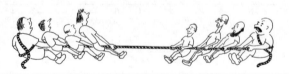

** In his *An Introduction to Medical Statistics*, Bland evokes a picture of people of normally distributed height, randomly allocated to stand upon boxes of normally distributed height. The sum RV of height of the individual above the ground will have a distribution which is the sum of these random variables; the mean height is the mean of the peoples' heights plus the mean box height. If they are randomly allocated (i.e. independent), the variability is the sum of the variability of each variable (person height and box height)—tall people on high boxes, short people on low boxes. For the difference RV, he describes people of normally distributed height standing in normally distributed holes in the ground. The RV for the difference is still the height above the ground; the mean height is the difference in the means (people and holes), but the variability is still the sum of the individual variabilities (variance); (short people in deep holes, tall people in shallow holes). Lifts, tugs-of-war, boxes, holes—choose whichever picture makes the idea most clear.

3.8.1 The rules of probability: conditional probability

Independent and compound events

- A probability is a number between 0 and 1; that is, it lies in the interval [0,1]. A probability is the *long-term relative frequency* of an event. The probability of throwing a six with a fair die is 1/6, because if we continue long enough, then a six will appear on approximately 1/6 of the throws. The longer we continue throwing, the closer will the relative frequency be to the expected value.
- An event with probability 1 is certain to happen: an event with probability 0 cannot happen.
- *The summation rule.* If two events are independent—the occurrence of one has no influence upon whether the other event occurs—then the probability of *either* event is the *sum* of the individual probabilities. This rule extends natural-ly to more than two events. If we ask what is the probability of throwing a six or a five with a single throw of a die, then the sum of the individual probabilities is 1/6 + 1/6 = 1/3.
- *The product rule.* If two events are independent, then the probability of occur-rence of *both* events is the *product* of the individual probabilities. What is the probability of throwing a six followed by a five? Each throw has an individual probability of 1/6 of showing the number we want; the probability of the compound event is therefore 1/36.

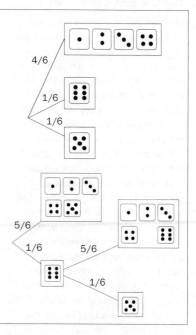

Probability rules in action: the probability tree and conditional probability

Difficult intubation (D) occurs in about 2% of the population at large. It occurs with a probability of approximately $p(D) = 0.02$; this means that intuba-tion is easy (E) in 98%; $p(E) = 0.98$. Numerous tests, all of them imperfect, have been devised to detect the condi-tion. Let us suppose that we have a test that may enable us to predict difficulty. The test is binary; that is, either positive (+) or negative (−). The possible outcomes of applying the test to an unselected group of patients are shown as a probability tree.

Random situations can be displayed as a probability tree—it can be viewed as a network of '*flows*' of probability. Probabilities 'flowing' into a box must equal those 'flowing' out. All patients are viewed as either easy or difficult. This is a modelling simplification—there are only two branches out of the box. This is the first binary split in the tree.

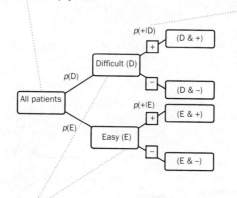

If the result of the test were uninfluenced by whether the patient was easy or difficult, then the test would be no better than guessing; that is, useless in dis-criminating easy from difficult. Since these are then independent events, the probability of (+ | D) would be $p(+)$; it is now uncondi-tional since it is the same whether intubation is easy or difficult:

$$p(D \ \& \ +) = p(D) \times p(+).$$

The probability of a positive test in a difficult patient is called the probability *conditional* upon the patient being difficult, $p(+ \mid D)$. The probability of any *unselected* patient arriving in the (D & +) box is the product of the individ-ual probability 'flows' on the pathway $p(D) \times p (+ \mid D)$. This is the product rule.

When the test is applied to these patients, the test can be either *positive* (+) or *negative* (−), which gives another binary split to each of these boxes. This gives us four result boxes: (D & +), (D & −), (E & −), and (E & +).

The probability of a positive test is

$$p(D \ \& \ +) + p (E \ \& \ +) = p(D) \times p(+ \mid D) + p(E) \times p(+ \mid E).$$

This sums the flows through the two pathways to positive test boxes. (Summation rule.)

3.9.1   **Predicting difficult intubation**

Clinical test performance

We have now encountered the idea of a conditional probability, where the test result is conditional on the presence or absence of a condition—here difficulty in intubation, D. Before we perform a test, there is a probability of D, $p(D)$, which is dependent upon the extent of prior information. If the patient is unselected, then $p(D)$ is that of the prevalence in the general population, 2%. If we already know that the patient has ankylosing spondylitis, then it will be higher than this. We will call the probability level before we do the test the *pre-test probability*. After performing the test, we hope that we have more information, so that the probability of the condition is different—either more or less probable. This is the *post-test probability*. If we do not change the $p(D)$, by doing it, the test is useless. A positive test is one that increases the probability of disease, $p(D|+) > p(D)$; a negative test decreases it, $p(D|-) < p(D)$.

We now fill out the details of the probability tree using the rules of probability and construct a function relating pre-test and post-test probabilities.

The post-test probability should be different from the pre-test probability; otherwise, the test is useless. The 'line of test uselessness' is $y = x$; pre-test = post-test probability. A positive test lies above this line, a negative one below it. For a good test, a *positive* test result should give a post-test probability of the condition being present near to unity (i.e. certainty). A *negative* result should give a post-test probability near to zero. Tests for difficult intubation are not good tests.

The performance of an ideal positive test would lie on this line; whatever the input probability, the occurrence of a positive test guarantees that the 'disease'—here difficulty in intubation—is present; that is, there is an output probability of unity.

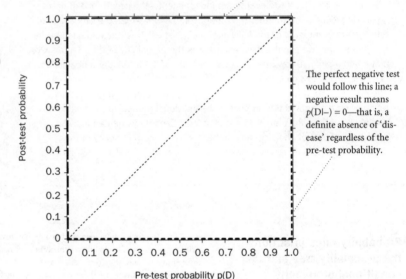

The perfect negative test would follow this line; a negative result means $p(D|-) = 0$—that is, a definite absence of 'disease' regardless of the pre-test probability.

This is the conditional probability of a positive test result in a difficult patient, $p(+|D)$. This is the True Positive Rate (*TPR*), or the *sensitivity*. The test is sensitive if it picks up most of the difficult patients. $p(D \ \& \ +) = p(D) \times TPR$.

This path has probability $p(D)$, the pre-test probability. This will depend upon what prior information we have. This will be our input variable.

This is $p(E)$, the pre-test probability of an easy intubation. $p(E) = 1 - p(D)$.

This is $p(-|E)$, the True Negative Rate (*TNR*), or the *specificity* of the test. $TNR = 1 - FPR$. A test is specific if a positive result is a reliable indicator of the condition—the *FPR* is small.

This is $p(-|D)$, the False Negative Rate (*FNR*) = $1 - TPR$.

This is $p(+|E)$, the False Positive Rate (*FPR*).

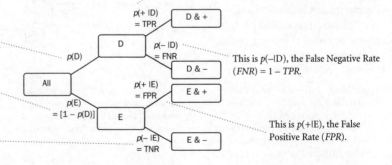

3.9.2   Pre- and post-test probabilities

Constructing the test function

What we really want to know from a test is $p(D| +)$. This is the probability that the patient is truly Difficult given (i.e. conditional upon) a positive test result. This is *not* the same as $p(+ |D)$, which is the probability that a difficult patient has a positive test (*TPR*). $p(D| +)$ means (D & +) as a proportion of *all* positive tests, true positives and false positives; that is, [(D & +) + (E & +)].

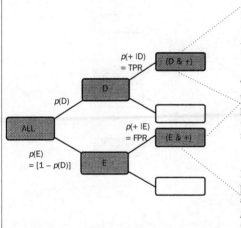

If we follow the path to the true positive box, the probability of arriving in this category is $p(D \& +) = p(D) \times TPR$ (product rule).

The probability of a positive test—either the true or false positive is $p(+) = p(D) \times TPR + (1 - p(D)) \times FPR$ (summation rule).

If we follow the path to the false positive box, the probability of arriving in this category is $p(E \& +) = (1 - p(D)) \times FPR$ (product rule).

The post-test probability $p(D| +)$ is the proportion of true positives from all positive tests. This is a result called Bayes' theorem, and it enables us to calculate the significance of a test result from knowledge of $p(D)$, the specificity (*TNR*), and the sensitivity (*TPR*):

$$p(D|+) = \frac{p(D \& +)}{p(+)}$$

$$= \frac{p(D) \times p(+|D)}{p(+)},$$

$$p(D|+) = \frac{p(D) \times TPR}{p(D) \times TPR + [1 - p(D)] \times FPR},$$

which can be rearranged as

$$p(D|+) = \frac{p(D) \times TPR}{p(D) \times [TPR - FPR] + FPR}.$$

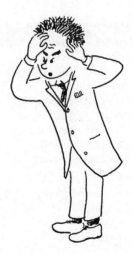

Note that when $FPR = 0$, the test is completely specific and $p(\mathrm{D}\mid +) = 1$ for all $p(\mathrm{D})$.

This is an equation of the form:

$$y = \frac{ax}{bx + c},$$

where x is the pre-test probability $p(\mathrm{D})$ and y is the post-test probability, $a = TPR$. $b = [TPR - FPR]$ and $c = FPR$. This is a rational function, the graph of which is a rectangular hyperbola (2.6.3).

A similar approach gives us an expression for the post-test probability after a negative result:

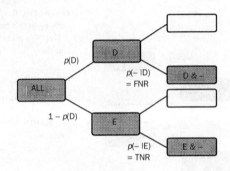

$$p(\mathrm{D}\mid -) = \frac{p(\mathrm{D}) \times FNR}{p(\mathrm{D}) \times [FNR - TNR] + TNR}.$$

When $FNR = 0$—that is, the test is completely sensitive—$p(\mathrm{D}\mid -) = 0$ for all $p(\mathrm{D})$: a negative test means a guarantee of no difficulty in intubation. Unfortunately, there is no such test.

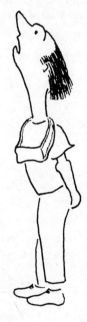

Notation

$p(\mathrm{D})$ = pre-test probability

$p(\mathrm{D}\mid +)$ = post-test probability (positive test)

$p(\mathrm{D}\mid -)$ = post-test probability (negative test)

$p(+ \mid \mathrm{D}) = TPR$ = sensitivity

$p(- \mid \mathrm{D}) = (1 - TPR) = FNR$

$p(- \mid \mathrm{E}) = TNR$ = specificity

$p(+ \mid \mathrm{E}) = FPR = (1 - TNR)$

3.9.3   **The test function**

We have used the rules of probability and derived expressions for the input and output probabilities for both positive and negative tests. What do these test functions look like?

The post-test probability is a function of *three* variables, $p(D)$, *TPR*, and *TNR*—that is, the pre-test probability, the test sensitivity, and the test specificity. The performance of any candidate test must be compared with some means of final decision—this means is usually called the 'gold standard test'. In this context, the gold standard test is whether the patient is classed as difficult when we actually attempt intubation. The point of the test procedure is to predict. Gold standard tests in other circumstances may be expensive, impractical, invasive, or only possible after death, necessitating the use of an inferior decision-making procedure. Or they may simply be too late: intra-operative tests for predicting a stroke after carotid endarterectomy must be compared with the gold standard—'*Did* the patient have a stroke?'

Fallible tests

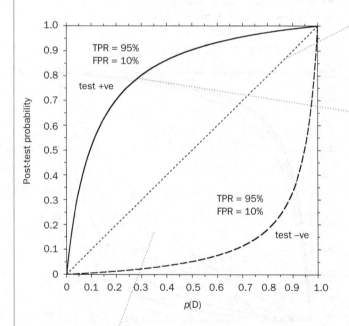

TPR = 95%
FPR = 10%

test +ve

TPR = 95%
FPR = 10%

test −ve

x-axis: $p(D)$
y-axis: Post-test probability

This is the line of identity—the 'line of test uselessness'. It is the line that defines a post-test probability identical to the pre-test probability: in other words, we have no more information after the test than before.

If the hypothetical test is not useless and we obtain a positive result, the probability of difficulty is greater than the pre-test probability, so the function must lie above the line of identity.

An ideal test would have a post-test (+) probability of 1 for all values of $p(D)$ and a post-test (−) probability of zero for all values of $p(D)$. (3.9.1)

The test function is shown for *TPR* = 95%/*FNR* = 10%. Even with a sensitivity of 95% and specificity of 90%, the post-test probability at low $p(D)$ is severely affected by the fact that a *FPR* of 10% is acting on a large proportion $(1 − p(D))$ of the population, and that false positives are 'diluting' the true positives. A positive test result greatly increases the probability of difficulty in intubation, but below $p(D) \approx 0.09$ (i.e. 9% of the tested population) most positives are still false positives. The tests that we have are much less useful than this hypothetical example.

If the test is not useless and we obtain a negative result, the probability of difficulty is less than the pre-test probability, and so the function must lie *below* the line of identity. Note that this is not a mirror image of the positive test curve.

3.9.4   **Specificity and sensitivity**

Effects of variation in *TPR* and *TNR*

The interpretation of a test will depend upon its sensitivity (*TPR*) and specificity (*TNR*). In tests involving measures rather than attributes (e.g. thyro-mental distance rather than the binary, 'Are the jaws wired together?', yes/no type of test), we are able to change the *FPR* and *TNR* (although not independently) by altering the threshold for a positive test. How does this variation affect the post-test probability?

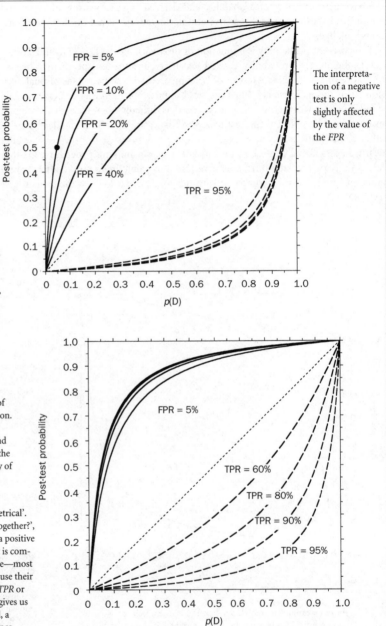

The interpretation of a negative test is only slightly affected by the value of the *FPR*

FPR $= 1 - TNR = 1 -$ specificity. The graph shows the post-test probability for tests with 95% sensitivity and various levels of specificity. If, for example, the *FPR* = 5% and the *TPR* = 95%, then when $p(D) = 0.05$, only half of the positive results will be true positives, because 5% of 95% is the same as 95% of 5%. The interpretation of a *positive test result* is heavily influenced by the specificity of the test.

The sensitivity of a test (*TPR*) is a measure of its ability to detect true difficulty in intubation. The interpretation of a *negative test result* is most influenced by the level of sensitivity and much less so by the *FPR*. This graph shows the post-test probability for tests with specificity of 95% and various levels of sensitivity.

Interpretation of test results is usually 'asymmetrical'. For example, if the test is 'Are the jaws wired together?', the *FPR* is zero—intubation *will* be difficult—a positive test guarantees difficulty. *TNR* = 1 and the test is completely specific. However, it is not very sensitive—most truly difficult patients will not be difficult because their jaws are wired, but for other reasons entirely. *TPR* or $p(+|D)$ is thus very low. A positive result here gives us utterly reliable information; on the other hand, a negative result does not give us much reassurance.

The topic of medical diagnosis and decision-making is fascinating and involved; it can be surprisingly difficult to think about. For example, the optimum choice of threshold between a positive and negative test in a continuous measure can be difficult in balancing the effects of missing true positives and treating false positives unnecessarily. Further information is available from the books in the bibliography.

3.10.1   Location: the mean, the median, and the mode

When faced with a list of data, we naturally want to make sense of them, and this will involve making some sort of summary assessment of the data. We have seen a few examples of random phenomena and noted some of the features—the shape of the distribution of the data, whether we are dealing with discrete or continuous data, and so on. We need to describe summary measures of location of the data— where they are on the number line. This requires some measure of where the 'centre of gravity' of the data is—a measure of *central tendency*—and how spread they are about this central value—a measure of *dispersion*.

Measures of central tendency

One of the simulated Poisson data sets from (3.2.1) is shown in the bar chart and we can see that the data are clustered around the region 5–6.

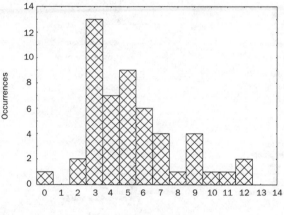

The mean of this data set is $\bar{x} = 5.38$. The mean, or average, is the most useful general measure of central tendency, and we shall see why shortly. In symmetrical distributions, the mean, median, and mode (if there is one) are likely to be quite close together. In skewed distributions, there may be considerable differences.

The peak frequency is 3; this outcome has occurred more often than any other single value and is thus the most 'typical'. The most frequently occurring outcome is the modal value. The *mode* is easy to see, needs no calculation, but has very limited value since it is only useful in circumstances in which repeated values arise—in discrete random variables. For those concerned with rubber glove utilization in operating theatres, it may be very useful—a limited number of sizes recur frequently; however, it is useless in formal statistical inference—that is, in reaching conclusions. We shall say no more about the mode.

The total number of observations is $n = 50$. If we arrange the data in order of magnitude and count to the halfway point—the middle value (for n odd) or the mean of the middle two values (n even)—this value is the *median*. The median in this case is 5, since the two middle values are both 5. The median is less valuable than the mean in mainstream statistical analysis, but comes into its own when we cannot find a convincing probability model for the data and need to use methods based on ranking data in order. We will explore one method of this type, the Mann–Whitney test (3.20).

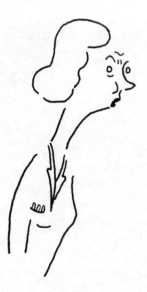

Sources of uncertainty

We have encountered variables in which we are counting events and those in which we are measuring something. We can, in principle at least, count events in a Poisson process, say, without any error and the variability we notice is entirely due to the random nature of the underlying process. In the SVP example we were estimating an unvarying quantity with an imperfect measurement technique, so that measurement error is a source of uncertainty. This measurement error can be either an error of accuracy or of precision (or both).

We are frequently interested in an inherently variable quantity (eg Cerebral Blood Flow) which we measure by an imperfect method so that we now have two sources of uncertainty in our attempt to estimate the mean value of the variable.

When we are comparing one measured variable against one or more others we have a more complex circumstance still. Each variable can vary independently about its own mean, and the uncertainty is further compounded by any measurement error, so that establishing a true difference in mean value can be difficult.

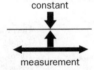

constant

measurement

Error of precision.
Method is accurate.

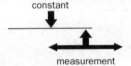

constant

measurement

Error of accuracy
and precision

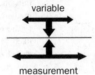

variable

measurement

Both variable and
measurement method
contribute to variation.
Method accurate.

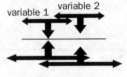

variable 1   variable 2

measurement

Comparison of means of two
samples. Despite accuracy, combination of natural variability and
imprecision of measurement
cause considerable overlap, so
identification of genuine difference in mean is difficult.

3.10.2   Dispersion: total error functions

The summary measures of mean, median, and mode are ways of describing the 'middle' or centre of gravity of the data. If there were no spread of the data, then we would not need any further measures. But we also need to describe how variable or dispersed the data are around this central figure. We may quote the *range*—where the data start and finish—but this is heavily influenced by any freak outlying values. The *interquartile range* is the interval which holds the central 50% of the data, so that 25% lie below and 25% above this interval. This concentrates upon the typical values in the middle, and the occasional wild outlier does not have disproportionate influence. Both of these are useful in basic description of the data and to enable us to gain an initial feel for them, but we need something more subtle for analysing data. We will now meet the idea of an error function, which shows the connection between measures of central tendency and dispersion. This topic may require some considerable thought, but it is worth spending some time on this, since the ideas introduced are central to statistical analysis.

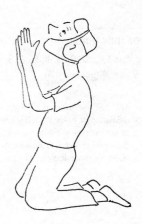

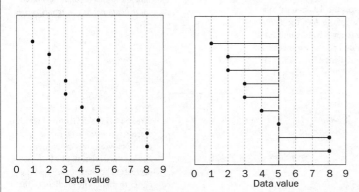

A measure of dispersion must involve some means of encapsulating how 'far' the data points are from their 'centre of gravity'. The distance of any datum point from a candidate central value must form the basis of a measure of dispersion—this is the *deviation* from the central value. The diagram shows the deviations of the data points from the arbitrary value $x = 5$ as an example. We can sum all of the deviations for each point from the x value in question to provide a measure of total dispersion from the x value. Here the total sum of deviations from $x = 5$ is 21—ignore the direction of deviation, and just add all of the line lengths.

Error functions

Consider another data list from Poisson $\mu = 5$: 1, 2, 2, 3, 3, 4, 5, 8, 8. The mean $\bar{x} = 4$ and the median is 3. The data are displayed as points on the number line, but have been vertically spaced only to allow us to see multiple points of the same value.

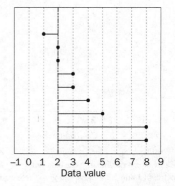

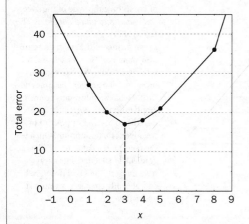

This is the graph that we obtain by carrying out the total dispersion sum for all values of x. In effect, we have 'swept' the dotted line (shown for $x = 5$ and $x = 2$ above) through *all* values of x and plotted the lengths of the summed deviations. The total dispersion is minimized at the value $x = 3$, when the total dispersion is 17. We will examine the graph in detail next.

Why have we chosen the value $x = 5$? There is no particular reason: we could try any other value that we choose and calculate the total length of lines—the sum of deviations—and see if we obtain a smaller value for the dispersion. This is the deviations of the points from the value $x = 2$. The sum of line lengths is 20. In fact, we can calculate the sum of deviations for *all* values of x by 'sweeping' the line across the data to create a function of x and *choose as a central measure that value of x which minimizes the sum of deviations*. If we minimize the dispersion measure, our central measure is the best 'fit' that we can make to the data.

3.10.3   Summing deviations: The *TEF* for the median

Error functions

Data list: 1, 2, 2, 3, 3, 4, 5, 8, 8.
$n = 9$. $\bar{x} = 4$ median $= 3$

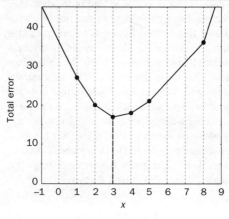

This *TEF* minimizes at $x = 3$, the median value of the data. It is not a smooth curve—it has corners, and these corners occur at x values at which there are data points.

The relationship of the total dispersion of the data points from any value of x is a *function*—we input an x value and obtain a value for total dispersion. We can think of this dispersion as a measure of the *error* that we make in summarizing the data by a single central measure. We will call this relationship a *total error function* (*TEF*). Because we want to minimize the error that we make in summarizing, we choose the x value that minimizes the *TEF*. The first *TEF* that we create is the function with the rule '*for any value of x, calculate the sum of absolute deviations of the data points (i.e. ignoring sign) from x*'.

We 'sweep' the vertical dashed line from left to right across the data and calculate the value of the *TEF* as we do so. If we are to the left of all of the data, the *TEF* is falling. As we move one unit to the right, the *TEF* value reduces by one unit for each datum point: we are approaching closer to *each* point because we are outside the range of the data. We have nine data points, so the gradient of the *TEF* is –9.

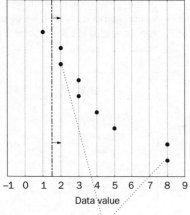

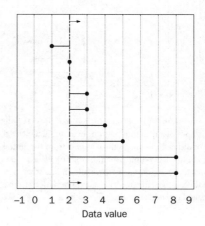

Between $x = 2$ and $x = 3$, there are three points the deviation of which is increasing as we sweep to the right—we are moving away from them—and six the deviation of which is decreasing because we are moving closer to them. The gradient of the *TEF* is –3: it is still falling.

As we sweep the line into the data range between 1 and 2, we move *nearer* to these eight points, as we are moving *away* from the point at $x = 1$. What we *reduce* from *one* (any one) of the points we are approaching, we are *adding* simultaneously to the deviation from the point at $x = 1$. The gradient of the *TEF* is thus –7 between $x = 1$ and $x = 2$. The gradient is determined by the balance of the *number* of data points to either side of the sweep line. Think hard about this—this *TEF counts* data points.

The total dispersion attributable to these four points does not change between $x = 6$ and $x = 8$, but we are moving away from the other five. The gradient is +5.

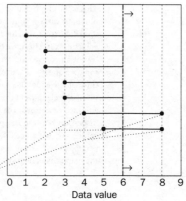

The value of the *TEF* reaches a minimum when we have equal *numbers* of points on either side of the sweep line—*the minimum point of this TEF is thus always the median*. As we sweep further to the right, there are now more points to the left and the total deviation—the *TEF* value—increases. The gradient becomes positive. To have a minimum point, a graph must change gradient from negative to positive or positive to negative at that minimum. Outside the range of the data, the *TEF* has a gradient of +9. Gradients always have integer values and these gradients abruptly change at x values at which there are data points.

3.10.4 Summing squared deviations: the *TEF* of the mean

A smooth error function

Data list: 1, 2, 2, 3, 3, 4, 5, 8, 8. $n = 9$ $\bar{x} = 4$ median = 3

We come across the word 'square' all over the place in statistics—variance is the *square* of standard deviation, least *squares*, chi-*squared*—Why do statisticians like to square everything? We shall find out. The *TEF* using the sum of absolute deviations had corners, and functions with corners are awkward to deal with. If we adopt the same approach with deviations from the sweep line, but change the rule for the *TEF* to '*calculate the deviations from x, square them and then sum them*' what happens?

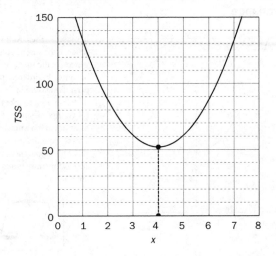

Using this rule for the *TEF* with the same data, we obtain a smooth curve—a parabola with its minimum at $x = 4$. The positions of the data points are no longer shown by abrupt changes in gradient. *The minimum point of this TEF is always the mean of the data set.* The demonstration of this is given in (2.13.1). Smooth functions such as this are easy to manipulate. Details of quadratic functions are given in (2.7.).

The *TEF* approach emphasizes that dispersion and central measures are intimately connected—we measure dispersion *from* the central value that we choose. The way in which we choose to quantify dispersion gives a function—we have seen two ways—and we choose the 'best fit' central value from the minimum of this function.

The parabolic error function

We use the new rule,

$$TEF = \sum_{i=1}^{i=n}(x - x_i)^2$$

where for our data list $i = 1, 2, 3, \ldots,$ 9, and $x_1 = 1$, $x_2 = 2$, $x_3 = 2$, ..., $x_9 = 8$. x is the position of the sweep line; x_i is the ith datum point. It is important to realize that anything involving x with a subscript refers to the *data*—and is therefore *fixed* for any data set. Anything with 'bald' x refers to the position of the sweep line, which is our independent *variable*. We are asking how the *TEF* varies with choice of x value for *this* set of data. The *TEF* value is thus a function of x:

$$\sum_{i=1}^{i=n}(x - x_i)^2 = \sum(x^2 - 2xx_i + x_i^2)$$
$$= nx^2 - 2x\sum x_i + \sum x_i^2.$$

Where $\sum x_i = 36$ $\sum x_i^2 = 196$. This is a quadratic function the graph of which is a parabola. For our data set, we have $TEF = 9x^2 - 72x + 196$, which has its minimum value at $x = 4$. The function value at this point is $TEF = 52$. This *TEF* can be written in completed square form (2.7.3) as $TEF = 9(x - 4)^2 + 52$.

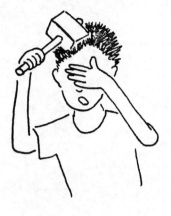

3.10.5 Total sum of squares, *TSS*: variance and standard deviation

Why are we concerning ourselves so much with this business of error functions? We have shown that the squaring-procedure *TEF* minimizes at the mean, and that this ensures the best central measure that we can make by fitting a single figure to the data—at least by using this particular rule for the *TEF*. We get a nice smooth, mathematically tractable function. The value of this *TEF* at its minimum point is the *total sum of squares about the mean*, which we abbreviate to *TSS*. The selection of the mean can be viewed as a *model* of the data—the simplest that we can have, since we are summarizing all of the data with a single figure. The idea of the mean as a model will seem a more sensible concept when we use more involved models such as linear regression later (3.18).

Coefficient of variation

The idea of the error function can be difficult to grasp, but we shall need to use the concept extensively, so it is worth allowing the ideas time to sink in.

The variance and standard deviation are scaled according to the number of data points to be measures of mean dispersion. The amount of dispersion relative to the location of the mean can be quantified as the coefficient of variation; if the mean $\mu = 100$ and the standard deviation $\sigma = 1$, then this is relatively much less dispersed ($\sigma/\mu = 1\%$) than if the mean $\mu = 10$ with the same standard deviation ($\sigma/\mu = 10\%$). The coefficient of variation is σ/μ, the ratio of the standard deviation to the mean.

TSS and variance

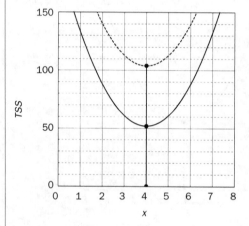

Because it arises from sums of squares, the variance, has units which are the square of the original units. In order to have a dispersion measure in the original units, we need to take the square root of the variance—the root mean squared (r.m.s.) deviation. This is the *standard deviation*. It should be apparent that the variance is the more fundamental quantity.

The $TSS = 52$ for our data set. If we had the same degree of dispersion but twice as many data points, then the value of the *TSS* would almost certainly be larger. Imagine if we had all of the data points duplicated; then $n = 18$, $\bar{x} = 4$ and the *TSS* would be 104, but the degree of dispersion would be no greater. In order to produce a dispersion measure independent of the size of the data set, we obviously need to scale our *TSS* to take account of the number of data points contributing to it—the size of the sample n. The scaled specific measure of dispersion which takes the number of points into account is the *mean squared deviation about the mean*, or the *variance*.

We would expect to scale by a factor n to obtain the variance. The reason why the scaling factor to obtain the variance from the *TSS* is not usually the sample size n but a *smaller* value, $n - 1$, will become apparent before long:

$$\text{sample variance} = \frac{TSS}{(n-1)} \qquad \text{sample standard deviation (s.d.)} = \sqrt{\frac{TSS}{n-1}}$$

For our sample, the variance = 36/8 = 4.5. The sample s.d. = 2.12.

The squaring procedure actually has little to do with getting rid of negative deviations from the mean, as is commonly supposed (although it does). Its purpose is to give us a smooth and easily manipulated *TEF*. Alternatively, we could just ignore the negative signs and deal with absolute deviations, in which case we obtain an error function that *counts* the data points as we saw, and minimizes at the median. This is a much less useful approach.

3.11.1 General features

It seems to be true that, however little students know about probability and statistics, they will be familiar with the essential features of the 'bell-shaped' normal distribution. The normal distribution made a short appearance as a model of measurement error when we were considering estimation of the SVP of a new anaesthetic agent (3.5.1). This model was essentially an empirical one, in that the pattern of measurement error had the same 'shape' as the normal. Why does the normal distribution have such pre-eminence in statistical method and where does it come from?

Origins of the normal distribution

The clue to the importance of the normal distribution lies in the example of sums or differences of the results of throwing dice (3.7). We sample from one distribution—in that case a uniform distribution—and the arithmetical process of summing independent observations results in a distribution with features that are not present in the sampled distribution; the distribution of the individual throws is uniform, but the distribution (i.e. the relative frequencies) of the sum shows a centralizing tendency, which tends to reduce the occurrence of extreme values. This is a consequence of the independence of the individual throws and the rules of probability (3.8.1).

The importance of the normal distribution can be summarized as follows:

- Many naturally occurring phenomena are determined by multiple additive factors. In biological variables for instance, genetic, nutritional, and other environmental factors will all contribute. This additive process acts just like the die example to produce a symmetrical bunching around a central value which, in a large population, appears as a normally distributed variable. Similar multiply additive error factors in measurement lead to a normally distributed error. Remember always that the normal distribution is a mathematical model of real-life phenomena; it may be a more or less good model.
- Calculation of means from data involves summation and, whatever the underlying distribution, in repeated sampling the distribution of those means tends towards a normal distribution. Much statistical activity is directed at making inferences based upon the mean of sets of data, and this necessarily requires use of the normal.
- There are other circumstances in which the combined effect of processes acts as the product rather than the sum of the individual contributions for example, in many metabolic processes the concentration of a product feeds in as the reactant in the next step in the chain, in a Law of Mass Action system. Such processes tend to produce positively skewed distributions of final products—that is, there is bunching at the low end with a long tail of high values. However, a log transformation of the data may well be normally distributed, since the multiplicative effect is converted into an summing process in logs.
- Convenience of analysis is an important reason: there is an enormous armoury of techniques based upon the normal distribution, which means that it can be expedient to apply normally based techniques to data that are not strictly normal. Appropriate transformations may render these data more nearly normal and suitable for such analyses. Surprisingly, sometimes it may not matter too much if the data are exactly normally distributed, so that useful inferences can still be made. These are matters of judgement that require expert statistical opinion. Tests which can still yield useful information in these circumstances are said to be 'robust' to non-normality.

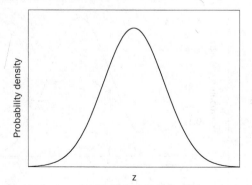

3.11.2 **The standard normal distribution**

The standard normal distribution is a basic pattern, like the functions that we discussed in part 2. Like them, we can apply transformations to turn it into other members of the family (2.5).

The standard normal formula

The standard normal distribution—the basic bell-shaped curve—is described by a rather complicated-looking formula:

$$f(x) = \frac{1}{\sqrt{2\pi}} \exp\left(-\frac{x^2}{2}\right)$$

Any general normal distribution of arbitrary mean and variance can be described by a (scaling and translation) modification of this basic pattern function.

    There is no need to memorize this. The integral of this function is the area under the curve of the normal distribution and is the cumulative standard normal distribution. The above expression cannot be integrated to give a function in terms of basic functions, and so has to be integrated numerically (2.16). Values of the cumulative normal distribution are tabulated and these are what we consult (either in a book of tables or by asking the computer to perform tests) when we need to determine the significance of a result or calculate a confidence interval from a normal distribution.

The normal pattern function

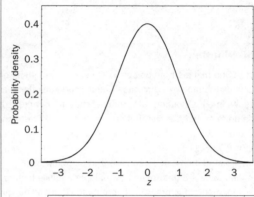

The standard normal has mean $\mu = 0$ and has the well-known symmetrical bell shape about this value. The distribution is continuous. The horizontal axis is conventionally denoted by z.

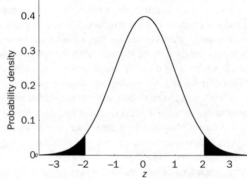

The spread of the distribution is governed by the value of the standard deviation, σ which is unity for the standard normal. The variance is therefore also 1. About 68% of the area lies within one standard deviation of the mean—that is, in the interval $[-1,1]$. About 95% lies within two standard deviations—in the interval $[-2, 2]$. Three standard deviations to either side of the mean encompass 99.7% of the distribution—there is a probability of $p = 0.003$ of encountering a value outside this range.

The vertical axis is the probability *density*. This is a necessary idea for continuous distributions: the probability of data from the distribution lying between two values, z_1 and z_2, is the *area* under the density curve between z_1 and z_2. The area under the whole curve is 1.

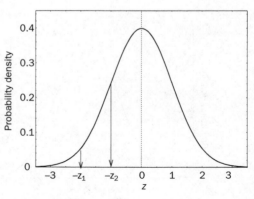

For a discrete distribution such as the Poisson, the probabilities are confined to certain specific values—in the Poisson case, these are integers. We can give a probability value for any specified discrete outcome. With a continuous distribution, we must specify an interval and calculate the area under the curve between these values to establish the probability that the variable will lie within the interval.

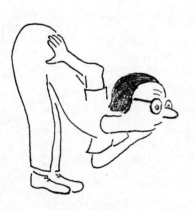

3.11.3 Transformations of the standard normal distribution

Translation and scaling

The standard normal distribution has a mean $\mu = 0$ and a standard deviation $\sigma = 1$. We can transform the standard normal into any other normal distribution, or vice versa, by simple transformations, as described in (2.5). Any other normal distribution has the same shape as the standard normal, but the spread (σ) may be greater or less than unity; and the central value, the mean μ, around which the data are dispersed, may be different.

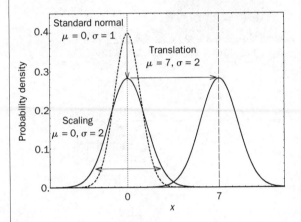

The standard normal $\sim N(0, 1)$ can be transformed into any general normal distribution $\sim N(\mu, \sigma^2)$ by multiplying (scaling) by σ the standard deviation and then adding μ (translation). The scaling stretches or compresses the unit standard deviation by the appropriate amount, and the addition or subtraction of μ shifts the whole curve so that it is symmetrical about the new mean μ. Random numbers from the standard normal, available in tables, can be used to simulate data from any other normal distribution by this procedure.

Note that the scaling procedure (here by a factor of two) spreads the distribution out, but also depresses the peak of the curve since the area under the whole curve must always remain 1. This is the same phenomenon we observed with the Poisson of increasing mean (3.2.3).

Transforming data from an arbitrary $\sim N(\mu, \sigma^2)$ back to the standard normal is accomplished by adopting the reverse procedure. We subtract the mean μ (translation) from each datum and divide by the standard deviation σ (scaling). This procedure is required, for instance, to refer any data obtained from the distribution $\sim N(\mu, \sigma^2)$ to tables of the standard normal for performing significance tests, and so on.

Approximation of Poisson and Normal

We have seen that the general shape of the Poisson becomes smoother and more symmetrical as the mean increases and more closely resembles a normal distribution. We can approximate the discrete Poisson distribution with the normal distribution of the same mean and variance, but because the Poisson only gives probabilities for integer values of x, the bars are centred on these x-values. For $\mu = 16$, the area under Poisson 'curve' ie the sum of the bar heights for $x \leq 16$ is actually the area for $x \leq 16.5$ because the $x = 16$ bar occupies a width of $x = 1$ symmetrically based on $x = 16$. When we are calculating areas under the matching normal curve, we need to account for this discontinuity in the discrete distribution and calculate the normal probability for $x \leq 16.5$ rather than 16. This is the continuity correction. The matching cumulative probability for the normal curve of the same mean and variance, $N(16, 16)$, for $x = 16$ is of course $p = 0.5$. The Poisson $\mu = 16$ cumulative probability is $p = 0.5659$. This is an error of about 11%. Using the continuity correction, the cumulative normal for $x = 16.5$, we obtain an approximate probability of $p = 0.5498$, an error of about 3% which is commendably close. As the mean increases and typical individual probabilities decrease (because of the increased variance), the use of a continuity correction in matching the discrete and the continuous becomes less important.

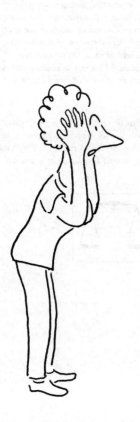

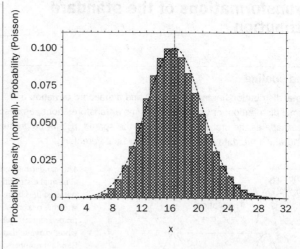

The discrete Poisson $\mu = 16$ and the normal $N(16, 16)$ are quite well matched although the asymmetry of the Poisson is still evident.

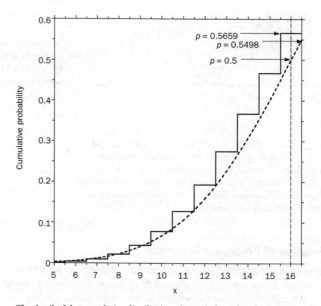

The detail of the cumulative distributions (3.11.4) show that the function values (areas under the respective Poisson and normal graphs) are matched most closely at the end of the Poisson intervals.

3.11.4   The cumulative normal distribution

Areas under the bell curve

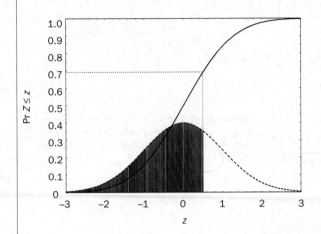

The cumulative standard normal distribution is a graph of the area under the curve of the standard normal distribution. Its value for any z is the area under the curve to the left of z: this means the probability that a standard normal variable takes a value less than z and it is entirely analogous with the cumulative distribution of any other family—for example, Poisson or binomial. It can be transformed to the cumulative distribution of any normal distribution by the same methods.

The cumulative standard distribution is symmetrical about $z = 0$ because the standard normal is symmetrical about this figure. It has value 0.5 at $z = 0$ because half of the area under the curve lies to the left of $z = 0$.

The cumulative function has value 0.1587 at $z = -1$. This means that 15.87% lies below $z = -1$. Because of the symmetry of the function, 15.87% of the area lies above $z = +1$. Thus 31.74% of the distribution lies further than 1 away from the mean, and hence $100 - 31.74 = 68.26$% of the distribution lies within $z = \pm 1$. These proportions are preserved in transformed distributions, as we would expect. 68.26% of any normal distribution lies within one standard deviation of the mean. The exact z value for encompassing 95% of the distribution is ± 1.96.

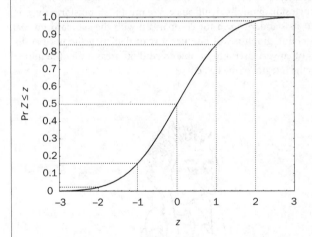

The cumulative function has value 0.0228 at $z = -2$. 2.28% of the area lies below $z = -2$ and hence 4.56% of the distribution lies further than two standard deviations away from the mean. Thus 95.44% lies within $z = \pm 2$.

The probability that a standard normal variable takes a value between any particular z values is simply the difference in the areas—the difference in the cumulative function value for each. For instance, the probability that a standard normal variable takes a value between $z = -1$ and $z = +2$ is $p = 0.9772 - 0.1587 = 0.8185$.

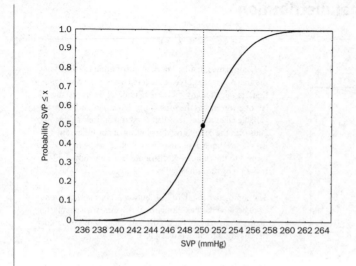

The cumulative distribution for the SVP measurement with $\sigma = 4$ mmHg is shown. This is just a scaled and translated version of the standard curve. We just relabel the horizontal axis appropriately.

The cumulative standard normal distribution is what appears in statistical tables as normal probabilities. It enables us quickly to determine the probability associated with any observation from a (null, i.e. hypothesized) normal distribution, so that we may reach a conclusion about its significance. We must first transform the normal observation to its standard form for comparison with the standard normal. The cumulative function graph is just another way of depicting the normal distribution, and it is often very useful to be able to read off areas under the normal curve directly. It is the integral of the bell curve.

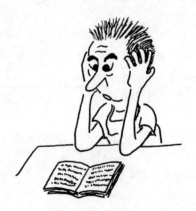

3.12.1   **Population and sample**

Two key concepts that we shall need repeatedly are those of population and sample. A population may be some circumscribed group—the number of children under eight years admitted to a particular ITU in in a particular year, for example—or some more abstract collection. In the anaphylactoid reaction example, the random variable was the observed number of severe reactions annually. The observed values of the RV form a *sample* from all the possible observations that we might make—the *population*. Although we can actually only make a limited number of observations, we view these observations as arising from some larger collection, the population. It is usually quite clear what the population comprises in any given problem. We shall simply mean the larger possibly infinite group of possible observations from which our actual ones are drawn. The distribution of the population is called the parent distribution—the samples are its children, in a sense. The samples are then used to calculate measures—statistics—which have related but distinct distributions. These are the sampling distributions of the statistics.

μ, σ^2, $\bar{x}$ and s^2

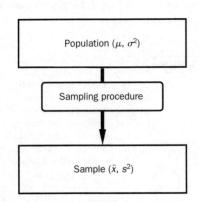

Population (μ, σ^2)

Sampling procedure

Sample ($\bar{x}$, s^2)

The measurements of SVP of the new anaesthetic agent form a sample from an infinite population: in principle, we could go on measuring the SVP for ever, acquiring more and more data. We consider the population to be characterized by a form of distribution (for SVP, normal because we expect measurement errors to be normally distributed) with mean μ and variance σ^2. Population values for mean and variance are given Greek symbols. Remember that μ might not be the same as the actual SVP if the method is not accurate. μ is the mean of the *measurement* method.

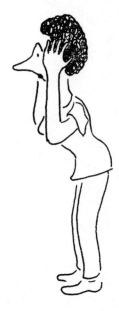

The sample data are used to make an inference about the population and we will usually want to *estimate* the values of μ and σ^2. There may be prior information on either of these, but this is unusual. Otherwise, they must be estimated from the data themselves and we calculate the sample mean $\bar{x}$ and sample variance s^2, for example. Sample statistics are given Roman symbols. A statistic is any quantity calculated from the data. We need to ensure that samples are representative of the population from which they are drawn.

Statistical inference involves a two-part process: probability models of the population, based upon modelling assumptions, form the basis for predicting the behaviour of random samples from this population. This predicted behaviour is used to make inferences from actual samples about the populations from which they are drawn. The process of inference is liable to error because of random variation. The probability and likely magnitude of the errors are predictable from the theory, which enables us to quantify the confidence that we have in our conclusions.

3.12.2   Estimation and decision-making

We use the theoretical results of probability theory to make inferences about a parent distribution by studying a sample from that population. Statistical inference, for our purposes, is concerned with two closely related processes; decision-making or significance testing, and estimation. We are usually trying to make up our minds about some problem—'Is there evidence that anaesthetic agent *A* releases plasma peptide *B*?'—or we are estimating a quantity—'What is the SVP of this substance?'

The former emphasis on significance testing has been changed by the easy availability of computing, since it is now easy to obtain exact probabilities for observed results, and the need for binary (accept/reject) decisions at arbitrary levels of significance is disappearing.

Statistical inference

The process of statistical inference is a two-way one. The theory tells us how a particular statistic—something such as the sample mean, $\bar{x}$, calculated from sample data—varies in repeated samples. from a parent population of known characteristics (distribution and parameters). This is the sampling distribution of the statistic. We then 'look back' from the sample statistics and infer what the characteristics of the parent population might plausibly be.

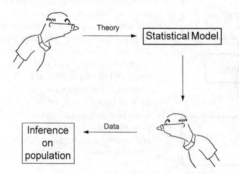

Using this theoretical foundation, we can work back from the data from our single sample and make a statement about our estimated value for the SVP and how close we think we are to μ, the mean of the measurement method. We clarify the details of how this is done next.

The SVP example led us to take a probability model (measurement errors are usually normally distributed). Further theory tells us that when we take samples, the sample mean $\bar{x}$ is an unbiased estimator of the population mean μ and that this is also normally distributed. The standard error of the mean which we meet soon is a measure of how variable is the estimate of the μ by the sample mean $\bar{x}$. If our physical chemistry is correct, μ should be close to the true SVP.

The estimation of a constant quantity by a measurement method of known precision is a highly unusual circumstance. Most problems in medicine and biology are much more uncertain than this one. This has been deliberately chosen to be nearly the simplest possible example of estimation. We shall look at more realistic problems and identify the sources of uncertainty involved and how these uncertainties lead us to be less confident in our estimates.

This approach is only slightly modified by those circumstances in which we have no convincing probability model for the parent distribution. We then cannot estimate parameters of the underlying distribution (because we cannot suggest one) but we may still be able to construct meaningful statistics, and they *do* have sampling distributions that enable us to perform significance testing. These are the non-parametric methods; for example, the sign test (3.15.2) and the Mann–Whitney test (3.20.).

3.13.1 SVP measurement again: estimation from the mean of a sample

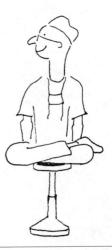

We met the example of SVP measurement (3.5.1) as an instance of the normal distribution in action; measurement errors are normally distributed. The manufacturer knew from past experience that the precision of his estimation was such that 95% of measurements occurred within 8 mmHg to either side of a central mean value. Now that we have encountered the standard normal distribution, we know that, for a normally distributed variable, 95% of observations will lie within about two standard deviations (1.96 exactly) of the central, mean value. The standard deviation σ of the SVP measurement method is thus 4 mmHg. σ is a measure of precision.

The SVP problem is therefore one of estimating the unknown mean of a normal distribution of known standard deviation.

Sampling error of the mean

The standard deviation $\sigma = 4$ mmHg means that this is how widely *individual* determinations of SVP are expected to vary. If we make a number of n separate determinations, we have a sample of size n. Each of these measurements is an independent observation from an infinite population with distribution $\sim N(\mu, 4^2)$ (parent distribution).

What happens when we calculate the mean of such samples? To calculate the mean we:

- sum the individual observations and
- divide (scale) by the sample size

We know from the dice-throwing experiment (3.7) that there is a centralizing tendency at work when we sum independent observations from a random variable—extreme values become less probable because of the 'ironing out' process of the addition. The division by the sample size n gets us back to the scale of the individual data. Since the calculation of the mean involves a summation, we expect the means of samples of a number of observations to be less variable than the individual observations. The larger the sample, the more likely are any occasional extreme values to be swamped by the more 'ordinary' ones.

We therefore expect means of samples to be closer to the mean of the underlying parent distribution μ than the individual observations themselves. The means of large samples will tend to be closer to μ than those of small samples.

The less precise the measurement method is, the more variable we expect the means of such samples to be.

A large number of determinations (large n) with a precise determination method (small σ) will ensure a sample mean $\bar{x}$ close to the true mean μ. Small, imprecise samples will plainly be more liable to give a sample mean $\bar{x}$ well away from μ.

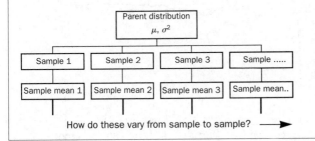

If we could (theory) take repeated samples of a given size n from the same distribution and calculate a mean for each one, the means would vary from sample to sample. If we were to do this for a very large number of samples, we could describe a *sampling distribution of the mean*. The variability of the sample mean determines how confident we can be in any mean $\bar{x}$ calculated from the particular single sample we have (practice).

3.13.2 SVP estimation: the sampling distribution of the mean

Expected value and standard error of the sample mean

Usually, we only have a single sample to study. Statistical theory allows us to predict the behaviour of a statistic such as the sample mean in repeated samples and describe a sampling distribution. This allows us to make an inference about the population from which the sample (the one we actually have) arises—the parent distribution.

If we are sampling from a normal distribution—that is, the parent distribution is normal $\sim N(\mu, \sigma^2)$—then the distribution of the means from such samples is also normal with mean μ. The mean of the sample means (the expected value of the sample mean) is thus the true mean: the sample mean $\bar{x}$ is a statistic which is said to be *unbiased* because it 'homes in' on the correct value, the population mean μ. In the long run, the average value for $\bar{x}$ in repeated samples is μ. Even if we are sampling from a non-normal distribution, such as the Poisson, then the expected value of the sample mean is still μ, and the sampling distribution will still be approximately normal because of the operation of the centralizing tendency.

The other fact that we need to know about the sampling distribution of $\bar{x}$ is its variability, its standard deviation. As we have noted, the variability of the sample mean depends upon the variability of the parent population (σ) and how large the sample is, sample size n. The standard deviation of the distribution of the sample mean is the *standard error of the mean SEM*:

$$SEM = \frac{\sigma}{\sqrt{n}}.$$

The *SEM* thus is larger for larger σ and diminishes as the square root of the sample size, n.

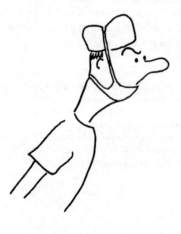

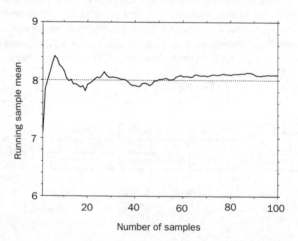

100 samples of size $n = 10$ from Poisson $\mu = 8$ have been simulated. We calculate the means of all samples and, taking them in any order, calculate the 'running mean' of all the samples. For instance, for sample 20 we have added all the sample means 1–20 and divided by 20 and plotted this value. We can see that after an erratic start (a small number of samples, with each sample having a proportionally large influence), the fluctuations settle down as each new sample has progressively a smaller proportional effect. The 'long-run' behaviour is for the sample means to approach the true value $\mu = 8$ quite closely. It homes in on the true value.

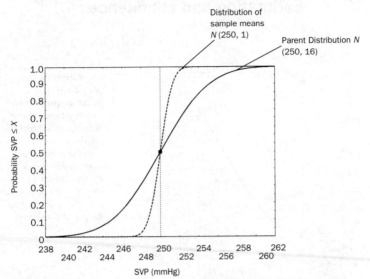

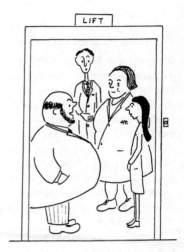

If we have a sample of $n = 16$ SVP determinations, then, for $\sigma = 4$ mmHg, the standard error is $SEM = 1$ mmHg. The cumulative distributions of the parent distribution and the sampling distribution of the mean of samples of this size are shown. The mean of both distributions is the same—the sample mean is unbiased. The spread of the sampling distribution of the mean is 1/4 that of the parent distribution for $n = 16$.

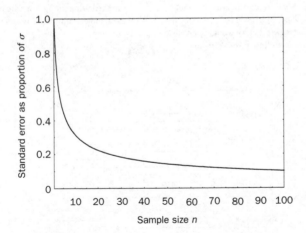

If the manufacturer wanted to make a more reliable (i.e. precise) estimate of the SVP, he could take a larger sample (increase n) or improve the performance of his instrument (decrease σ).

The 'law of diminishing returns' applies to sample size: if we want to halve the standard error, we need a sample four times as large.

3.13.3   **Estimation and confidence**

Point and interval estimates

Since we know that in the long run (i.e. if we take repeated samples and take the 'mean of means') the sample mean $\bar{x}$ 'homes in' on the parent population mean μ, our best estimate for μ is $\bar{x}$. This is a *point estimate*, since we specify a single figure as our 'best guess'. We can, however, be more informative if we quote a range within which we expect the true value for μ to lie with a specified degree of certainty.

    For the SVP example, the sampling distribution of $\bar{x}$ is normal and has a standard deviation, $SEM = 1$ mmHg, so we know that about 95% of the sample means will lie in the interval $\mu \pm 2$ mmHg. We can thus quote a 95% *confidence interval* (CI)—a range within which 95% of sample means will lie. This is 4 mmHg wide, and we centre it on the sample mean $\bar{x}$ which is our best point estimate of μ. The 95% CI is thus $\bar{x} \pm 2$ mmHg. Calculated in this way, 95% of intervals that we quote in such samples would contain the true mean μ (We should really use ± 1.96 mmHg for the 95% intervals, but 2 is near enough).

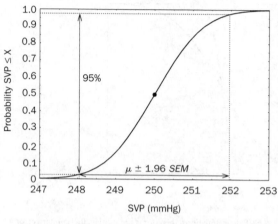

The shape of the sampling distribution is exactly normal if we are sampling from a normal distribution and approximately so even if we are sampling from some other distribution. It is always centred on μ, since $\bar{x}$ is an unbiased estimator of μ, whatever the parent distribution.

95% of the sampling distribution lies within 1.96 SEM of the true mean μ. The absolute size of the interval depends upon the size of the SEM, which in turn depends upon sample size and population variability: $SEM = \sigma/\sqrt{n}$. In our example, $SEM = 1$ mmHg. We thus have an interval about 4 mmHg wide, which will contain 95% of the sample means that we would calculate in repeated sampling from $\sim N(\mu, 16)$.

A 99% CI would be wider than a 95% CI. 99% of a normal distribution lies within 2.58 standard deviations of the mean. Our 99% CI for the SVP would thus be $\bar{x} \pm 2.58$ mmHg. Confidence intervals for other levels of significance can be constructed using the appropriate point on the standard cumulative normal distribution.

Twenty 95% confidence intervals for μ have been simulated in this way from $\sim N(250, 16)$. We *expect* 19 of these CIs to include the true mean, $\mu = 250$; in fact, two of the simulated intervals fail to include the mean. Since the simulation is itself a random variable we are not surprised if we do not always obtain the expected value; in the long run, however, we will average one 'miss' in every 20. [This simulation RV is distributed as a binomial variable $\sim B(20, 0.05)$; in other words 20 trials with a $p = 0.05$ of missing the mean μ].

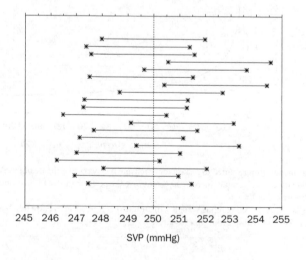

All of the intervals are of the same width since we know the SEM (σ and n are both known quantities): only the position varies.

3.14.1   Samples of unknown mean and variance

The SVP example was quite easy to deal with because the manufacturer knew the precision of the measurement method, $\sigma = 4$ mmHg; he was attempting to determine the unknown mean of a normal distribution of known variance. If he had no information on the value of σ, then he could still make a point estimate of μ from the sample mean $\bar{x}$, but he could not quote a CI because he would need to know the precision σ to calculate the *SEM* (3.13.2). Such prior knowledge of the variability of the parent population is very unusual indeed in practical studies; it is far more common to have no information about either mean or variance. Usually the only information that we have is contained within the sample itself and we have to use this to estimate the population standard deviation to be able to calculate a value for *SEM* and hence a CI for μ. We can, however, easily calculate a *sample standard deviation*, *s*, and use this to calculate a value for *SEM*. But how do we proceed to calculate a CI from this?

Narrow CIs mean precise estimation; broad CIs mean less precise estimation. *Estimation* of σ from the samples rather than *firm knowledge* of its value must have the effect of making our CIs for estimating μ broader. In the SVP example, prior knowledge of the value of $\sigma\ (= 4$ mmHg) and the form of the distribution (normal) enabled us to go straight to tables of the normal distribution, and extract the factor 1.96 as a multiple for the *SEM* in order to calculate the width of a 95% CI for μ to either side of the sample mean $\bar{x}$.

We therefore need a distribution which is more spread out than the standard normal, so that we multiply the *SEM* calculated from *s* by a larger factor than we need when we do know σ. This distribution is the famous Student's *t*-distribution. We shall explore the *t*-distribution in more detail later (3.16) when we have studied how we estimate *s* from sample data.

The t_5-distribution and standard normal

The details of the *t*-distribution can wait until later. At the moment, all we need to note are a few features. The *t*-distribution has a mean of $\mu = 0$ like the standard normal and has a similar symmetrical shape, although is 'squashed' so that it is flatter and more spread out than the normal. Although it is very closely related to the normal, unlike the normal the *t*-distribution is completely specified by just one parameter—ν the *degrees of freedom*. The number of degrees of freedom is closely related to the sample size; large samples enable us to estimate σ better than do small samples. The *t*-distribution approximates to the standard normal as the degrees of freedom increase.

The standard normal distribution (dotted line) is shown, as well as the *t*-distribution for $\nu = 5$. The *t*-distribution is more splayed out, so that the 95% limits occur at $t = \pm2.57$, rather than $z = \pm1.96$ for the standard normal. This is the factor that we need to multiply the *SEM* by in order to obtain a 95% CI for estimation of μ in a sample of size $n = 6$.

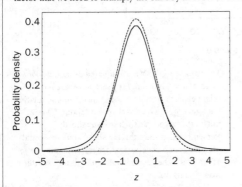

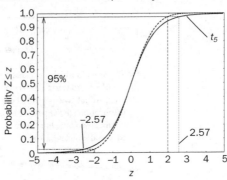

These features are shown in the cumulative distributions of the standard normal and the t_5-distributions. Tables are available which give the values of the cumulative *t* for different values of ν.

3.14.2 **Sampling distribution**

We now need to explore the estimation of population variability from sample data. We will do this with a Poisson variable to remind ourselves of the existence of distributions other than the normal and also to demonstrate the generality of the ideas involved. The fact that Poisson variance is 'built in' will be useful too. We will need the ideas that we met in the section on error functions and the *TSS* (3.10).

Sampling from Poisson $\mu = 8$

We will simulate a Poisson variable of mean $\mu = 8$. It might help to imagine some Poisson process—for example, the annual number of inadvertent dural taps during epidural placement in an obstetric unit—as motivating the simulation. We know that a Poisson distribution has a variance equal to its mean (3.2.4), so σ^2 = 8. We simulate 100 samples of size $n = 10$ (i.e. ten independent observations from Poisson $\mu = 8$)—this is a simulation of 100 decades, a millennium worth of dural taps. Simulation is a useful tool and can save some waiting around for real data.

For each of the samples, we calculate a mean $\bar{x}$ and a *TSS* about this value; that is, the sum of squared deviations from the mean $TSS = \Sigma_{i=1}^{i=10}(x_i - \bar{x})^2$. We plot the running mean of these *TSS* against the number of samples: for each sample in turn, we calculate the mean *TSS* of this and all preceding samples. This sounds complicated, but all we are doing is showing the long-run behaviour of the *TSS* in repeated sampling. We adopted a similar process with the same data in (3.13.2) to show the long-run behaviour of the mean in repeated samples.

After an erratic start, the *TSS* eventually settles down at a value of around 73. The early behaviour is erratic because of the small sample numbers, and thus each individual sample has a large influence. As we average more sample *TSS*s, each new sample has proportionately less influence—yet another example of the 'ironing-out', centralizing process.

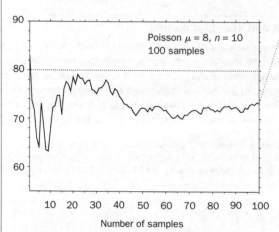

Poisson $\mu = 8$, $n = 10$
100 samples

Number of samples

The order in which we take the samples is arbitrary; a different order would give us a different graph, although the pattern would be similar and the final point at which all samples had been included would be identical.

The variance—the average squared deviation—of Poisson $\mu = 8$ is 8 and, for a sample of size $n = 10$, we might expect a *TSS* = 80. What we get in a simulation is a figure quite a bit less than this (about 73)—it misses the target. We shall see why shortly. Remember that since this is a simulation, we would get a different result on another run with another set of samples—the details would differ, but the pattern would be similar.

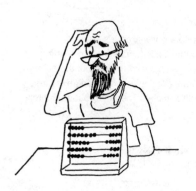

3.14.3   Expected value

Expected value of sample variance

It looks from the simulation as if we underestimate the variability of the population by looking at the sample *TSS*. The average long-run *TSS* should be about 80
($\sigma^2 = 8$, $n = 10$), but it actually seems to be settling near 73. This is indeed a
real effect, explained below. It can be shown that if we divide by $n - 1$ rather than
n, we enlarge our estimate of σ^2 and the sample variance will in the long run
home in on the correct value σ^2. The average value that we obtain by calculating
the sample variance in this way is σ^2; $TSS/(n - 1)$ is an unbiased estimator of σ^2.

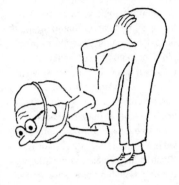

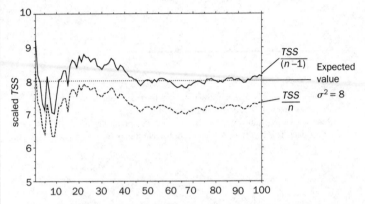

Division of the *TSS* by $n - 1 = 9$ brings the long-run average sample variance nearer to the
true value $\sigma^2 = 8$. This is not a proof it is a simulation, but it can be shown that division by
$n - 1$ will give us the unbiased estimator. This is an important graph; it shows that individual samples very quite widely in the sample variance s^2, causing the marked fluctuations
when we have averaged only a few samples, but 'in the long run' aiming for the correct
value σ^2. Division by n misses the mark.

Distribution of the sample variance

We have an unbiased estimator for
σ^2. On average, $s^2 = TSS/(n - 1)$ will
home in on the right value for σ^2, but
this does not tell us anything about
how confident we can be in any particular estimate of variance that we
make from an individual sample or
the shape of the distribution of sample variance. For this, we need a
sampling distribution for s^2.

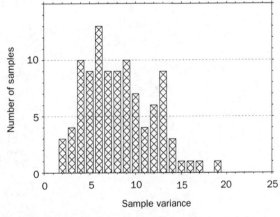

We know that the 100
samples that we simulat-
ed from Poisson $\mu = 8$
come from a distribution
with $\sigma^2 = 8$ and the simulation showed a mean
s^2 of about 8.1 overall.
This shows a histogram
of the spread of sample
variance s^2 in the 100
samples.

The histogram shows a distribution of values of s^2 which is skewed to the right—there is a tail of higher values. s^2 is always a positive quantity, since it is a sum of squared deviations scaled to sample size. We can never have values less than zero, but there is no
upper bound—the sampling distribution is liable to be asymmetric. We might guess that larger sample sizes would have a more   .
symmetrical distribution because we are summing more deviations, and this allows the centralizing tendency to work.

Why $n - 1$?

The scaling of the sample *TSS* to obtain the sample variance using a factor of $n - 1$ rather than n often occasions surprise. We have a sample of data from a population of unknown mean μ and what we want to know is how the data are dispersed around μ. But we do not know μ—that is usually what we want to estimate from the data—all we have is our 'best guess' for μ, which is the sample mean $\bar{x}$. But we obtain $\bar{x}$ from the same data, and we know that choosing $\bar{x}$ is the best possible fit to those particular data; the sum of squares is greater around any other value. Since our value for $\bar{x}$ will generally be different from μ, (sampling distribution of $\bar{x}$ (3.13.2)) the dispersion of the data about μ will be greater than that around $\bar{x}$. It is for this reason that we divide by a value less than n, i.e. $(n - 1)$—this expands the mean squared deviation, so that the estimate of the variance:

$$\frac{TSS}{(n-1)} = \frac{\sum(x - \bar{x})^2}{(n-1)}$$

is an unbiased estimator of σ^2.

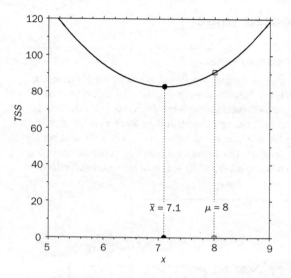

The *TEF* of one of the Poisson samples above has been plotted. The sample is from $P(\mu = 8)$ [14, 8, 4, 10, 5, 5, 8, 6, 6, 5], $\bar{x} = 7.1$, $TSS = 82.9$. It minimizes at the mean of the data $\bar{x}$, but the dispersion around $\mu = 8$ is $TSS = 91$.

The sample mean $\bar{x}$ is generally different from the true population mean μ. Estimating *TSS* about $\bar{x}$ underestimates the *TSS* about μ (which is what we really want to know) because $\bar{x}$ is specifically 'fitted' to those data. This is why we needed to study error functions.

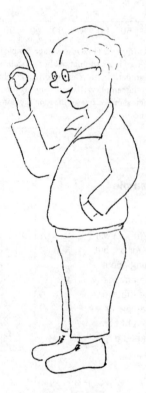

3.14.4 The chi-squared (χ^2) distribution

How might we go about constructing a sampling distribution for the variance? Let us return to the standard normal distribution $N(0, 1)$ (3.11.2) which is the basis for many of our probability models. We saw the importance of the idea of *summing squared deviations* in (3.10.5) and this is how we calculate variance from a sample; sample variance $s^2 = TSS/(n-1)$. The chi-squared distribution χ arises quite naturally from the standard normal and is of immense importance in statistical models. A general idea of where it comes from and why it is logical is all that we seek at present.

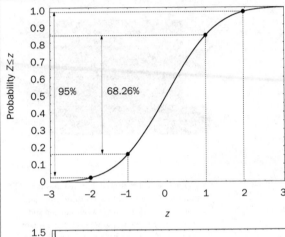

Since all squares are positive, all of the distribution of a *squared* standard normal deviate lies above zero. About 68% of the standard normal lies between −1 and +1. If we square a deviation in this range, we obtain a number which lies in the interval [0, 1]; that is, a positive fraction. About 68% of the distribution of the squared deviation will therefore lie in the interval [0,1].

Squared normal deviates

We can deduce some features of the distribution of squared normal deviates from the mean when we are sampling from the standard normal. The cumulative standard normal distribution shows us directly the probabilities associated with deviations (i.e. from the mean) of a given magnitude. To calculate a variance, we determine the deviations from the mean, square the result, and sum all such deviations. We therefore first need to know how the distribution of a single squared deviate behaves. This is the χ^2-distribution for a single deviate, the χ^2-distribution with one degree of freedom, $\nu = 1$.

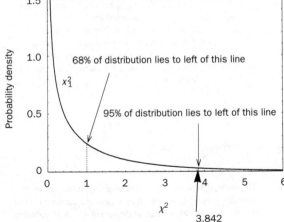

Since the variance of the standard normal is unity, the average squared deviation from the mean of the standard normal is 1. This is what the variance means. Thus the mean of the χ^2-distribution for a single deviate is 1.

95% of the standard normal lies less than ±1.96 from the mean. Thus 95% of the χ^2_1-distribution lies below $(1.96)^2 = 3.842$. 5% of the distribution lies to the right of this. The distribution is clearly highly skewed to the right.

The cumulative function for χ^2 is shown. It is the graph of the area under the curve of the probability density function.

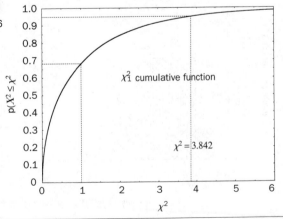

3.14.5 Adding squared deviates: more members of the chi-squared (χ^2) distribution

More χ^2-distributions

We have constructed the simplest member of the χ^2-distribution—that which describes the distribution of a single squared standard normal variate with *one degree of freedom*, $\nu = 1$. This is a very important distribution in its own right, as it is required for testing in a 2×2 contingency table (3.17.3). For sample variances, we need to know the distribution of *sums* of squared standard normal variates. The χ^2-distributions form a family like our other distributions, and the members are characterized by a single parameter, the degrees of freedom, ν. The χ^2-distribution for $\nu = 1$ is the building block for the rest of the family.

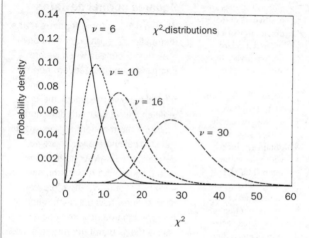

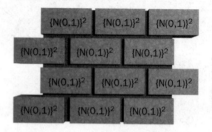

As the mean ($= \nu$) increases, the distributions shift along the horizontal axis. Note that the more skewed they are, the further proportionally the peak is from the mean value ν. The sample variances from our Poisson simulation histogram, (3.14.2) had the appearance of a skewed distribution like these. The sample size was $n = 10$, and the appropriate distribution actually $\chi^2(\nu = 9)$; even though these were Poisson variables, the χ^2 ($\nu = 9$) is still a good approximate model.

$\chi^2(\nu = 1)$ is highly skewed, but we know that summing independent observations from any random variable produces a centralizing and normalizing tendency, so we expect χ^2 for larger values of ν to look increasingly like the normal symmetrical bell shape. $\chi^2(30)$ is fairly symmetrical and bell-shaped. Skewness decreases as the value of ν increases, but dispersion increases, as we might expect (the variance of a sum of RVs, is the sum of the variances).

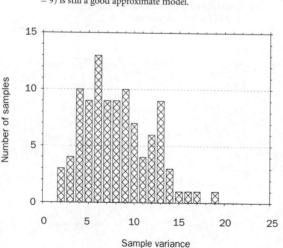

The rest of the family of χ^2-distributions is constructed from summation of $\chi^2(1)$ variates. If z^2 is a squared standard normal deviate, then the distribution of the sum of ν such independent variates $z_1^2 + z_2^2 + z_3^2 + z_4^2 + \ldots + z_\nu^2 \sim \chi^2_\nu$. Since the mean of χ^2 ($\nu = 1$) = 1, then the mean of $\chi^2(\nu) = \nu$. The mean of a sum RV is the sum of the means of the constituent RVs if they are independent. (3.7.1).

Sampling distribution of the variance

The form of the sampling distribution of the variance is χ^2, and for a sample of size n of unknown mean, the appropriate χ^2 has $\nu = n - 1$ degrees of freedom. For small samples (n small and hence small values of ν), because the distribution is markedly skewed, although the expected value of s^2 is the correct one—that is, σ^2—we still underestimate it most of the time.

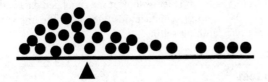

The mean of a distribution is the 'centre of gravity'. If the distribution is symmetrical, then the mean is in the middle. With a highly positively skewed distribution, the long tail means that most of the observations will be below the expected value; the few much higher values pull the mean up. The only cure for this is larger samples.

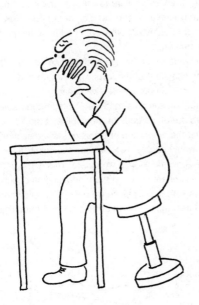

Sampling distribution of the variance: degrees of freedom

$$(n-1)\left[\frac{s^2}{\sigma^2}\right] \sim \chi^2_{(n-1)}$$

The expression in the square brackets is the ratio of the sample variance s^2 to the true value σ^2. This has the expected value of 1 for an unbiased estimator (which s^2 is). It is multiplied by $n - 1$: the mean of $\chi^2(n-1)$ is $n - 1$, so this looks sensible.

The same expression looked at differently

$$\frac{[(n-1)]s^2}{\sigma^2} = \frac{TSS}{\sigma^2} \sim \chi^2_{(n-1)}$$

shows that the ratio of the TSS to the population variance is distributed $\chi^2(n-1)$. This has a mean value $\nu = n - 1$, as we would expect.

The idea of degrees of freedom DOF is quite difficult to grasp. If we have only one piece of information, we cannot even begin to estimate a deviation. The basic concept is that, to estimate a variance at all, we need at least two pieces of information—this can be a known mean μ and a single datum point, or two data points. The mean μ is fixed and only the datum point represents a random quantity—two pieces of information, but only one free to move. If we do not know the mean, then we have to estimate it from the data. If we have a sample of size n, then for any figure for the sample mean $\bar{x}$, once $n - 1$ of the data points have been specified, the final value is already determined, since $\bar{x} = \Sigma x_i / n$. We then have $n - 1$ degrees of freedom. If we had a value for the true mean μ in addition, then all n would be free to vary. *Degrees of freedom* refers to how many independent pieces of information we have; when we calculate a mean from the data, then this is using the same information as that which we need for estimating dispersion in the sample.

3.15.1   **A simple test of significance**

Suppose that we are investigating the release of a plasma peptide after administration of an intravenous induction agent. We have a sample of ten patients and for each we have a pre-administration and a post-administration plasma peptide level. Thus we have a collection of ten data pairs. How can we decide whether there is evidence of release of the peptide by the agent? We shall see later one method—the paired t-test (3.16.3)—but first let us look at the simulated data with a rough and ready method—the sign test. This demonstrates all of the important features of significance testing in a simple setting.

The sign test

We can look at the data pairs, disregard the *magnitude* of any change, and simply record the *direction* of the difference and award a '+', say, if the peptide level is higher post-administration than pre-administration and a '−' if it is lower. Thus we obtain a single list of ten positive and negative signs. By ignoring the size of any difference, however, we have not used all of the information in the sample.

If all of the patients showed an increase (ten +ves), then we would probably be quite confident (how confident?) that there was a genuine release of peptide by the agent. Similarly, if all levels were lower after the induction, we would probably conclude that there was even a suppression of peptide. How would we interpret nine positives or eight positives? What we need is some model system which would mimic the situation.

If there were *no* tendency of the agent to release peptide, then we would expect there to be an even chance that the level would go up or down. We will ignore the possibility that the level is unchanged—we cannot measure very precisely, so this is unlikely. This situation could be modelled by repeatedly selecting beads, ten at a time, from a large barrel of beads in which 50% of the beads are red and 50% white, and recording the proportion of occasions when each of 0, 1, 2, …, 10 beads is red. This would enable us to assess the significance of the particular outcome of our study—how many +ves we obtain. This is the same idea as our model of the exam success, where we used the binomial distribution (3.4). The particular binomial we need is $\sim B(10, 0.5)$ since we have a sample of size $n = 10$ and $p = 0.5$ on the null assumption of an even chance of obtaining a '+' or '−'.

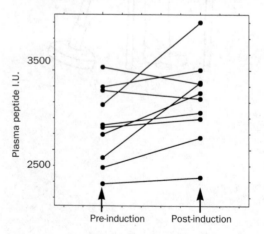

Paired sample data for peptide levels (International Units)

Before	After	Difference	Sign
3293	3504	211	+
3247	3143	−104	−
2402	3349	947	+
2279	2654	375	+
2813	2969	156	+
3069	4101	1032	+
2781	2888	107	+
3539	3332	−207	−
2692	3215	523	+
2074	2154	80	+

(Simulated data)

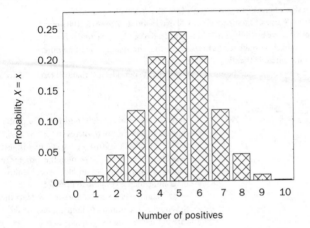

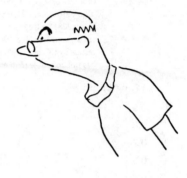

The expected (i.e. mean) number of beads in each sample is five, but of course we expect there to be some variability due to random sampling factors. The probability associated with each possible outcome is easily obtained from tables of the binomial distribution. The graph shows this distribution. Since $p = 0.5$, it is symmetrical (3.4.3).

The probability of all ten samples being positive if there were no real tendency to peptide release is $p(x = 10) = 0.0010$; that is, 1 : 1000. The probability of nine positives is $p(x = 9) = 0.0098$, and of eight $p(x = 8) = 0.0439$.

The distribution $\sim B(10, 0.5)$ allows us to assess the significance of our test result by reference to the behaviour of a model in which no difference (i.e. no tendency to peptide release) exists—the null distribution.

3.15.2   **The sign test**

A binomial model

We have made an assumption of no difference in the levels, and identified an appropriate distribution upon this assumption to quantify the probability of any particular outcome. Suppose that we had obtained seven positives in our sample of ten. What would we conclude? $p(x = 7) = 0.1172$: there is nearly a 12% chance of obtaining this exact result. This means that on average, out of 100 such samples even if there is no difference, we will obtain 7 positives on about 12 occasions purely by chance.

In fact, the question that we are asking is really 'What is the probability of this number of positives or even more?', since we are wanting to know how extreme is the result we obtain. We will be convinced by results which are unlikely to occur under the assumption of no difference. This is easily answered by reference to the cumulative version of the model distribution.

The probability of seven or more is the sum of $p(x \geq 7) = p(x = 7) + p(x = 8) + p(x = 9) + p(x = 10) = 0.1172 + 0.0439 + 0.0098 + 0.0010 = 0.1719$: one of these outcomes will occur about 17 times in 100 samples. This is obtained from the cumulative curve by finding the value for $p(x \leq 6)$ and subtracting it from 1. $(1 - 0.8281) = 0.1719$. This is not really unlikely enough for us to conclude that the assumption of no difference is unreasonable. We would therefore conclude that this test gives no convincing evidence of peptide release by this agent. This is not the same as saying that the agent does not release peptide; just that this test has not been able to demonstrate it.

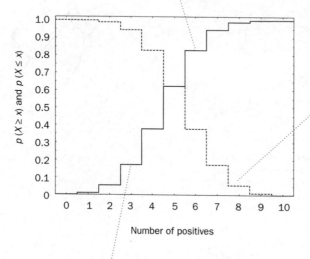

Actually, we obtained eight positives. The probability of eight or more positives is $p(x \geq 8) = 0.0439 + 0.0098 + 0.0010 = 0.0.0547$; that is, just over 5%. This can also be seen on the 'other way round' or mirror-image cumulative probability diagram, which gives probabilities for $p(X \geq x)$ rather than the $p(X \leq x)$ we are used to. Note that the equality is common to both curves, so take care in interpreting the graphs.

The individual probabilities from the binomial model distribution have been stacked in the usual way to give a cumulative distribution. This enables us to answer the question 'What is the probability of observing at least x positives (i.e. x or more)?'

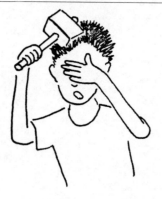

We decide a level of probability for an outcome which we consider unlikely under the assumption of no difference. We compare what we actually observe with this model and conclude whether or not the result is plausible under this assumption. This method is the sign test.

The sign test is rather crude and does not use all of the information in the sample. It has the disadvantage that the binomial is a discrete distribution and (particularly for small samples) has large steps between adjacent values. However, it is a quick and simple method for preliminary assessment of paired data and can be quite useful.

3.15.3   **General concepts**

Significance testing

A significance test is a process of rational decision-making which has a number of essential components. These stages are compared with the peptide example.

- We have a practical problem that we wish to make a decision about. (Does the administration of the induction agent cause a rise in plasma peptide?.)
- We perform the experiment and obtain the raw data (levels of plasma peptide before and after administration of the induction agent).
- We obtain a *statistic* from the raw data: a statistic is any quantity derived from the data—for example, sample mean, sample standard deviation, and so on (number of subjects in which the peptide levels rose, i.e. number of positives out of ten subjects).
- We identify a probability model of the statistic based on some postulate which arises from the situation in question. The postulate is the null hypothesis (NH or H_0) and the probability model that follows from it is the null distribution. The postulate of *no difference* in plasma levels caused by the agent (NH) means no difference in *either* direction; the postulate of *no rise* (i.e. a fall is irrelevant) is a different NH, although the null distribution is the same, $B(10, 0.5)$. What we do with the null distribution differs, that is all.
- The null distribution gives us a probability of obtaining the observed statistic (or a more extreme value) if the NH is true (the probability of obtaining eight or more positives if there is no real peptide release).
- We determine a level of probability below which we decide that the chance of this arising under the NH is so small that we reject the NH. If the probability is larger than this value, we continue to accept the NH. The size of this probability threshold of acceptance/rejection is the *significance level* of the test and is essentially arbitrary—we choose. Frequently, a value of $p = 0.05$ (i.e. 1/20) is taken (the probability of eight or more positives under the NH was 0.0547). This *could* arise by chance if the NH is true, but is rather close to the 5% level for rejection; we would still accept the NH, but we realize that we are close to the threshold. There is insufficient evidence of peptide release by the agent in this test by our acceptance criteria.
- The values of the statistic for which we accept the NH form the *acceptance region*. Values of the statistic outside the acceptance region fall within the *critical region*, in which case we reject the NH and accept the *alternative hypothesis* (AH, H_1). If the statistic falls within the critical region, the test result is said to be *significant*. (There is a not quite significant rise in peptide levels at the 5% level, since the probability of obtaining $x = 8$ or even more extreme is 0.0547.)
- The exact question asked is important in calculating probabilities and hence the acceptance region. 'Is there evidence of a *rise* in plasma peptide?' means that we ignore evidence of a significant fall in peptide—in other words, a significant excess of negatives. We are then only interested in one end of the null distribution—an excess number of positives. This is the way in which we calculate our critical region for the peptide data. This is called a *one-tailed test*, since only one end (tail) of the null distribution is used for the critical region. If we were just as interested in a significant fall as a rise, then we would sum probabilities at both ends of the distribution—a *two-tailed test*.

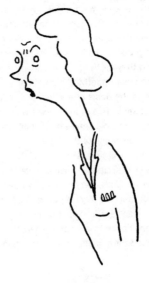

3.15.4 **Errors**

The null distribution of the sign test

There is an important point to be made about the sign test null distribution. This is always binomial $B(n, p)$ with $p = 0.5$ (even chance of +ve or –ve) and n the sample size. Unlike the exam success example, where the binomial was a direct model of the real-life situation, what we have done here is ask how the *statistic* derived from the data (the number of positives) will vary by chance. We have assumed nothing about the distribution of the data themselves, and only observe whether the value goes up or down. The idea of constructing statistics by ranking data in order of magnitude (in this case which side of zero they are) without assuming any particular underlying distribution forms the basis of a whole branch of statistics. This is the *non-parametric* approach. We shall explore just one more example of this—the Mann–Whitney test (3.20)—later. Null distributions which are continuous (smooth) are more easily dealt with than the discrete ones such as the sign test. An exact point for given significance levels can be determined for a continuous distribution.

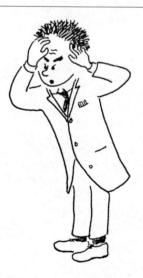

Errors in decision-making

Although the significance test is a quantitative approach to decision-making, it does not guarantee that we reach the right conclusion. There are two sorts of error that we can make:

1. We can obtain a value for the statistic within the critical region by chance even if the NH is true—in fact, this is how we construct the test. We would then reject the NH falsely. This is a *type 1 error*. The probability of making a type 1 error is the significance level of the test ie the size of the critical region. (We might obtain nine positives in the peptide example by chance ($p = 0.0098$, i.e. about 1%) even if the agent does not release peptide. We would then reject the NH by a type 1 error.

2. The second type of error that we can make is when we obtain a value for the statistic within the acceptance region when the NH is actually false. Unsurprisingly, this is a *type 2 error*. The probability of a type 2 error is much more difficult to determine than the type 1, and depends upon the size of the sample and the magnitude of the effect that we are seeking. (For example, the precision of the measurement method, the true extent of rise in mean peptide levels, and the sample size will all affect the ability of the test to detect a genuine effect.) The *power* of a test is defined as the probability of rejecting the NH. Power = $(1 - p$ (type 2 error)): the smaller the level of type 2 error, the more the test is able to detect a genuine difference. The sign test is not inherently a powerful test; we can usually do better.

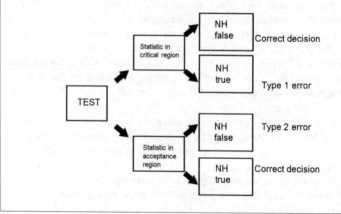

3.15.5   Test power

The power of a test is a measure of its ability to detect when the NH is false. We set up the test in such a way that we attempt to control the level of type-1 error, the probability of rejecting the NH when in fact it is true. The size of type-2 error measures how likely we are to accept the NH when it is false—there is a true difference, but we fail to detect it. The *power* of the test is the complement of this. Power = $1 - p$(type 2 error). Let us see how this is explained in the case of detection of a difference in means of two samples of a normally distributed variable. Power is the probability that the test will give a significant result at a given level of difference in means. The power function of a test describes how the value for the power varies with the magnitude of the true difference in mean between the populations compared.

This is our null distribution; it is the sampling distribution of the difference of means of two samples. Under the NH, $\mu_A - \mu_B = 0$, so it has a mean value of zero—the samples have the same mean. It is normal and symmetrically disposed about zero.

The variability in this statistic (the difference in sample means) is given by the *standard error of the difference in mean*. This depends upon the variance of the population that we are sampling from and the size of each sample. Large samples make the absolute value of this interval smaller.

The power function

We consider a two-tailed test for a difference in means of two samples A and B of a normally distributed variable. The NH is that the sampling distribution of the difference in means (3.16.4) has a mean zero—that is, the expected value of the difference is zero, $\mu_A = \mu_B$. The expected variation in the sampling distribution of the mean is given by the standard error of the difference in means.

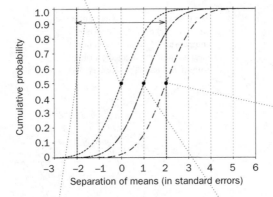

Separation of means (in standard errors)

If the difference in means is + 2 standard errors, then 50% of the distribution lies in the critical region for the test. The power is 50% and the type 2 error is 50%. We can carry out the same process for a difference in the other direction.

This is the acceptance region for the NH. We keep faith with the NH of no difference ($\mu_A = \mu_B$) if we observe a difference in sample means ($\bar{x}_A - \bar{x}_B$) which falls within this interval. For a significance level of 5% in a two-tailed test, this is 1.96 standard errors to either side of zero for large samples. For small samples we need a wider interval derived from the *t*-distribution (3.16).

If there *is* a real difference in means, the sampling distribution is the same shape (normal) and spread (standard error of difference) as the null distribution, but is located away from zero. If the real difference in means is +1 standard error as shown here, only 15.87% of the distribution lies within the critical region for the test. The power is thus 15.87% at this degree of separation. The type 2 error is 84.13%. We would correctly reject the NH on only 15.87% of occasions.

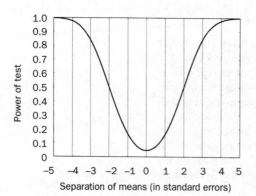

Separation of means (in standard errors)

If we construct a function relating the power to the difference in the means, we obtain a symmetrical graph. The greater the true separation in the means is, the more likely we are to detect a difference of course. This is for a two-tailed test $p = (0.05)$ for a difference in either direction $\mu_A > \mu_B$ or $\mu_B > \mu_A$

Note that when the difference is zero, the power is the significance level of the test. The power function gives us the probability of rejecting the NH. The NH is only true when the difference in means is actually zero—that is, at one point on this graph—and at this point the probability of rejecting the NH is the type 1 error. At all other points, the NH is false.

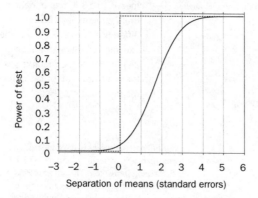

Separation of means (standard errors)

The power function for a one-tailed test $(\mu_A > \mu_B$ say) $p = 0.05$ is shown for comparison. The dotted line shows the ideal test function. Note the analogy with clinical testing procedures (3.9).

3.16.1   The *t*-distribution family

The distribution of $(\bar{x} - \mu)/\sigma$ is ~$N(0, 1)$, so that we can refer a result from any normal distribution $N(\mu, \sigma^2)$ to our standard normal distribution (3.11.2). Where the variance is unknown, it must be estimated by s^2. The distribution of $(\bar{x} - \mu)/s$ is ~ $t_{(n-1)}$ (3.14.1). We now look at the *t*-distribution family in general, so that we are equipped to use it in making inferences on the means of small samples of unknown population variance, σ^2.

The standard normal and *t*-distributions

Like the other distributions we have met, the *t*-distributions form a family. These are defined by a single parameter, the degrees of freedom, ν. The value of ν required for any application depends upon the sample size(s) n and how many parameters have been estimated from the data. We shall see particular examples of this. In general, the larger the sample size, the greater the value of ν is, and the more nearly does the *t*-distribution become like the standard normal.

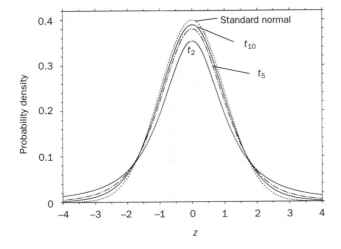

The *t*-distributions for $\nu = 2$, 5, and 10 are compared with the standard normal. In general, the spread of the t is greater than that of the normal, but this effect is less marked as the value of ν increases. This means in practice that we obtain a wider spread of plausible values about the mean when we calculate a *SEM* using sample data to estimate σ^2. This wider spread comes from the fact that we tend to underestimate the value of σ^2 by using sample data (3.14); this in turn arises from the asymmetry of the χ^2-distribution.

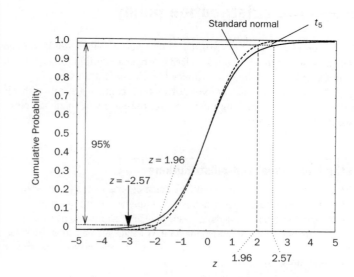

The cumulative functions for t_5 and the standard normal show the 95% points.
The t-distribution arises by calculating the distribution of the statistic obtained when a
standard normal variate (variation about μ) is divided by the square root of an independent
χ^2 variate (estimation of σ).

Flow diagram for t and normal

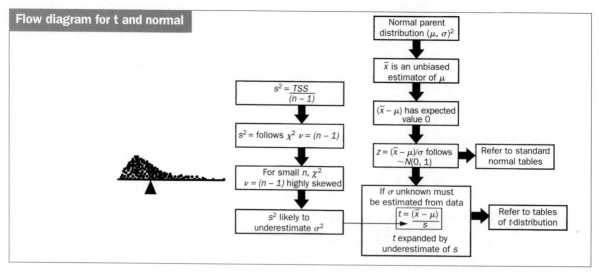

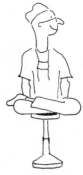

3.16.2 Inference on means of small samples: estimation and significance testing

The t-distribution provides us with the model distribution when we have small samples from normal populations with unknown variance. If we have large samples—say, $n > 30$—the t-distribution with $v = 30$ and the standard normal are so similar that it is not necessary to use the t; if the value for is σ^2 known, then we can use the normal even for small samples. For small values of v (small samples), the t is substantially different from the standard normal and we must use t for estimation and significance testing.

The single sample t-test is the simplest of the t-tests, and may be used for producing a CI for the mean of a single sample or, alternatively, performing a significance test for a hypothesized mean.

Single sample t-test: worked example

We have a sample of 16 SVP measurements and we wish to produce a CI for the mean μ; that is, an interval estimate of the value of SVP. This time, the measurement precision is unknown. The sample mean $\bar{x} = 252.0$ and the $TSS = 154.5$,

SVP measurements (mmHg)

256.4	252.5	251.5	253.0
256.0	254.6	246.6	248.6
251.8	252.3	249.8	252.6
248.2	258.3	250.7	249.0

(Simulated data)

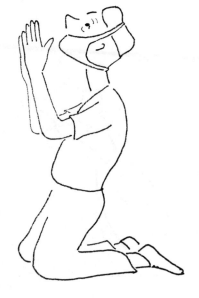

$n = 16$, $s^2 = TSS/(n-1) = 10.3$, $s = 3.2$, and $SEM = s/\sqrt{n} = 0.8$. This is referred to t for $v = n - 1 = 15$, where we find a figure for 95% of 2.1314. This is the factor by which we must multiply the SEM to obtain the 95% CI. The normal distribution would have given us a figure of 1.96 for this factor.

So the 95% CI for the SVP is $252.0 \pm 2.1314 \times 0.8 = 252 \pm 1.705 = 250.3$–$253.7$ mmHg.

These were simulated data from $N(\mu = 250, \sigma = 4)$. This CI does *not* include the true mean $\mu = 250$. This will occur on 5% of occasions; we have experienced a type 1 error.

The significance test approach might ask whether the value of the SVP might plausibly be 250 mmHg. Since the 95% CI does not include this value, then the test result is significantly different from the hypothesized mean at the 5% level. However, if we construct a 99% CI, the appropriate multiple of the SEM is the 99% point for $t_{(15)} = 2.6025$, now giving the 99% CI for the SVP as $252.0 \pm 2.6025 \times 0.8 = 252 \pm 2.082 = 249.9$–$254.1$. This now does include the true mean $\mu = 250$ mmHg. Greater degrees of confidence need wider intervals for the same data.

Summary data

Count :	$n = 16$
Mean :	252.0
TSS :	154.5
Sample variance; $s^2 = TSS/(n-1) = 10.3$	
Sample SD; s	$\sqrt{10.3} = 3.2$
SEM : $= s/\sqrt{n}$	0.8
95% $t_{(16-1)}$:	2.1314 $t \times SEM = 1.705$
95%CI of mean	$= 252.0 \pm 1.705 = 250.3 - 253.7$

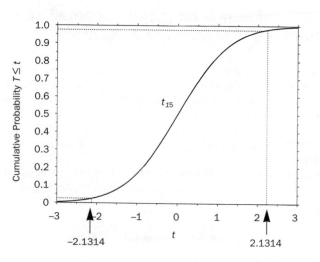

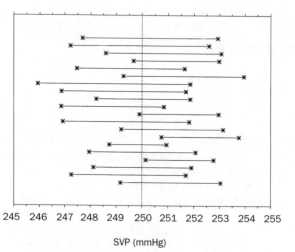

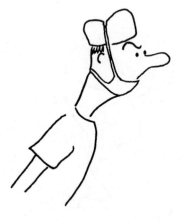

As in (**3.13.3**), twenty 95% confidence intervals have been simulated. Note that this time the width of the CI varies with each sample, since we are estimating σ from the sample s; not only does the location vary, so also does the estimate of the dispersion. The use of the t-distribution ensures that on average we will still encompass the true mean μ on 95% of occasions. In this simulation, again two of the CIs do not include μ.

3.16.3 The paired *t*-test: the CI for a difference in means

Let us return to the peptide release problem (3.15). We studied this in the context of a simple test of significance, the sign test. This made no distributional assumptions about the data themselves, and was an example of a distribution-free or non-parametric test. We will now use the same data and use a test which does make the assumption that the data are normally distributed.

The paired *t*-test: worked example

It may be an obvious point, but we decide if there is any difference between two figures by subtracting one from the other and seeing whether or not we obtain the answer zero. If we have a series of paired data and we wish to know whether they are significantly different, we can subtract (say) the first datum from the second for each of the pairs and obtain a third data list—the signed differences—in other words, positive or negative, depending upon whether they rise or fall. It does not matter which order we choose to make the subtraction provided that we remain consistent and always subtract 'before' from 'after'. This time we shall use information about both the direction *and* magnitude of the change.

The paired *t*-test simply asks whether the confidence interval for the mean of the list of differences contains the value zero: Is it reasonable to believe that the mean difference could be zero? If the mean difference could plausibly be zero, then we would conclude that there is no evidence of peptide release. The *sign test* tells us that the probability of such a result (two negatives) arising by chance under the NH of no difference is $p = 0.0547$.

Paired sample data for peptide levels (International Units)

Before	After	Difference	Sign
3293	3504	211	+
3247	3143	−104	−
2402	3349	947	+
2279	2654	375	+
2813	2969	156	+
3069	4101	1032	+
2781	2888	107	+
3539	3332	−207	−
2692	3215	523	+
2074	2154	80	+

Summary data of difference column

Sample size:	$n = 10$
Mean:	312
TSS:	1542 915
Variance:	1 542 915/9 = 171435
SD:	$\sqrt{171435} = 414$
SEM:	$\dfrac{414}{\sqrt{10}} = 131$
90% $t_{(10-1)}$:	1.8331
SEM $\times$ t	$1.8331 \times 131 = 240$
90% CI of Mean:	$312 \pm 240 = 72 - 552$

This test is one-tailed since we are asking if there is an increase in peptide level.

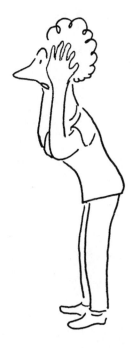

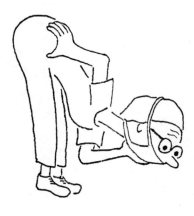

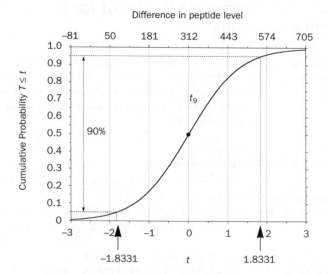

The 90% CI for the difference in mean [72–552] leaves 5% in each tail, and since the interval does not encompass the value zero—ie no difference—we have a one-sided 5% threshold level for a significance test at $-1.8331\,SEM$s. We therefore reject at 5% level the NH of no difference.

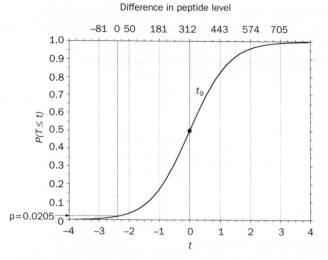

A computer statistics package gives us an exact probability level for the observed result arising under the NH of $p = 0.0205$; that is about 2% probability that the observed result is a chance event.

For the paired t-test, because the raw data are subjected to a subtraction process, the centralising tendency mechanism (3.7.2) has a chance to act and even if the original data are not strictly normally distributed, then the distribution of the *differences* will be more nearly so. Note that the paired observations across the groups are *not* independent because the data are from the same subject. *Within* the 'before' or 'after' groups, the data are independent because they originate in different subjects.

3.16.4 Differences in means of independent samples: the two-sample *t*-test

We commonly have data which arise from two or more groups where there is no natural pairing of data. A typical example might be the measurement of CBF under anaesthesia in a normocapnic control group and a group in which the $PaCO_2$ has been reduced. We are interested in the difference, if any, of mean CBF in the two groups. This is a problem requiring the two-sample *t*-test for comparison of means. The two-sample test requires a modification of the single sample *t*-test.

Problems involving comparison of means of more than two groups require an extension of the principles involved in the *t*-tests, but we do not cover these here.

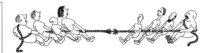

The two-sample *t*-test

We have two groups of unknown mean and unknown variance, and we wish to decide whether the mean CBFs of the two groups are different. The sample means are as follows: group A, $\bar{x}_A = 58.80$; group B, $\bar{x}_B = 51.46$. We are liable to conclude that the means of the two groups are different if the *sample means are far apart* and the *dispersion within the two groups is small*, and that there is, as a consequence, little overlap of the two groups.

At this stage, we make two modelling assumptions:

1. We assume that the measurements of the CBF are *normally distributed*—this is likely to be reasonable, because the CBF itself is likely to be normally distributed. In addition, some of the variability in the CBF measurement will be due to measurement error. Measurement error is normally distributed and even if the CBF were not quite normal, the *sum* of these random variables (CBF and measurement error) will be subject to the normalizing effects of adding RVs.

2. We further assume that *the variance of the two groups is equal*.

   To be able to make inferences from any particular result that we obtain, we need to determine the *sampling distribution of the difference of two means*. Each of the *sample means* separately has a sampling distribution:

$$\sim N\left(\mu_A, \frac{\sigma_A^2}{n_A}\right) \sim N\left(\mu_B, \frac{\sigma_B^2}{n_B}\right), \qquad \text{where } SEM_A = \sqrt{\frac{\sigma_A^2}{n_A}} \quad \text{and } SEM_B = \sqrt{\frac{\sigma_B^2}{n_B}}.$$

We know from the dice example that the distribution of a difference in RVs is that the mean of a difference is the difference of the means ($\mu_A - \mu_B$), but the variance of the difference is the sum of the variances.

The variance of the *difference in means* is

$$\left(\frac{\sigma_A^2}{n_A} + \frac{\sigma_B^2}{n_B}\right)$$

Note that this is not the same as saying that the standard deviation of the sum is the sum of the standard deviations*. To decide whether there is a difference in means between the groups, we need to determine whether the CI (at the level we choose) for the difference in the means includes the value zero; in other words, no difference.

---

* This relationship is the same as that of the sides of a right-angled triangle. If the triangle has base σ_A and perpendicular σ_B, then the standard deviation of the difference (or sum) RV of independent variables with these standard deviations is the length of the hypotenuse. We add variances (the squares of the sides, σ_A and σ_B) to obtain the square on the hypotenuse (Pythagoras). This is the variance of the sum or difference RV. The standard deviation of the sum RV is the square root of this.

Cerebral flood flow ml/100 g/min. (simulated data).

Group A	Group B
66.12	59.11
65.37	58.46
53.04	46.64
51.91	44.90
59.41	52.39
62.69	55.96
58.95	51.94
69.55	62.55
58.56	50.69
49.18	42.04
54.66	47.70
56.21	49.27
	53.18
	45.61

$\mu_A = 55$
$\mu_B = 48$
$\sigma_A = \sigma_B = 7$
(simulation values)

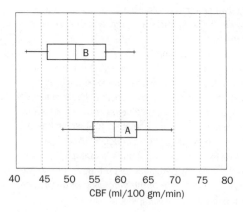

The boxplot is a way of displaying the features of data location and spread. The range is shown by the 'whiskers' emerging from the box. The box itself shows the spread of the central 50% of the data and the bar denotes the median. Some appreciation of location, spread and symmetry is possible with this display.

CBF (ml/100 gm/min)

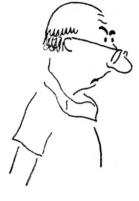

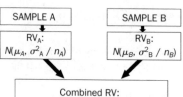

SAMPLE A

RV_A:
$N(\mu_A, \sigma^2_A / n_A)$

SAMPLE B

RV_B:
$N(\mu_B, \sigma^2_B / n_B)$

Combined RV:
$N(\mu_A - \mu_B), [(\sigma^2_A / n_A) + (\sigma^2_B / n_B)]$
Distribution of difference of two means

Estimation
Significance test

Difference of two means
Expected value = $(\mu_A - \mu_B)$

Variance = $[(\sigma^2_A / n_A) + (\sigma^2_B / n_B)]$

3.16.5 Two-sample *t*-test

Standard error of the difference in means: pooling the variance estimates

We create a new RV—the sampling distribution of the difference in the two means. The expected value of this difference is $\mu_A - \mu_B$, and we wish to see if this could plausibly be zero, but we need a value for the *standard error of the difference in means*, SE_{diff}. We make the assumption that the variances of the two groups are equal—which is often reasonable—so that we can pool the variance estimates from each group. Inspection of the data in a boxplot, for instance, will reveal whether this is reasonable. We calculate the *TSS* about the mean for each group; TSS_A and TSS_B. Since we have used two means, each estimated from the data, we lose a degree of freedom for each and the pooled variance estimate (*TSS/DOF*) is

$$s^2 = \frac{TSS_A + TSS_B}{(n_A - 1) + (n_B - 1)}, \qquad s = \sqrt{\frac{TSS_A + TSS_B}{(n_A - 1) + (n_B - 1)}}.$$

The estimated individual *SEM*s are thus $SEM_A = s/\sqrt{n_A}$ and $SEM_B = s/\sqrt{n_B}$.

   Using the fact that the variance of a difference is the sum of the individual variances, the standard error of the difference, SE_{diff}, is as follows:

$$SE_{diff} = \sqrt{\left\{\frac{s^2}{n_A} + \frac{s^2}{n_B}\right\}} = s\sqrt{\left\{\frac{1}{n_A} + \frac{1}{n_B}\right\}}.$$

Under the NH of no difference in mean, the statistic $(\bar{x}_A - \bar{x}_B)/SE_{diff}$ follows a *t*-distribution with $n_A + n_B - 2$ DOF. This is referred to tables or directly carried out by computer package.

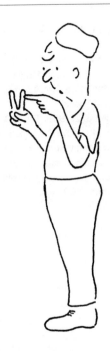

Two-sample t-test worked example

**Cerebral blood flow ml/100g/min
(simulated data)**

CBF$_A$	CBF$_B$
66.12	59.11
65.37	58.46
53.04	46.64
51.91	44.90
59.41	52.39
62.69	55.96
58.95	51.94
69.55	62.55
58.56	50.69
49.18	42.04
54.66	47.70
56.21	49.27
	53.18
	45.61

The two-sample *t*-test

	Sample A	Sample B
Count:	n_A=12	n_B=14
Mean:	58.80	51.46
TSS:	424.96	463.56

Difference in means = 58.80 − 51.46 = 7.34

Pooled estimate of variance, $s^2 = (TSS_A + TSS_B)/(n_A + n_B - 2)$

$$= 888.5/24$$
$$= 37.02$$
$$s = \sqrt{37.02} = 6.08$$

$$SE_{diff} = 6.08 \times \sqrt{\left(\frac{1}{12} + \frac{1}{14}\right)} = 6.08 \times (0.393) = 2.39$$

$$t = 7.34/2.39 = 3.069$$

Two-tailed. $t_{(24)}$ 95% = 2.0639 (The normal gives $z = 1.96$, so the distributions are quite close)

95% CI for difference in means = $7.34 \pm 2.0639 \times 2.39 = 7.34 \pm 4.93$

$$= 2.41 \text{ to } 12.36$$

This 95% CI does not contain the value zero. The result is therefore shows a significant difference at a $p = 0.05$ level.

The (two-tailed) $t_{(24)}$ 99% point is 2.7969. The 99% CI is thus $7.34 \pm 2.7969 \times 2.39 = 7.34 \pm 6.68 = 0.66$ to 14.02. So this result is also significant at $p = 0.01$ level. In fact the result is given a two-tailed probability $p = 0.0053$ of arising under the NH—such a result would only arise about 5 times in 1000 by chance if there were no difference in mean; $\mu_A = \mu_B$. We would therefore feel quite confident to conclude that the mean CBF in group A is larger than that in Group B.

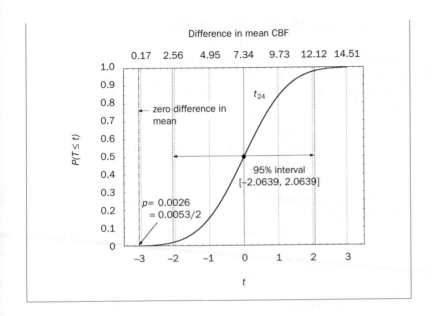

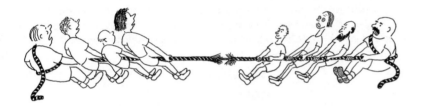

3.17.1   Cross-classifications

Suppose that we have a new intravenous anaesthetic agent Zapidate. This causes pain on injection in some patients and an investigation is conducted to examine the effect of the addition of local anaesthetic, 'Wondercaine', on the incidence of this. 261 patients are randomly allocated to one of two groups to receive Zapidate with or without addition of Wondercaine. We count the number of patients who experience pain on injection in each of the two groups. Suppose that the incidence of pain is lower in the Wondercaine group. How do we decide whether the effect of Wondercaine is significant?

Treatments and responses
Observed values.

	Zapidate alone	Zapidate + Wondercaine	Total
No pain on injection	93	117	210
Pain on injection	31	20	51
Total	124	137	261

Look at the table of results (simulated data). The *column totals* show the numbers in each of the groups. These totals are determined by the random procedure which allocates patients to *treatment* group. This is one way in which the 261 patients are classified; it has nothing to do with the observed *response* of the patients. The column totals are not really of great interest in themselves, since they arise from the randomization procedure. (They should simply be a realization of a RV ~$B(261, 0.5)$—that is, a binomial variable with an equal probability of allocation to each group.)

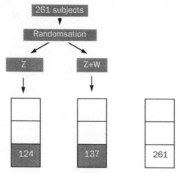

If we now look at the *row* totals, these tell us the numbers in each *response* group—that is, whether or not they experienced pain; the rows have nothing to do with the *treatment*. The column and row marked 'Total' simply tell us the overall numbers in each of the treatment groups and response groups respectively. These are the *marginal totals*. Note that each of the entries in the table is a *count* of the number of subjects falling into a particular category: the 261 patients have been classified in two ways according to treatment and response.

We concentrate first on the marginal totals and ignore what is going on in the body of the table. The row marginal totals enable us to estimate the proportion of the subjects experiencing pain *assuming no difference due to the treatment*—the null hypothesis, NH. The estimated probability of pain on injection $p(pain)$ = $51/261 = 0.195$. Since we have no more information than is in the table, all of our analysis must rest upon the way in which the actual *observed marginal totals* could arise from variation in the entries in the cells in the body of the table. We cannot consider any change in the marginal totals themselves.

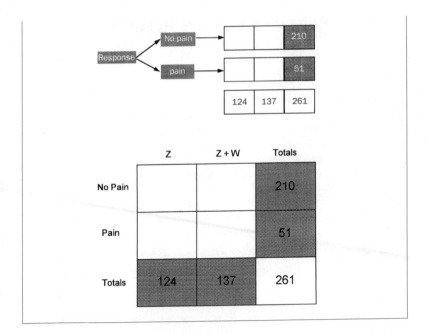

	Z	Z + W	Totals
No Pain			210
Pain			51
Totals	124	137	261

We have two treatment groups; $n_Z = 124$ and $n_{Z+W} = 137$. We need to see how the fixed marginal totals might arise for different entries in the body of the table. With an estimated $p(\text{pain}) = 0.195$, we should really use the binomial distributions $B(124, 0.195)$ and $B(137, 0.195)$, but large binomials are tedious to deal with, and we use the Poisson approximation instead which, for large n, is very close to the binomial and much more easily handled. For small numbers in the cells, we need the exact distribution, and Fisher's exact test which uses the 'proper' binomials is the one for the job. Details are in Bland (see bibliography).

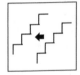

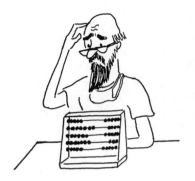

3.17.2 Poisson processes again

Normal approximation to the Poisson

We saw in (3.11.3) the conditions for a normal approximation to the Poisson. At low expected values, the Poisson is markedly skewed and not very 'smooth', since it is discrete with small variance and the total probability is distributed through only a small number of plausible values. At higher expected values it is smoother and more nearly symmetrical (because of the operation of the centralizing, normalizing tendency), and it is a much better approximation to a normally distributed variable of the same mean and variance.

The analysis of cross-tabulations by using the χ^2-distribution which arises from the normal is only valid if the *expected* values in the cells are large enough for a normal approximation to be reasonable. A minimum expected value of 5 is often adopted—although we know that Poisson $\mu = 5$ is still quite skewed. The method is thus always approximate.

The approximation can be improved by the *Yates' correction*, where the statistic calculated is not (observed − expected)^2/expected but $(|\text{observed} - \text{expected}| - \frac{1}{2})^2$/expected. Because the Poisson is discrete, we have seen that the best fit with a normal distribution approximation is obtained by using a continuity correction which effectively reduces some of the variability, because we can count events only in whole numbers. We reduce each of the absolute deviations by 1/2 before squaring. Continuity corrections were introduced in (3.11.3) Details are available in Bland or other standard texts.

Observed and expected values

The occurrence of pain on injection is a random process—we know that some patients will experience this, but not how many or which ones. This is an analogous circumstance to the anaphylactoid example (3.2), which was a Poisson process. In the same way as we calculated the mean number of reactions annually, we have here a proportion $p(\text{pain}) = 51/261$, and this gives us an expected number, under the NH, for each of the two treatment groups. The marginal totals still sum as before; they are fixed. The expected values that we calculate in this way for the pain row are the means of the associated null Poisson distributions ($n_z \times p$) and ($n_{z+w} \times p$). They only differ because the sizes of the treatment groups differ. For the no-pain row, the entries are (n_z) ($1 - p$)) and (n_{z+w}) ($1 - p$)).

Expected numbers under the NH of *no treatment difference*.

	Zapidate alone	Zapidate + Wondercaine	Total
No pain on injection	99.77	110.23	210
Pain on injection	24.23	26.77	51
Total	124	137	261

We have *expected* values (from our NH assumptions) and *observed* values, and we also have a probability model—the Poisson distribution. We also know that a Poisson distribution conveniently has a variance which is the same as the mean or expected value.

For a *normally distributed* RV ~ $N(\mu, \sigma^2)$, $(x - \mu)/\sigma$, is a standard normal variate and $(x - \mu)^2/\sigma^2$—that is, (observed − expected)^2/variance—is a squared normal deviate. Sums of independent squared normal deviates are distributed as χ^2. If the Poisson is a good approximation to the normal, then the statistic (observed − expected)^2/variance will be approximately a squared standard normal deviate. Sums of such statistics will follow a χ^2 distribution (3.14.3). For large values of μ, the normal is a good approximation to the Poisson.

We base our model on the observed marginal totals and ask whether the observed values in the cells are compatible with the assumed NH model of no difference due to the treatments. If the marginal totals are fixed, then the contents of only one cell is sufficient to determine all of the other three cells. There is thus only one degree of freedom and we must refer the statistic to the χ^2-distribution with 1 DOF. This method is the chi-squared test, and it is an approximate method which is valid only if the assumptions of reasonable approximation are valid—this boils down to large numbers in the cells. We have actually approximated a binomial by a Poisson, used the convenient property of equality of mean and variance in this distribution, and then further approximated this Poisson by the appropriate normal. The chi-squared test is an approximate method.

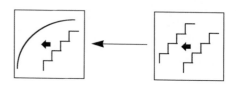

3.17.3 The χ^2-test for association

	Z	Z + W	
NP	93	117	210
P	31	20	51
	124	137	261

Performing the test

We are now in a position to carry out the test.

The statistic that we calculate is $\Sigma \dfrac{(|O - E| - 0.5)^2}{E}$ for each of the four cells.

This is referred to the χ^2-distribution with 1 DOF. (|O – E|) means the absolute magnitude of the difference (i.e. ignoring the sign).

	Zapidate alone	**Zapidate + Wondercaine**
No pain on injection	$\dfrac{(|93 - 99.7| - 0.5)^2}{99.77}$	$\dfrac{(|117 - 110.23| - 0.5)^2}{110.23}$
Pain on injection	$\dfrac{(|31 - 24.23| - 0.5)^2}{24.23}$	$\dfrac{(|20 - 26.77| - 0.5)^2}{26.77}$

	Zapidate alone	**Zapidate + Wondercaine**
No pain on injection	0.394	0.357
Pain on injection	1.622	1.469
$\Sigma = 3.842$		

We obtain $\Sigma \dfrac{\left(|O - E| - \dfrac{1}{2}\right)^2}{E} = 3.8417$. (Remember that in (3.14.4) we

deduced the 95% point (one-sided) of the χ^2- as $1.96^2 = 3.8416$). This has a probability of $p = 0.05$ under the NH of no difference in occurrence of pain in the two groups. We would probably conclude that there was quite good evidence of a genuine effect of Wondercaine in reducing pain on injection. The number of subjects was large and all of the cell contents are 20 or above and we are quite justified in using the χ^2-test. This is a one-tailed test; we are only interested in large values of χ^2.

What do we do if the numbers are much smaller, so that the conditions for use of the χ^2-test are not fulfilled? There is an exact test (Fisher's test) that analyses the way in which the marginal totals can arise under the binomial distribution and assigns an exact probability to the observed values under the NH. Fisher's test is appropriate for 2×2 tables with small numbers. This is quite straightforward and can be performed by any statistical software package, but there is insufficient space here to explain the way in which it works. It should however be apparent why we need a different test if numbers are small.

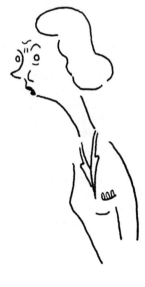

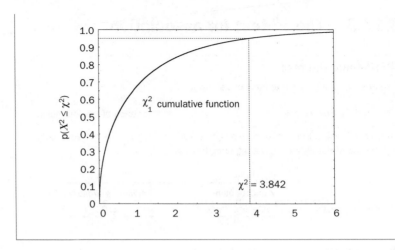

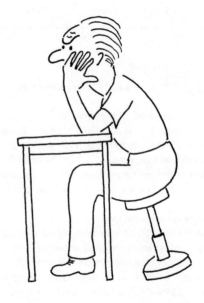

Larger cross-tabulations

This example has used a table with cross-classification into 2×2 groups. We might easily be interested in more groups than this—for instance, a four-level classification of a pre-operative grading of predicted difficulty of intubation—and the grade (1–4) of subsequent view at laryngoscopy would give us a 4×4 table. The χ^2-test can be used in such cases, provided that the expected values in any cell are greater than, say, 5. The appropriate DOF for a table of r rows and c columns are $(r-1)(c-1)$—in the case of a 4×4 table, nine DOF. This means that large numbers of subjects will be required if particular gradings are rare. Groups can be combined—for example, Laryngoscopy Grades III&IV—if necessary to achieve high enough expected values. Fisher's exact test is only possible with 2×2 tables.

3.18.1   Linear relationships between variables

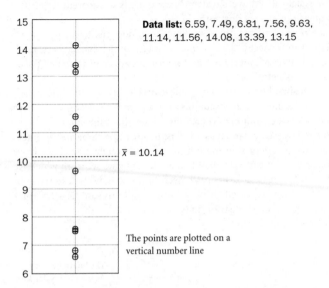

Data list: 6.59, 7.49, 6.81, 7.56, 9.63, 11.14, 11.56, 14.08, 13.39, 13.15

$\bar{x} = 10.14$

The points are plotted on a vertical number line

Look at the data list (simulated data) and the plot of these points. If this is all the information that we have, then we can calculate a mean $\bar{x} = 10.14$ and $TSS = 75.79$ for the data and hence derive a value for the sample variance and standard deviation. We know from our study of error functions that we cannot make the TSS about a chosen 'fit' any smaller than that about the mean value. Using the techniques of (3.16.2) we can calculate a CI for the mean at a chosen level, and this is about all we can do.

If, however, we know that these are $PaCO_2$ values in kPa from a single subject undergoing apnoeic oxygenation and we have a value for the duration of apnoea when each measurement is taken, then our view of the data may be rather different.

Time (mins)	$PaCO_2$ (kPa)
0	6.59
2	7.49
4	6.81
6	7.56
8	9.63
10	11.14
12	11.56
14	14.08
16	13.39
18	13.15

When the $PaCO_2$ data are plotted against the duration of apnoea, although it is obvious that the points do not lie *exactly* on a straight line, we discern a definite trend that the $PaCO_2$ rises with the duration of apnoea (and this is of course what we expect it to do). We might reasonably believe that this trend is linear. The fit of the data pairs to a straight line is evidently not as good as the genuine data in (1.8.1), but this might be simply because we have a poor quality gas analysis system, or have not timed the samples very carefully. These errors are not sufficient to obscure the underlying trend.

The data are not as convincingly linear as those in (1.8.1) because they are more scattered, around even the best line we might fit. A line could be fitted to the data in (1.8.1) quite satisfactorily 'by eye' since the linear trend is so apparent.

A number of questions arise at this point:

- We feel that a *straight line* 'fits' the data better than does the best *single figure* (the mean). How can we decide upon a 'line of best fit' so that the data are as little dispersed as possible? Minimization of dispersion is an 'error function' problem; this question has a familiar ring.

- If we have fitted the best line we can, how can we decide whether this line is convincing evidence of a linear relationship between the variables? This must have something to do with the amount of remaining scatter about the line.

- The best fit line to any particular data set will be defined by a slope and an intercept—we need two pieces of information to define a straight line (2.5). If we perform a similar experiment, we will obtain a different data set from which we would obtain a different best fit line. We need to know how the estimates of slope and intercept are expected to vary from sample to sample—In other words, what are their sampling distributions?

We will cover these points in turn.

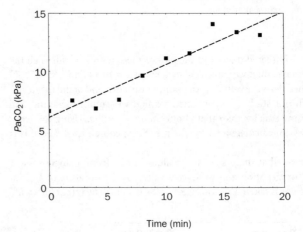

The line of best fit predicts a mean value for $PaCO_2$ at any time t. This prediction is based upon the data. The deviations of the data from the best-fit line are the *residuals*. They are evidence of irreducible random variation which the fitting of the line has not abolished—there is residual scatter.

Each datum point is defined by two numbers—a time at which the measurement is taken and a $PaCO_2$ value measured at that time. There is a fairly convincing linear trend despite the appreciable scatter. The line is the best fit that we can make. How do we choose the line and how do we decide if there really *is* a linear relationship?

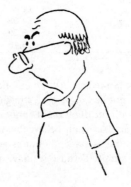

3.18.2   Finding the line of best fit: least squares

The concept of an error function, which we explored in (3.10), is the key idea to finding a line of best fit. In exactly the same way as we found the *single figure of best fit* (the mean of the data set) by minimizing the squared deviations (*TSS*) about this figure, if we suspect a linear relationship between variables, we use the same idea to find the *line of best fit*, by minimizing the squared deviations of the data points from the line. This is the *method of least squares*. The technique of studying linear relationships between variables is linear regression.

For consistency, we should call the variable plotted along the horizontal axis the independent variable and that along the vertical axis the dependent variable. But 'independent' has another technical meaning in statistics, so instead we term these the *predictor* (x) and *response* (y) variables respectively. We wish to use the duration of apnoea to predict the response of the $PaCO_2$.

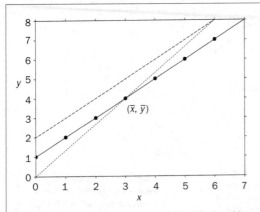

Seven points on the line $y = x + 1$ are shown. The dotted line passes through the point $(\bar{x}, \bar{y})$, which the best fit line always does, but has a gradient which is too steep. The dashed line has the right gradient, b, but the wrong position of intercept, a. The least squares method selects the values of a and b to minimize the dispersion, and would in this case select $a = b = 1$ for a perfect fit.

An error function of two variables

It is easy to lose sight of the main ideas in a lot of algebra, so as usual we will keep mainly to a graphical approach. In the error function for the mean, we minimized the sum of squared deviations from the mean. This minimum was the *TSS*. For a linear relationship, we need to pick a value for the slope b, and the intercept a, of a line $y = a + bx$ that minimizes the sum of squared deviations, *SS*, of the data from the line. It should be clear that choosing either an intercept or a slope (or both) away from the optimum value will cause the *SS* from the line to increase. We can find a function that describes the *SS* of the data about the line for any values of a and b and minimize this function by our choice of slope and intercept.

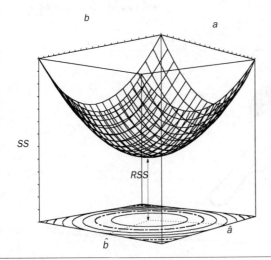

Varying the single figure around which we calculated the error function gave us a parabola that minimized at the mean; the *TEF* for the mean was a function of a single variable. We now need an error function of two variables, the slope b and the intercept a. This gives us a three-dimensional version of the parabola—a paraboloid. The vertical axis is the sum of squared deviations from the line. We choose values for a and b which minimize this *SS* in exactly the same fashion. The value of the function at this point is the residual sum of squares (*RSS*). It is always smaller than the *TSS* around the mean $\bar{x}$ if there is any dispersion of the data

3.18.3   **Building blocks**

Quantities in linear regression

The derivation of the least squares method involves techniques beyond our scope, and so is omitted; all we need to know is that there is an algorithm—a routine procedure—which will give us a 'best-fit' straight line to a set of x–y data points. The least squares procedure always gives a line that passes through the point $(\bar{x}, \bar{y})$, the mean value of the predictor (x) variable, and the mean value of response (y) variable. The gradient is then sufficient to define the line. All of the important results in linear regression and correlation can be expressed in terms of three quantities calculated from the data:

$S_{xx} = \Sigma\,(x_i - \bar{x})^2$. S_{xx} is the sum of squared deviations of the x values of the data points about *their* mean value $\bar{x}$. S_{xx} does not involve y. This can be thought of as the 'horizontal' sum of squares.

$S_{yy} = \Sigma(y_i - \bar{y})^2$. This is the sum of squared deviations of the y values of data points from the mean of the response variable $\bar{y}$. S_{yy} does not involve x, the predictor variable. *This is the quantity that we have called TSS—the sum of squared deviations ignoring any possible relationship with x—in other words, with the simplest model of a single mean value.* This can be thought of as the 'vertical' sum of squares.

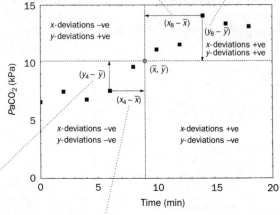

$S_{xy} = \Sigma\,(x_i - \bar{x})\,(y_i - \bar{y})$. S_{xy} is the sum of products of the x- and y-deviations of the individual data points from their respective means; that is, it involves both x and y. S_{xx} and S_{yy} are always positive because they are sums of squares. S_{xy}, on the other hand, is the sum of products of two quantities—the deviations from the respective means—which may be either positive or negative. S_{xy} may therefore be of either sign. If we multiply two deviations of the same sign, we obtain a positive product; if we multiply two deviations of opposite sign, we obtain a negative product. If the gradient of the regression line is positive as in the diagram, S_{xy} will also be positive. If the gradient is negative, S_{xy} will be negative. If there is no linear relationship, S_{xy} will have a value near zero. We might expect S_{xy} to appear in the determination of the least squares gradient b.

$\dfrac{1}{(n-1)} S_{xy}$ is called the sample covariance.

The regression line is our least squares fit—the best we can achieve. In most cases there will still be residual scatter of the data points around this line as evidence of random processes including natural variability and measurement error. These are in addition to any systematic linear relationship between the variables which accounts for some of the dispersion.

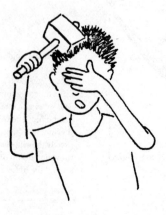

3.18.4 **Reducing the *TSS***

Accounting for variation

The gradient of the least squares best fit line is $b = S_{xy}/S_{xx}$. b has the same sign as S_{xy}. Having decided upon the best fit line that we can, we may then calculate how large is the residual scatter of the data points from the line. The sum of squared deviations from the *line* is the measure that we calculate as the residual sum of squares, *RSS*. The *TSS* around the overall mean $\bar{y}$ of the data (i.e. ignoring any linear relationship with x) is reduced by fitting a better model—the line. What we are left with is the *RSS*. The difference between the two is the explained sum of squares, *ESS*; the linear model 'explains' some of the variation around the overall mean $\bar{y}$:

$TSS = ESS + RSS$.

How can we decide if the linear fit is a convincing model? Two means come to mind:

- The degree to which the *TSS* is reduced by fitting the data to a line is an indication of how good the linear model is in explaining the variability—recall how we viewed the data list in (3.18.1) differently when we suspected a relationship with time of apnoea—much of the spread of the $Paco_2$ values became explicable as a function of time. We can compare the *ESS* and the *TSS* or *RSS* and ask whether the magnitude of *ESS*—the reduction attributable to the linear model—is sufficient not to have arisen by chance.
- The existence of a linear relationship implies a best-fit line which has a gradient significantly different from zero. A constant function has gradient of zero; the mean is the best constant we can fit by a least squares procedure. If we can determine a sampling distribution for the gradient b, we can find a CI and discover whether this CI contains the value zero. If it does, then we may decide that there is insufficient evidence of a linear relationship.

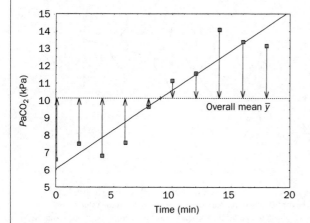

The dispersion of the data points about the overall mean $\bar{y}$ value is considerable. The sum of these squared deviations is the *TSS*.

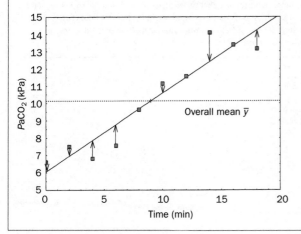

The dispersion of the data points about the best-fit line is much better. The sum of these squared deviations is the residual sum of squares, *RSS*. The difference between the *TSS* and *RSS* is the explained sum of squares, *ESS*. The linear relationship explains a large proportion of the variability around the overall mean. We do not need much convincing that there is a genuine linear relationship here.

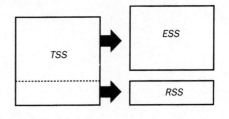

3.18.5   Completing the model and the RSS

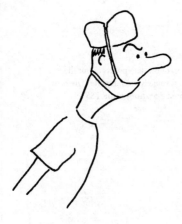

Defining the linear regression model

We have reduced the *TSS* by fitting a line and have residual scatter about the line. The *RSS* is the raw material for examining the irreducible variability (noise) in the data. We have a model which has the following features:

- There is a linear relationship between the predictor variable (x) and the response variable (y) such that the *mean* value of y for any x is determined by $y = a + bx$, where b is the slope of the line.
- The least squares procedure determines an estimated value for b, from the data. This estimate is $\hat{b}$. The least squares line always passes through the point $(\bar{x}, \bar{y})$, so that the intercept a is given by $a = \bar{y} - \hat{b}\bar{x}$.
- We need to make an important assumption about the remaining dispersion about the line that produces the *RSS*. The dispersion about the line is usually modelled as a *normally distributed variable of constant variance σ^2*.
- We need to estimate b from the data. Just like the sample mean, the value of the estimate, $\hat{b}$, will vary from sample to sample because of random sampling effects; it will have a sampling distribution. The variability of this estimate will depend upon the value of σ^2.

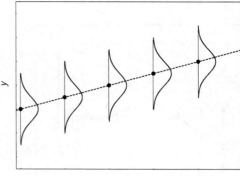

The model is now $y = a + bx + $ error, where the error term is a normally distributed RV $\sim N(0, \sigma^2)$. The mean value of the variable lies on the line, but the value of the response variable is subject to a random, normally distributed error about this mean. A frequent and convenient assumption is that the variance of this random error is constant through the range of x—this means that the scatter about the line does not change with the x value. This is often a reasonable assumption, and inspection of the data may give an indication whether this is justifiable.

Formulae in linear regression

All of the quantities that we need to calculate in linear regression and correlation can be expressed in terms of S_{xx}, S_{xy}, and S_{yy}. These are shorthand terms for expressions that can make formulae look quite complicated. We need to relate these to the two sums of squares and the sum of products. S_{yy} is the usual TSS about the overall mean $\bar{y}$.

The estimated slope of the regression line $\hat{b}$ is S_{xy}/S_{xx}. This estimate is subject to sampling variation and has a variance σ^2/S_{xx}. The standard error of the slope is thus $SE(\hat{b}) = \sigma/\sqrt{S_{xx}}$. We usually have to estimate σ from the sample RSS.

The *explained sum of squares*, ESS, is as follows: $ESS = \hat{b}S_{xy}$. This is the part of the TSS which can be 'explained' by the linear relationship with x. The size of the ESS is dependent upon the magnitude of the slope b. This makes sense because a steep gradient means that a change in x value makes us predict a large change in y. Conversely, a slope near zero implies that knowledge of x does not help us much to predict the value of y. Since $\hat{b}$ and S_{xy} always have the same sign, $\hat{b}S_{xy}$, the ESS, is always positive. A sum of squares must be positive.

The *residual sum of squares*, RSS, comes from the remaining dispersion around the least squares line. It is the result of unexplained random variation not attributable to a systematic linear relationship. $RSS = TSS - ESS = S_{yy} - \hat{b}S_{xy}$. The RSS is the basis for our estimate of population variance after the systematic linear relationship has been accounted for:

$$s^2 = \frac{RSS}{n-2} = \frac{S_{yy} - \hat{b}S_{xy}}{n-2}.$$

Estimating σ^2

The value of σ^2 is usually unknown and must be estimated from the data. The RSS is the total sum of squared dispersions about the line and a scaled (mean) squared deviation must be related to the number of data points contributing to it. Because in fitting the line we have had to estimate *two* quantities, we lose a degree of freedom for each, so we divide the RSS by $(n-2)$ to obtain the variance estimate.

Estimated $\sigma^2 = s^2 = RSS/(n-2)$
We have a normally distributed variable of unknown mean and variance, both of which must be estimated from the data. We expect the *t*-distribution to be involved (3.16).

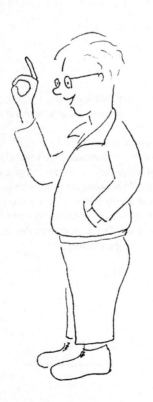

3.18.6   Worked example

Regression of Pa_{CO_2} on duration of apnoea

$\bar{y} = 10.14$ $\bar{x} = 9.00$

S_{yy}:   75.79

S_{xx}:   330.00

S_{xy}:   150.18

The least squares estimate of slope is

$\hat{b} = S_{xy}/S_{xx} = 150.18/330 = 0.455$ kPa/min.

The estimated intercept is

$a = \bar{y} - \hat{b}\bar{x} = 10.14 - (9 \times 0.455) = 6.045$ kPa.

The equation of the least squares regression line is thus $y = 6.045 + 0.455x$; that is,

$Pa_{CO_2} = 6.045 + 0.455t$ kPa,

where t is the duration of apnoea (minutes).

$RSS = TSS - ESS = 75.79 - \hat{b}s_{xy} = 75.79 - 68.35 = 7.44.$

Estimated residual variance $s^2 = RSS/(n - 2) = 7.44/8 = 0.93.$ $s = \sqrt{0.93} = 0.96.$

The standard error of the gradient estimate is se (gradient) $s/\sqrt{S_{xx}} = 0.96/18.17 = 0.053.$

What do we do with the standard error of the gradient? We have assumed that the random deviation about the line is normally distributed with constant variance. The deviations are $n = 10$ observations from $N(0, \sigma^2)$. We estimate σ from the data as s, so it should not be surprising that the estimate of the slope $\hat{b}$ by the least squares procedure follows a t-distribution. Fitting the line required two quantities (slope and intercept) to be estimated, so we have $n - 2$ degrees of freedom.

Thus

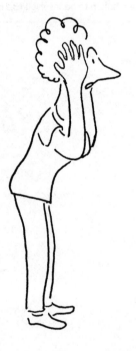

$$\frac{(b - \hat{b})}{SE(b)} \sim t_{n-2}.$$

We have $n = 10$, so we consult tables for, say, the 95% point of $t(8) = 2.306$ and it is this multiple of SEs that we need either side of our estimate of b to give us the 95% CI for the gradient.

The 95% CI for the gradient is thus $0.455 \pm 2.306 \times (0.0528) = 0.455 \pm 0.1218 = 0.333 - 0.577$. If the CI includes the value zero for the gradient, we cannot be confident that the gradient is not zero. A gradient of zero means that there is *no* linear relationship between the variables which gives us one way of concluding whether a relationship exists. It can be shown that this is entirely equivalent to the approach through comparing *RSS* and *ESS*. To demonstrate this would require the introduction of yet another offspring from the normal, the *F*-distribution (details in Bland), so we will abstain.

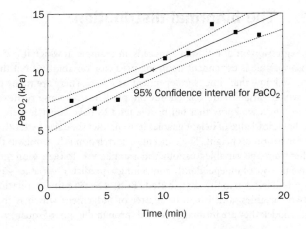

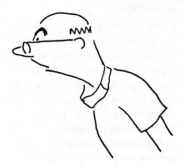

Confidence interval for y

The least squares regression line always passes through the point $(\bar{x}, \bar{y})$. This point acts as a 'pivot' for the regression line, the gradient of which is subject to sampling error. As we know, the mean of y will also be subject to sampling error. The combination of the uncertainty in the slope *and* the pivot point $(\bar{x}, \bar{y})$ means that the confidence interval for y will widen as we move away from the mean value of the predictor variable x. The CI for y is narrowest at the mean of x.

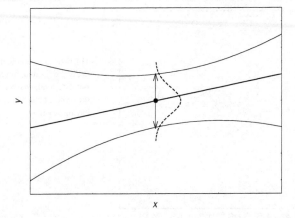

Linear functions are extremely important in modelling. We have seen ways of transforming non linear relationships into linear plots which can then be analyzed by techniques of linear regression. We have seen also that fitting a line to set of points can be viewed as a way of explaining or accounting for some of the variation in the data. Linear regression is an example of an analysis of variance method (ANOVA), which should probably be called analysis of sums of squares since we have apportioned the *TSS* between *ESS* (ie 'explained' by the linear model) and the residual, 'unexplained', *RSS*. The two-sample *t*-test for example, can similarly by viewed as a method of analysis of sums of squares by calculating the reduction in *TSS* (ie the *ESS*) by treating the data as one sample dispersed around the 'grand mean' of all of the data (for the *TSS*) and then the dispersion about the two sample means (for the *RSS*). This approach extends to problems involving more than two sample groups. Further details are available in the texts listed in the bibliography.

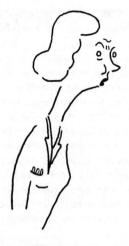

3.19.1   The binormal distribution

The $PaCO_2$ regression on duration of apnoea is an example in which it is clear that the response variable is dependent upon the predictor variable and not the other way round; we know that time is independent of $PaCO_2$. There are many circumstances in which variables are related but the predictor/response relation is less clear. For instance, we know that tall people tend to have larger feet than short people, so that knowledge of height enables us to predict shoe size better than if we have no information on height. The concept of correlation is based upon the ability to predict from one variable to another in a similar way to regression but where we may have no way of independently controlling a 'predictor' variable—the related variable is itself normally distributed. Both describe linear relationships between two variables, and it can be matter of judgement which is the more appropriate model; they are intimately related through the sum of squares.

Bi-variate normal distributions: vital capacity and height

Tall people tend to have a larger vital capacity (VC) than short people; we can predict vital capacity better if we know a person's height. VC also declines gently with age, but we shall ignore this. The scatter diagram shows the results of (simulated) measurements of height and VC in 50 individuals. It is evident from the plot that the greater the height, the greater is the tendency to have a larger VC, although there is plenty of scatter. Both height and VC are normally distributed quantities and we would like to describe a *joint distribution* to model how they vary together.

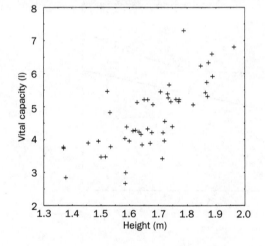

The two variables are normally distributed, but are not independent since we see the trend of taller individuals having larger VCs.

We can describe a *joint probability distribution* of both normal RVs together. This gives a 3-D distribution diagram which can also be displayed as a contour plot. This shows how the RVs vary together. Parallel to any axis we can see the familiar shapes of the normal bell curve, but the mean value is 'slewed' according to the position along the axis of the other variable. Just as the area under the univariate normal curve sums to 1, the *volume* under the surface of the bi-variate distribution totals to 1. The contour plot shows a shape similar to the height–VC scatter plot. There is still a linear relationship between the variables.

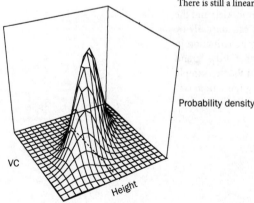

Probability density

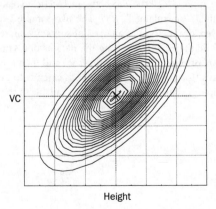

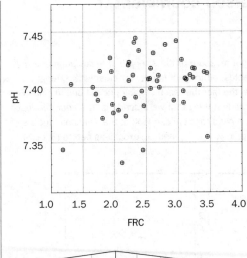

Both FRC and plasma pH are normally distributed, but we do not expect them to be related. If we made simultaneous measurements of both, we would not expect any co-variation and the scatter plot of these data pairs would show no particular pattern. Knowledge of one variable gives us no information about the other.

The joint distribution of uncorrelated variables is shown in contour and in 3-D bivariate distribution form.

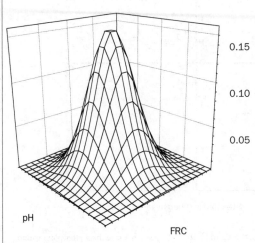

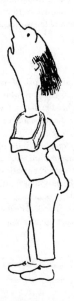

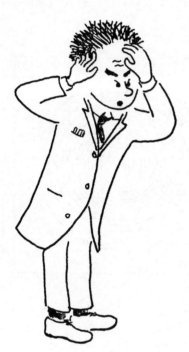

3.19.2   **The Pearson coefficient, *r***

Measuring correlation

Correlation is often viewed as a measure of the *strength of association* between two normally distributed variables, although it is not very clear what strength means. We need to cope with the fact that each variable, height and VC, has its own mean and variance, so the first thing that we must do is to *standardize* each variable. We have a list of (x,y) pairs, and we can look at the x variable and y variables separately and calculate $\bar{x}$, $\bar{y}$, S_{xx}, S_{yy}, and S_{xy} exactly as before (3.11.3).

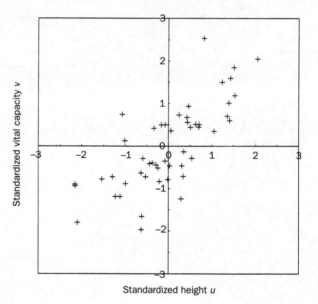

Standardized height *u*

We subtract the value of $\bar{x}$ from the x's and $\bar{y}$ from the y's to relocate the scatter plot around the origin, and we divide the relocated x and y values by their respective standard deviations (usually estimated from the data) to obtain standardized deviations that is, observations from the standard normal distribution. This gives us a scatter plot of standardized deviations which is independent of the particular units that we use for measurement of the two variables.

Each point is now a pair of standardized observations (u_i, v_i), where u_i is the standardized x; that is, $\{(x_i - \bar{x})/s_x\}$ and v_i the standardized value $\{(y_i - \bar{y})/s_y\}$.

For any general point, if the point lies in the first or third quadrants, the product $u_i v_i$ will be positive, and if it lies in the second or fourth quadrants the product will be negative. We can calculate the sum of $u_i v_i$ products for all points.

x negative *y* positive	*x* positive *y* positive
x negative *y* negative	*x* positive *y* negative

The correlation coefficient, *r*

The correlation coefficient

$$r = \frac{1}{(n-1)} \sum u_i v_i,$$

is the sum of *uv* products, scaled to the number of points and will be positive if most points lie in the first and third quadrants and negative if most points lie in the second and fourth. If the points lie approximately equally in all quadrants, the sum will be near zero. It can be shown that *r* always lies between −1 and +1.

The Pearson correlation coefficient, *r is a measure of how far points from the two variables occupy similar positions in their respective normal distributions.* If all of the points lie on a line *v = u*, each point is occupying the same position on each of its constituent distributions (perfect positive correlation, when *r* = 1). If all of the points lie on the line *v = −u*, then they occupy equivalent symmetrical points at the *opposite* ends of their respective distributions (perfect negative correlation, when *r* = −1). Correlation measures a linear relationship between two normal variables.

If the points lie on this line, they occupy the symmetrically *opposite* positions within the respective distributions *u* and *v*. This is perfect negative correlation, *r* = −1.

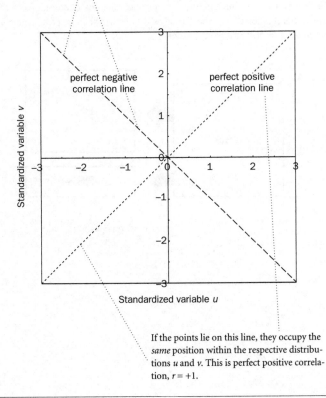

perfect negative correlation line

perfect positive correlation line

Standardized variable *v*

Standardized variable *u*

If the points lie on this line, they occupy the *same* position within the respective distributions *u* and *v*. This is perfect positive correlation, *r* = +1.

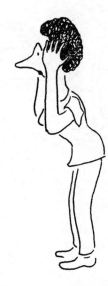

3.19.3   **Correlation and regression**

Linear relationships between variables

There are a number of ways of considering the meaning of a correlation:

* Correlation is often described as a measure of *strength of association* between two variables. This can seem to imply a cause–effect relationship which is not necessarily the case. Strength of association is not the most fruitful way to consider correlation.

* We can think of the correlation coefficient r as measuring the *extent to which the data points occupy equivalent positions in the respective two normal variables*. After all, this is how the measure is constructed.

* The expression $r^2 = ESS/TSS$ tells us that r^2 is the *proportion of the TSS which is explained by taking into account the linear relationship between the variables*. A correlation of $r = 0.5$ means that 25% of the *TSS* is explained by the relationship and that 75% remains unexplained.

Regression and correlation are really two different views on linear relationships between two variables. The apnoea example is inappropriate for the correlation approach because time is not normally distributed and the $Paco_2$ is clearly in a dependent (response) variable position. Correlation is about related normal RVs.

However, it is quite appropriate to view the height–VC relationship from either angle.

Caution should be exercised in confusing high degrees of correlation with cause–effect relationships—there may be a 'third variable' involved which is affecting each of the others independently.

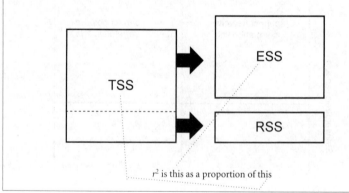

r^2 is this as a proportion of this

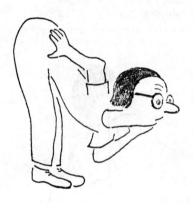

Vital capacity and height

The scatter plot of vital capacity and height was of simulated data.[*] We correlate: vital capacity with height

Count: $n = 50$

	Sum of squares	Mean
Vital capacity y	51.71 (S_{yy})	4.69
Height x	0.97 (S_{xx})	1.67
$(n - 1) \times$ covariance:	5.27 (S_{xy})	

$$r^2 = (S_{xy})^2/(S_{xx})(S_{yy}) = (5.27)^2/(51.71) \times (0.97)$$

$$= (27.86)^2/(50.24)$$

$$r^2 = 0.553$$

$$r = 0.74$$

The r value, the Pearson correlation coefficient that we obtain, is 0.74. $r^2 = 0.55$.

This means that 55% of the variation in VC considered as a 'lone variable' is explained by the association with height when we consider these how these quantities vary together in these simulated data.

[*] Such data are simulated by generating a random sample for one variable, height, say (using appropriate mean and variance for height) and then, using these values as input variables into a linear function. The output from this procedure has then another randomly generated normally distributed variable added to represent the random variation of VC about the line. using the appropriate (unexplained, residual) variance of VC—the *mean* VC is now already determined by the linear relationship.

3.19.4   **The normal plot**

We often need to determine whether a particular set of data is normally distributed. We can display the data as a bar chart, box plot or some other inspection method, but it may be difficult, especially with small data sets, to decide whether the normal is a reasonable model. We can use the idea of correlation to help us.

Is it normal?

Suppose that we have a sample of size $n = 5$ from a putative normal distribution and we arrange the data in order of size. We would expect the data points to occupy positions on the cumulative normal distribution, symmetrically disposed about the mean value. On average, 10% of the parent distribution will lie below the lowest datum point in such samples and 10% above the highest: 20% of the distribution will lie between each of the points. In general, for n data points the proportion of the distribution lying outside the data will be $1/n$, and this will be split into two equal parts, $1/2n$ above and $1/2n$ below. Between each pair of adjacent data points, there will be $1/n$th of the distribution.

We take the standard normal distribution and apportion its cumulative distribution in the same way and obtain the z values associated with these positions on the cumulative distribution by reading the graph backwards. We then plot these z values against the actual data so that we have, for each datum point, a predicted z value from a known normal distribution. If the data truly arise from a normal distribution, these data points should lie close to a straight line, because the joint distribution (data and standard normal) should have a correlation of close to 1. Statistical packages on computer will perform a normal plot of data very rapidly.

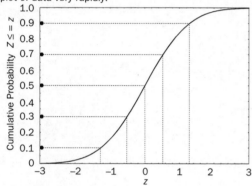

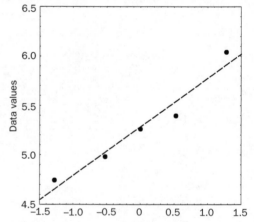

The number of data points splits the cumulative standard normal distribution symmetrically. Above the highest and below the lowest data points (taken together), the total proportion of the distribution is the same as between the individual points. The z values can be read off the horizontal axis when the positions have been fixed. We plot these z values against the actual data. This is shown for $n = 5$.

Table:

%pt	z value	Data from ~$N(5.5, 0.75^2)$
10%	−1.28	4.74
30%	−0.5244	4.98
50%	0	5.26
70%	0.5244	5.39
90%	1.28	6.04

(Simulated data)

This is the normal plot for the data in the table. Although there are only five data points, it is very plausible that these lie on a straight line and represent normally distributed data. $r = 0.975$.

This has been a very brief consideration of correlation and much has been omitted. The sampling distribution of r^2, for instance, is rather intractable and a confidence interval for r is not easily obtained. How this problem is tackled, together with a more extensive discussion of the pitfalls in correlation and further information concerning related variables, should be obtained from more comprehensive treatments.

3.20.1   **The non-parametric approach**

Imagine that we are conducting a study to compare the effectiveness of two analgesics in pain relief after minor surgery. Suppose that we have randomly allocated seven patients to two groups; three to receive drug A and four to drug B. Pain relief can be measured by asking patients to use an analogue pain score. It is not obvious how results of individual pain scores might be distributed, so we will use a technique which does not make any assumptions about the distributional origin of the data. Since we have no postulated distribution, we shall not be able to estimate parameters, but we can decide whether there is evidence of a difference in the effectiveness of the two analgesics. Of course, with such pathetically small numbers, we could not reach any very firm conclusions, but we can more easily see how the test works.

Rank order

We can rank the pain scores in order of magnitude, noting which group the score belongs to, so that we obtain a sequence of three A's and four B's. If all of the scores in group A are smaller than all of those in group B, we would obtain the sequence AAABBBB, and we might be tempted to conclude that A is a more effective analgesic. Conversely, if all of the scores in group A are larger than any in group B, we would obtain the sequence BBBBAAA and conclude that B is superior to A. How strong is the evidence if we do observe either of these results and what about outcomes containing mixed A's and B's as we go up the sequence? Suppose that we observe AABBABB. Is there any evidence of a difference in median pain score; we are ranking the data, so that the median, which involves counting to the middle point in a data set, is the appropriate central measure?

If there is a preponderance of A's at one end and hence B's at the other, there is more likely to be a difference in median than if the mixture is more homogeneous. How can we measure this?

AAABBBB	ABABABB	ABBBAAB	BAABABB	BABBBAA	BBABBAA
AABABBB	ABABBAB	ABBBABA	BAAABBB	BBAAABB	BBBAAAB
AABBABB	ABABBBA	ABBBBAA	BABABBA	BBAABAB	BBBAABA
AABBBAB	ABBAABB	ABBBBAA	BABAABB	BBAABBA	BBBABAA
AABBBBA	ABBABAB	BAABBBA	BABABAB	BBABAAB	BBBBAAA
ABAABBB	ABBABBA	BAABBAB	BABBABA	BBABABA	

There are 35 distinguishable ways in which three A's and four B's can be arranged. If the two groups have the same median, then all of these 35 sequences are equally likely.

N distinguishable objects can be arranged in $N!$ ways. The first can be chosen in N ways, the next in $(N-1)$ ways, the next in $(N-2)$, and so on. If there are only two kinds of object (such as A's and B's), then there are fewer distinguishable sequences. There are then

$$\frac{N!}{n_A! n_B!}$$

where n_A is the number of A's and n_B is the number of B's. $N = n_A + n_B$.

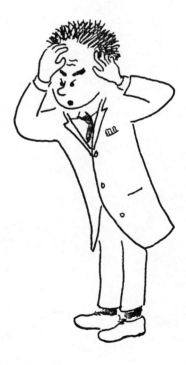

3.20.2   The Mann–Whitney test for difference in median

> ### The Mann–Whitney U test
>
> We would suspect a difference in median pain score if there were a marked 'bunching' of the groups. We need a scoring system to measure the preponderance of the A's at one end and the B's at the other for all possible sequences. This can then be used to produce a sampling distribution of these scores under the NH of no difference in the median. This gives us a means of determining a critical region for rejection of the NH. This is simply a significance test, like any other (3.15).
>
> Sample: AABBABB
>
> We enumerated the different sequences ($n_A = 3$, $n_B = 4$) for illustration; there were 35 of them. If we had groups of size ($n_A = 8$, $n_B = 10$) say, then there would be 18!/ (8! × 10!) = 43 758 distinguishable sequences. We do not want to write all of these down.
>
> A simple scoring system enables us to decide quite easily. We pick A's, say, and move up the sequence and note, under each A, how many B's precede it in the sequence. We add all of these to obtain a score, the U value. Here we have 0 + 0 + 2 = 2: $U = 2$.
>
> | A | A | B | B | A | B | B |
> |---|---|---|---|---|---|---|
> | 0 | 0 | | | 2 | | |
>
> Alternatively, we might choose the B's and note, for each B, how many A's precede it in the sequence. We sum these and obtain $U^* = 2 + 2 + 3 + 3 = 10$.
>
> | A | A | B | B | A | B | B |
> |---|---|---|---|---|---|---|
> | | | 2 | 2 | | 3 | 3 |
>
> We have obtained two scores $U = 2$ and $U^* = 10$ from the same sequence. What we have done, in essence, is to compare each of the B's with each of the A's. There are ($n_A = 3$) × ($n_B = 4$) = 12 comparisons to be made; for each A we have asked how many B's are smaller than it and similarly for each B how many A's are smaller than it. The U value is a sum of the measures of position of the A's in comparison to the B's, and the U^* value is the sum for B's compared to A's. The sum of the two, $U + U^* = (n_A = 3) × (n_B = 4) = 12$, as we have then made all comparisons. The value of U (or U^*) is the Mann–Whitney statistic for the test for difference in median.

The null distribution for ($n_A = 3$, $n_B = 4$)

We have described a method of scoring, but we need a null distribution; that is, a model distribution based upon the NH of no difference in median between two groups to compare our score with. Under the NH, all of the 35 described sequences are equally probable, but the associated U and U^* values are not equally probable. All we do is calculate a U value in the same way for each of the sequences shown. The relative frequency bar chart for the U values 0–12 is the graph of the null distribution. We can use this in the same way as the null distribution for any other statistic to construct acceptance/critical regions and perform one or two-tailed tests as appropriate.

The Mann–Whitney U test is easily performed by hand, even for quite large samples. The critical values for one- and two-tailed tests for equal and unequal sample sizes are available in tables or computer package—that is, the null distribution characteristics are easily available.

The probability distribution for $U(n_A = 3, n_B = 4)$ is discrete—the probability values are in 35ths—and symmetrical. The symmetry means that it does not matter whether we calculate U or U^*: we will obtain the same probability value, since $U = 12 - U^*$.

The distribution has a superficial similarity to the binomial distribution that we need for the sign test, but since we always have three A's and four B's, each slot is *not* filled independently, and so it is not binomial.

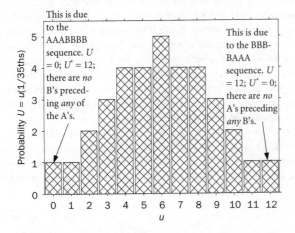

This is due to the AAABBBB sequence. $U = 0$; $U^* = 12$; there are *no* B's preceding *any* of the A's.

This is due to the BBB-BAAA sequence. $U = 12$; $U^* = 0$; there are *no* A's preceding *any* B's.

The discrete nature of the distribution means that we cannot make the critical region any size we choose: we must choose integer values of U and the jumps in the graph make smooth adjustment of the critical region impossible. We can choose values at one end or the other (two-tailed, large U^*, *or* large U) if we are looking for a difference in either direction. Or we can choose a critical region at one end only (say, large U and small U^*) for a difference in a specified direction.

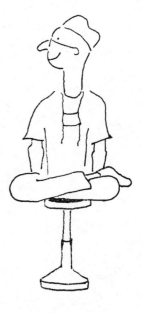

This is a very brief introduction to the non-parametric, distribution-free, or rank order methods. They are used when distributions cannot be assumed or are likely to be appreciably skewed and the normality assumption underlying the t-tests, for example, is not fulfilled. The Mann–Whitney test is the distribution-free equivalent of the two-sample t-test (3.16.4) and is surprisingly powerful. There is a non-parametric equivalent of all of the standard normal-based tests and they are generally very easy to perform. Further details are available in the works listed in the bibliography.

3.21.1 **Queues**

In many of the models developed in this book, you may have been tempted to question the assumptions made or have felt that the model could be improved in some way by taking account of other factors which may behave differently from the assumptions. For instance, we blithely took a respiratory quotient of unity in all of our respiratory models simply because it made things easier. This does not mean that the *RQ* actually is unity—it is usually about 0.8. The predictions of our models will not therefore match reality exactly; the general pattern will not usually be affected by such simplifications, but the precise predictions will. It is open to you to improve the models. That is what they are there for.

There are many directions in which the material in this book can be taken, and we will mention just one. We started with the IOP, and in all of the models in which this was used, the inputs and outputs were *deterministic*—there was no random element in them. We might consider an IOP model in which inputs and outputs are subject to some stochastic (random) process. Imagine the patients waiting in the emergency department to be seen. The number waiting to be treated will involve random processes and the arrival (input) of patients will be unpredictable in detail, although certain patterns will be observable—Friday evenings are generally busier than 5 a.m. on Sunday. The rate at which these patients can be treated and transferred (dead, discharged home, or admitted to a ward) out of the department (output) will also be subject to random factors (staff absence because of illness, complexity of condition, admission of very urgent cases, and so on). Such circumstances can be modelled by an IOP approach using appropriate probability distributions to model random arrivals and departures. This is the subject matter of queuing theory and has been applied to the provision of anaesthesia services—patients waiting for anaesthesia and surgery are in a queue. In this example there will be a great deal of non-random influence—staffing levels, prioritisation of urgency of the cases, for instance—which mean that simple Poisson-type processes are usually insufficient to model the problem.

The availability of computing has enabled random simulations of such processes to be carried out quite easily once the model has been constructed; but, as always, the assumptions upon which any model is based must be examined very carefully, the predictions compared with reality, and the model modified as required.

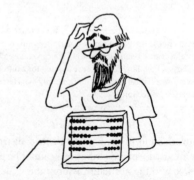

Bibliography

General

Barrow, J. D. (1992). Pi in the sky. Penguin, London.
McLeish, J. (1992). Number. Flamingo, Harper Collins, London.
These are both readable and informative paperbacks about numbers and the development of mathematics in understanding the real world from ancient times to the computer age. They are of no direct relevance to physiology, but they provide excellent background for the curious.

Wells, D. (1995). You are a mathematician. Penguin, London.
This is an inexpensive paperback that aims to entice the reader into greater appreciation of the enjoyment that can be derived from mathematics. It is readable and thought-provoking, and contains in Chapter 10 a discussion of mathematical modelling.

Physiological and pharmacological models

Caro, C. G., Pedley, T. J., Schroter, R. C. and Seed, W. A. (1978). The mechanics of the circulation. Oxford University Press: Oxford.
This book contains an introduction to Newtonian mechanics applied to the function of the circulation. Although it is quite old, much of the material is still useful, especially in the comprehensible presentation of dimensions, fluid mechanics, and mass transfer in the first section of the book.

Eger, E. I. (1974). Anesthetic uptake & action. Williams and Wilkins, Baltimore.

This is a well-illustrated treatment of anaesthetic pharmacology, particularly of inhalational agents. It is less good on non-inhaled drugs. Despite its age, it is still well worth reading selectively.

Hull, C. J. (1991). Pharmacokinetics for anaesthesia. Butterworth–Heinemann, Oxford.

This fills a similar role to Nunn for pharmacological models. It is the standard reference work in pharmacokinetics in anaesthesia, although too comprehensive for examination candidates.

Nunn, J. F. (1994) Applied respiratory physiology (4th edn). Butterworth–Heinemann, Oxford.

This is and will probably remain for the forseeable future, the 'bible' for anaesthetists studying respiratory physiology, although not without some surprising omissions. I have consulted it extensively in successive editions over the years. This is the first source for further background and refinement of the respiratory models presented in Part 1.

Riggs, D. S. (1963). The mathematical approach to physiological problems. MIT Press, Cambridge, Massachusetts.

This is a beginner's guide to mathematical modelling in physiology and pharmacology. Although the presentation now seems rather dated, the essence of the material is as valuable as ever. It has no treatment of probability or statistics, but discusses very thoroughly topics such as dimensional methods and approximation in generating usable physiological models. This book is full of common sense and should be read by all students and teachers of physiology.

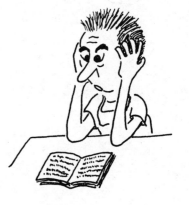

Mathematical background

Collinson, C. Anderson, J. and Holmes, P. (eds). Modular mathematics. Edward Arnold, London.
This is a series of titles for first-year maths undergraduates and is accessible to anybody with A-level mathematics or equivalent. The books are strictly for the enthusiast in search of deeper explanation, but the series includes titles on differential equations, analysis, and calculus. The title on 'mathematical modelling' by J. Berry and K. Houston is particularly relevant.

Graham, L. and Sargent, D. (1980). Countdown to mathematics, Vol. 2. Addison-Wesley, Reading, Massachusetts.

This is a revision manual of school maths and covers simple graph work, algebra, geometry, and trigonometry. It is intended for resuscitation of moribund numeracy. Numerous exercises are included. An anaesthetist who needs the very elementary Volume 1 should not be in practice.

Mayor, E. (1994). *e*: the story of a number. Princeton. University Press, Princeton New N. Jersey.

This is written for the general reader and explains the emergence of the constant *e* as a fundamental quantity in mathematics. It is readable and fascinating, although it will not help you pass the exam. Read it afterwards.

Probability and statistics

Armitage, P. and Berry, G. (1987). Statistical methods in medical research. Blackwell Oxford.

This is the standard methods text for those involved in research projects. It is long, comprehensive, and provides accessible explanation of how the methods work, but assumes a knowledge of the fundamentals of probability and statistical inference. It is not a first text, but it is invaluable for practical guidance.

Bland, M. (1995). An introduction to medical statistics (2nd edn). Oxford University Press, Oxford.

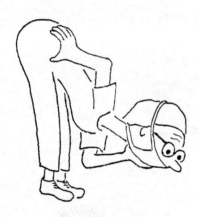

This is the standard background text that I have used. It is an inexpensive but quite extended treatment of principles and methods, covering a much greater range than attempted here. Examples are generally from epidemiology and general medicine, with few of direct inspiration to anaesthetists. The treatment is friendly and even occasionally humorous. It is probably the best introductory treatment available.

Cobb, G. W., Witmer, J. A. and Cryer, J. D. (1997). An electronic companion to statistics. Cogito, New York (Available through Oxford University Press).

This is a workbook with attached CD-ROM. This contains animations, graphical displays, and so on, and is intended for use with any standard text. The material covers all of the important concepts and techniques and is excellent for learning by doing, but omits most of the theoretical background. It is more alive to the difficulties experienced by students of this subject than are other texts—with the exception of Gonick and Smith (1993).

Gonick, L. and Smith, W. (1993). The cartoon guide to statistics. Harper Perennial, New York.

This is a light-hearted but far from trivial introduction to probability and statistical inference. It covers all the fundamental concepts through a comic format, showing that statisics can be fun—unbelievable but true! Examples require a familiarity with American culture and delicatessen produce (normally distributed dill-pickled cucumbers), but this is the book to go to for an introduction to the subject. It is excellent and inexpensive.

Milton, J. S. and Arnold, J. C. (1990). Introduction to probability & statistics. McGraw-Hill, New York.

This is actually a textbook for engineering and computer science students, but it provides a fundamental background in probability theory accessible to those with sound knowledge of maths and calculus. It is not for the casual or faint-hearted reader.

Index